Study Guide for

Fundamentals of Nursing
Human Health and Function

SEVENTH EDITION

RUTH F. CRAVEN, EdD, RN, BC, FAAN
Professor Emerita
Department of Behavioral Nursing and Health Systems
University of Washington School of Nursing
Seattle, Washington

CONSTANCE J. HIRNLE, MN, RN, BC
Clinical Education Specialist
Virginia Mason Medical Center
Seattle, Washington

Senior Lecturer
Biobehavioral Nursing and Health Systems
University of Washington School of Nursing
Seattle, Washington

SHARON JENSEN, MN, RN
Instructor
School of Nursing
Seattle University
Seattle, Washington

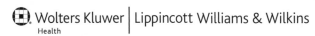

Wolters Kluwer | Lippincott Williams & Wilkins
Health

Philadelphia · Baltimore · New York · London
Buenos Aires · Hong Kong · Sydney · Tokyo

Vice Publisher/Editor: Julie Stegman
Product Manager: Michelle Clarke
Editorial Assistant: Jacalyn Clay
Senior Designer: Joan Wendt
Illustration Coordinator: Brett MacNaughton
Manufacturing Coordinator: Karin Duffield
Prepress Vendor: Aptara, Inc.

7th Edition

ISBN 978-1-60547-783-1

Care has been taken to confirm the accuracy of the information presented and to describe generally accepted practices. However, the author, editors, and publisher are not responsible for errors or omissions or for any consequences from application of the information in this book and make no warranty, express or implied, with respect to the content of the publication.

The author, editors, and publisher have exerted every effort to ensure that drug selectin and dosage set forth in this text are in accordance with the current recommendations and practice at the time of publication. However, in view of ongoing research, changes in government regulations, and the constant flow of information relating to drug therapy and drug reactions, the reader is urged to check the package insert for each drug for any change in indications and dosage and for added warnings and precautions This is particularly important when the recommended agent is a new or infrequently employed drug.

Some drugs and medical devices presented in this publication have Food and Drug Administration (FDA) clearance for limited use in restricted research settings. It is the responsibility of the health care provider to ascertain the FDA status of each drug or device planned for use in his or her clinical practice.

Preface

This Study Guide was written by Sophia Lichenstein-Hill and Wendy Rychwalski for the seventh edition of *Fundamentals of Nursing: Human Health and Function,* by Ruth Craven, Constance Hirnle, and Sharon Jensen. The study guide is designed to help you practice and retain the knowledge you've gained from the textbook, and it is structured to integrate that knowledge and give you a basis for applying it in your nursing practice. The following types of exercises are provided in this study guide.

LEARNING OBJECTIVES

The first section of each Study Guide chapter lists the Learning Objectives of the textbook chapter, to remind you of the goals of the chapter as you work your way through the exercises.

ASSESSING YOUR UNDERSTANDING

The second section of each Study Guide chapter concentrates on the basic information of the textbook chapter and helps you to remember key concepts, vocabulary, and principles.

- Fill in the Blanks
  These questions correlate very closely with the textbook and focus on important information in each chapter.

- Matching Exercises
  Matching exercises help you to distinguish among several key terms, drugs, or adverse reactions.
- Ordering Exercises
  Ordering exercises ask you to remember particular orders, for instance testing processes and prioritizing nursing actions.
- Short Answer Questions
  Requiring more critical thinking than the exercises in the assessing Your Understanding section, these short answer questions offer an exciting and practical means to challenge you and "stretch" your application of the concepts.

APPLYING YOUR KNOWLEDGE

These case studies challenge you to reflect on the critical thinking and blended skills developed in the classroom and apply them to your own practice.

PRACTICING FOR NCLEX

Each chapter contains a section of multiple choice questions presented in NCLEX exam format.

Enjoy your studies, and know that this study guide is a tool that will help you better understand the sometimes complicated world of pharmacology.

Contents

CHAPTER 1

The Profession of Nursing

SECTION I: LEARNING OBJECTIVES

Upon completion of this chapter, the student will be able to do the following:

1. Discuss how nurses have developed more independent practice during the last 50 years.

2. Identify how critical thinking is integral to nursing education and practice.

3. Discuss the influence of nursing's historical development on contemporary views of professional nursing.

4. Identify distinct pathways for entrance into and continuation of professional nursing practice.

5. Identify roles and responsibilities of professional nursing within the healthcare delivery system.

6. Describe the purpose and function of professional nursing organizations.

7. Recognize major nursing theories and their relevance to nursing practice.

8. Identify the four major concepts of nursing theories.

9. Discuss the relationship between nursing theories and non-nursing theories.

10. Explain the relationship of functional health pattern typology to nursing.

SECTION II: ASSESSING YOUR UNDERSTANDING

Activity A FILL IN THE BLANKS

1. The _____ defines nursing as "Nursing is the protection, promotion, and optimization of health and abilities, prevention of illness and injury, alleviation of suffering through the diagnosis and treatment of human response, and advocacy in the care of individuals, families, communities, and populations."

2. The _____ degree nursing program is considered the entry for professional nursing practice.

3. The American Nurses Credentialing Center states that _____ validates nursing specialty knowledge.

4. The board of nursing in each state sets requirements for _____.

5. Sigma Theta Tau International provides leadership and _____ in practice, education, and research to enhance the health of all people.

6. Nurses engage in physician delegated actions as well as _____ interventions, which include repositioning a patient every 2 hours.

7. Nurses act as patient _____ when they communicate the needs and concerns of patients and ensure that patients understand their treatments.

8. _____ hierarchy provides a framework for recognizing and prioritizing basic human needs.

9. Unfreezing, movement, and refreezing are the three states of Lewin's theory of _____.

10. One way to organize nursing information in a holist way is to use Gordon's concept of functional health _____.

Activity B MATCHING

Match the nursing role in Column A with the definition in Column B.

Column A

____ 1. Licensed practical nurse

____ 2. Registered nurse

____ 3. Nurse practitioner

____ 4. Clinical nurse specialist

____ 5. Nurse researcher

Column B

A. A nurse with advanced experience and expertise in a specialized area of practice who can educate, manage, and consult other nursing professionals.

B. An individual who has met the ANA's requirements for beginning professional and technical practice in nursing.

C. A nurse with advanced education who functions with more independence and autonomy and who is highly skilled at doing nursing assessment, performing physical examinations, counseling, teaching, and treating health problems.

D. A professional who provides patient care after completing a 1-year program that prepares them to perform technical skills under the supervision of registered nurses.

E. A nurse who is responsible for development and refinement of nursing practice through the investigation of nursing problems.

Activity C ORDERING

1. Place the levels of proficiency a nurse passes through when acquiring and developing nursing skill in the order in which they occur:

   a. Advanced beginner: The advanced beginner can demonstrate marginally acceptable performance. He or she has had enough experience in actual situations to identify meaningful aspects or global characteristics that can be identified only through prior experience.

   b. Proficient: The proficient nurse perceives situations as a whole rather than in terms of aspects and manages nursing care rather than performing tasks.

   c. Novice: A beginning nursing student or any nurse entering a situation in which he or she has not previous experience. Behavior is governed by established rules and is limited and inflexible.

   d. Expert: The expert nurse no longer relies on rules or guidelines to connect understanding of a situation to an appropriate action. The expert nurse, with an enormous background of experience, has an intuitive grasp of the situation and zeroes in on the problem.

   e. Competent: Competence is reflected by the nurse who has been on the same job for 2 or 3 years and who consciously and deliberately plans nursing care in terms of long-range goals.

   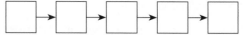

2. Place the events of historical significance for the profession of nursing in the order in which they occur:

   a. Clara Barton organized the American National Red Cross.

   b. Dorothea Dix establishes the Army Nurse Corps.

   c. Lillian Wald and Mary Brewster found the Henry Street Settlement.

   d. Florence Nightingale is named Superintendent of Nursing and cares for soldiers in the Crimean War.

   e. Esther Lucille Brown advocates that nursing education belongs in college and universities.

   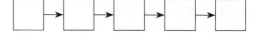

Activity D SHORT ANSWER

1. How does a new graduate become licensed as a registered nurse? Who sets the requirements for licensure? How is licensure transferred from state to state?

_____

_____

_____

2. Who are the members of the American Nurses Association and what are the organization's main functions?

_____

_____

_____

3. Describe how the four components of nursing theory (person, environment, health, and nursing) are applied in Florence Nightingale's theory Notes on Nursing: *What It Is, What It Is Not.*

_____

_____

_____

4. According to Maslow's hierarchy of needs, what are the two types of esteem needs and how do they differ?

_____

_____

_____

5. Describe how the nursing scope of practice has changed in the last 50 years.

_____

_____

_____

SECTION III: APPLYING YOUR KNOWLEDGE

Activity E CASE STUDY

Answer the following questions, which involve the nurse's role in assessing the needs of this patient.

John Rubenstein, age 37, is a quadriplegic who has just been transferred to a new long-term care facility. John confides in you that he believes his roommate is stealing from him. He also tells you that he has not eaten for 2 days because the facility has been including non-kosher pork products, which he does not consume because of his religious beliefs, in many meals. He has been feeling lonely since his arrival 1 week ago.

1. Based on Maslow's hierarchy of needs, which of John's concerns is most pressing?

_____

_____

_____

2. Why should his sense of loneliness not be dismissed?

_____

_____

_____

SECTION IV: PRACTICING FOR NCLEX

Activity F MULTIPLE CHOICE

Answer the following questions.

1. Matt has been a nurse for 17 years. He pursued a degree in nursing by attending a junior college for 2 years and successfully took the NCLEX-RN upon completion. Since getting his degree he has worked in an inpatient setting on a transplant floor. Based on the information given, which of the following degrees does Matt have?
   a. Associates degree
   b. Diploma
   c. Baccalaureate degree
   d. Licensed practical nurse

2. Which of the following contributors to the nursing profession established two missions; sick nursing and health nursing?
   a. Clara Barton
   b. Lillian Wald
   c. Dorothea Dix
   d. Florence Nightingale

3. Which of the following describes the role of the nurse practitioner?
   a. Is responsible for the continued development and refinement of nursing knowledge and practice through the investigation of nursing problems.
   b. Function independently, is skilled at doing nursing assessments, performing physical examinations, counseling, teaching, and treating health problems.
   c. Provides general anesthesia for patients undergoing surgery.
   d. Manages and controls patient care while being responsible for specific nursing units.

4. Which of the following defines the practice of nursing within each state?
   a. The National League of Nursing
   b. The American Nurses Credentialing Center
   c. The American Nursing Association
   d. Nurse Practice Act

5. Which of the following is not one of the four central concepts in nursing practice?
   a. Person
   b. Environment
   c. Spirituality
   d. Nursing

6. Oxygen, food, water, and rest are all examples of what type of human need as described by Maslow?
   a. Physiologic
   b. Safety
   c. Esteem
   d. Self-actualization

7. Mark is a 50-year-old man who has smoked one to two packs of cigarettes for the last 20 years. He has decided that he is ready to quit smoking but is not sure how best to go about it. He knows that it will be hard for him to do. Which of the following states of change, according to Kurt Lewin is Mark in?
   a. Refreezing
   b. Unfreezing
   c. Movement
   d. Contemplation

8. Marjory Gordon developed the concept of functional health patterns to help organize nursing information in a holistic way. Which functional health pattern focuses on health values and beliefs?
   a. Health perception–health management
   b. Elimination
   c. Cognitive-perceptual
   d. Self-perception

9. Nancy is a 13-year-old patient with cystic fibrosis. She has just recovered from a superimposed respiratory infection and is going home tomorrow. She confides in you that her home life is not the greatest right now. Her parents are fighting a lot. Sometimes, her mother has too much to drink and starts throwing things at people. At times she gets scared her mom will hurt someone. She feels as if she is causing her parents to fight and her mom to drink because she is always in the hospital. According to Maslow's hierarchy of need, which of the following issues should take priority when caring for Nancy?
   a. She feels as if she is the cause of her family's dysfunction.
   b. Her home life is not good right now.
   c. She feels scared that her mother will hurt someone.
   d. Her parents are fighting a lot.

10. Jordana is a nurse on an adult medical floor. She is taking care of Martin who is a 66-year-old man with congestive heart failure. Jordana is taking into account the fact that Martin will most likely go home on a diuretic and that he should be monitoring his weight daily. She provided education accordingly. According to Brenner, which of the following levels of proficiency is Jordana demonstrating?
   a. Competent
   b. Advanced beginner
   c. Proficient
   d. Novice

11. Which of the following nursing theorists
    created a theory whose purpose it was to
    develop an interpersonal interaction between
    patient and nurse?

    a. Nightingale
    b. Henderson
    c. Rogers
    d. Peplau

Health, Wellness, and Complementary Medicine

SECTION I: LEARNING OBJECTIVES

Upon completion of this chapter, the student will be able to do the following:

1. Define *wellness, holism, and health promotion.*

2. Compare and contrast selected models of the concept of health.

3. Identify the connections among mind, body, spirit, and symptoms.

4. Explain the differences among allopathic medicine, complementary and alternative medicine (CAM), and integrative healthcare.

5. Explain the role of holistic healthcare in nursing.

6. Give examples of some commonly used holistic interventions.

7. Reflect on how you will incorporate wellness, health, and integrative healthcare into your patients' care and your own.

SECTION II: ASSESSING YOUR UNDERSTANDING

Activity A FILL IN THE BLANKS

1. The World Health Organization has defined "health" as "a state of complete physical, mental, and _____ well-being, not merely the absence of disease or infirmity."

2. In the health belief model, a relation exists between a person's beliefs and _____.

3. Holism acknowledges and respects the interaction of a person's mind, body, and _____ with the environment.

4. Immunizations are a prime example of _____ prevention.

5. In Pender, Murdaugh, and Parsons' health promotion model, a spiritual assessment is made which includes beliefs and _____.

6. Holistic healthcare emphasizes humanism, choices, self-care activities, and a _____ relationship between healthcare provider and patient.

7. Integrative medicine is healing-oriented medicine that takes account of the whole person (body, mind, spirit, and community), including all aspects of _____.

8. Meditation, deep personal thought and _____, may be one of the most basic and powerful self-care activities that people can incorporate into their lives.

9. The term botanicals represent _____ with medicinal properties.

10. Therapeutic Touch is a "consciously directed process of _____ exchange during which the practitioner uses the hands as a focus of facilitating healing."

Activity B MATCHING

Match the Mind–Body Interventions in Column A with their characteristic(s) in Column B.

Column A

___ 1. Acupuncture

___ 2. Reflective meditation

___ 3. Receptive meditation

___ 4. Expressive meditation

___ 5. Traditional Chinese medicine

Column B

A. Deep personal thought and reflection focusing on the deep interconnection between mind and body.

B. Based on the basic principle of inserting very fine needles into various areas of the body to stimulate the meridians and promote harmony within the system.

C. Deep personal thought and reflection that includes movement or expression with the concentrative methods of whirling, shaking, or dancing.

D. A complete healing system. Includes acupuncture, massage, herbal treatments, nutrition, moxibustion, movement, and meditation.

E. Deep personal thought and reflection focusing on a chosen theme, question, or topic to gain insight into significant questions or concepts.

Activity C ORDERING

1. Place the stages that a patient moves through in their search for effective wellness behavior in order from ineffective to most effective. *Write the correct sequence in the boxes provided below:*

   a. Action

   b. Preparation

   c. Precontemplation

   d. Maintenance

   e. Contemplation

   f. Termination

   [ ] → [ ] → [ ] → [ ] → [ ] → [ ]

Activity D SHORT ANSWER

1. According to the Health Belief Model, what factors can affect a person's response to illness?

   _____

   _____

   _____

2. How has holism and the Holistic Health Model influenced nursing?

   _____

   _____

   _____

3. Describe the differences between allopathic medicine, CAM, and integrative healthcare.

   _____

   _____

   _____

4. Describe the Theory of Integral Nursing that was developed by Barbara Dossey.

   _____

   _____

   _____

5. What are some of the issues surrounding safety, standardization, and regulation of botanicals?

   _____

   _____

   _____

SECTION III: APPLYING YOUR KNOWLEDGE

Activity E CASE STUDY

Answer the following questions, which involve the nurse's utilization of holistic healthcare.

Cynthia Listman is a 65-year-old woman with a history of hypertension and depression. She is a new patient to the clinic. You are the nurse assigned to perform her intake interview.

1. As a nurse who is aware of CAM, how are you going to approach this patient so that you are able to gather all pertinent information for this intake interview?

   _____

   _____

   _____

2. What are some key questions that you will want to ask her?

   _____

   _____

   _____

3. Choose one CAM modality that might be appropriate to suggest to this patient and state why.

   _____

   _____

   _____

SECTION IV: PRACTICING FOR NCLEX

Activity F MULTIPLE CHOICE

Answer the following questions.

1. Gregory Smith is a 35–year-old man who comes in to the clinic for a follow-up appointment. One month ago he was complaining of a productive cough for 1 week and was diagnosed with acute bronchitis. He is a smoker and was given information on smoking cessation as well as a prescription for antibiotics at that time. Today he states that he no longer has any symptoms of bronchitis and, in general, is feeling good. According to which model of health is Gregory completely healthy at this visit?
   a. The Clinical Model
   b. The Health Belief Model
   c. High-Level Wellness Model
   d. Holistic Health Model

2. Which of the following is an example of tertiary prevention?
   a. Sam is prescribed an antihypertensive medication to control his newly diagnosed high blood pressure
   b. Linda is having her first colonoscopy because she just turned 50
   c. A school nurse is giving a talk about good hand washing to a first-grade class
   d. A pamphlet on nutrition for children is given to all patients in a pediatric clinic
   e. A hearing test is done on a newborn in the hospital

3. Which of the following is not a principle that encompasses the basic goals of integrative medicine?
   a. Reject allopathic medicine and embrace CAM practices
   b. Establish a partnership between client and practitioner
   c. Facilitate the body's innate healing abilities
   d. Focus on promoting health and preventing illness, as well as treating disease

4. A chant is a form of which category of meditation?
   a. Concentrative
   b. Receptive
   c. Reflective
   d. Expressive

5. As identified by the National Center for Complementary and Alternative Medicine, which of the following is not a major domain of CAM?
   a. Biologically based therapies
   b. Whole medical systems
   c. Integrative systems
   d. Energy medicine

6. In which CAM modality are the concepts of Yin and Yang important for diagnosis?
   a. Meditation
   b. Traditional Chinese medicine
   c. Therapeutic touch
   d. Botanicals

7. Martha Jimenez is a 32-year-old obese woman. She tells you that she has been exercising and trying to eat healthier for the last 2 months and is feeling healthier. But, she is frustrated now because during the first month she lost 5 pounds and in the last month she only lost 1 pound. She is worried that the stress she is feeling over her frustration is going to lead her to overeat again. Martha is in which stage of behavior change?
   a. Precontemplation
   b. Action
   c. Preparation
   d. Maintenance
   e. Termination

8. Sarah Stevens is an 85-year-old woman who is in the hospital recovering from hip replacement surgery. She is scheduled to go home in 2 days. According to the Health Belief Model, which of the following factors would be important to assess before Sarah goes home? Select all that apply.
   a. Her expectations for recovery
   b. What she has heard about recovering from this procedure
   c. How she has recovered from previous procedures
   d. Her living environment
   e. Whether or not she feels safe in her home

9. Which of the following are examples of "doing" therapy as discussed by Dossey? Select all that apply.
   a. Prayer
   b. Concentrative meditation
   c. Imagery
   d. Emptying a colostomy bag
   e. Changing a wound dressing

CHAPTER 3

Healthcare in the Community and Home

SECTION I: LEARNING OBJECTIVES

Upon completion of this chapter, the student will be able to do the following:

1. Discuss what is meant by community-based healthcare.

2. Identify three levels of healthcare and the services under each level.

3. Identify the role of various settings for community-based healthcare.

4. Explain how social, professional, and financial considerations have influenced the growth of community-based healthcare.

5. Determine the focus of nursing care in all settings and situations.

6. Discuss forms of community-based nursing practice, both traditional and more recent.

7. Identify the importance of continuity of care and discharge planning.

8. Describe the management of healthcare needs in the home from a systems perspective.

9. Identify factors that influence the patient's ability to manage healthcare within the home.

10. Explain the major areas requiring assessment by a home care nurse.

11. Describe nursing roles and responsibilities in home care.

12. Identify the importance of community resources in the care of patients receiving home care services.

SECTION II: ASSESSING YOUR UNDERSTANDING

Activity A FILL IN THE BLANKS

1. Emergency care, acute and critical care, diagnosis, and treatment are all fall under the category of _____ healthcare.

2. Community-based healthcare is the design, delivery, and evaluation of healthcare services developed in partnership with _____.

3. The main difference between community-based nursing and community health nursing is that community health nursing focuses on patient and _____ as community and community-based nursing focuses on individuals and families with the community.

4. Occupational health nursing is a common community-based setting where nursing care delivered in the _____.

5. Currently the focus of nursing care in home healthcare is on complex _____ health situations or acute care assistance.

6. Adding to the trends affecting home healthcare, Medicare now requires home health agencies to collect and report _____ information.

7. A person's environment comprises his or her physical, psychological, and _____ surroundings.

8. A systems view suggests that the individual, family, and community continually interact and influence on another by exchanging _____ and energy.

9. Injury potential, altered health maintenance, and knowledge deficit regarding _____ procedures are important considerations in home management.

10. Continuity of care is provision of health services without _____, regardless of movement between settings.

11. Assessment should encompass the functional abilities, strengths, and _____ of the patient, family, home, and community.

Activity B MATCHING

Match the discharge elements for the nurse or patient in Column A with the correct definition in Column B.

Column A

____ 1. Negotiation

____ 2. Continuity of care

____ 3. Collaboration

____ 4. Transition

____ 5. Facilitation

Column B

A. The act of assembling and directing activities to provide services harmoniously

B. When people's assumptions about themselves change and they develop new assumptions that allow them to adapt

C. The process by which the patient, nurse, and family determine goals

D. The provision of health services without disruption, regardless of the patients movement between settings

E. Making something easier and smoother, eliminating problems and barriers

Activity C ORDERING

1. Place the phases of the nursing home visit in the order in which they occur. *Write the correct sequence in the boxes provided below.*

   a. Previsit phase

   b. Postvisit phase

   c. Termination phase

   d. Initiation

   e. In-home phase

Activity D SHORT ANSWER

1. Describe the differences between primary, secondary, and tertiary levels of healthcare.

   _____

   _____

   _____

2. Who is community-based nursing care directed at?

   _____

   _____

   _____

3. Why is discharge planning so important?

   _____

   _____

   _____

4. Why do nurses need to know about community resources in the care of patients receiving home care services?

   _____

   _____

   _____

5. What are the major areas requiring assessment by a home care nurse.

   _____

   _____

   _____

SECTION III: APPLYING YOUR KNOWLEDGE

Activity E CASE STUDY

Answer the following questions, which involve the nurse's role in home healthcare.

You are a nurse providing an in-home visit to a new patient. Daren Ramirez is a 75-year-old man who had a cerebral vascular accident 1 month ago. Prior to the accident, he was living independently at home with his wife. He was discharged 2 days ago with an order for in-home nursing care.

1. What are the main things that you want to assess about this gentleman?

   _____

   _____

   _____

2. How would you organize the first in-home visit with this patient and his wife?

   _____

   _____

   _____

3. How would you approach patient education with Daren and his wife?

   _____

   _____

   _____

SECTION IV: PRACTICING FOR NCLEX

Activity F MULTIPLE CHOICE

Answer the following questions.

1. Which of the following is a safety deficit?
   a. Safety bars in the shower of an 86-year-old
   b. Rear-facing car seat for a 1-year-old
   c. Electrical outlet covers in the house of a 9-month-old
   d. An elevated toilet seat for a person who has recently had hip surgery
   e. Multiple area rugs in the house of a 95-year-old

2. Which of the following is not a cognitive or sensory deficit?
   a. Chronic severe pain
   b. Dementia
   c. Asthma
   d. Substance abuse
   e. Blindness

3. Referring a smoker to a smoking cessation program is a nursing intervention for which level of discharge planning?
   a. Primary referral
   b. Basic referral
   c. Complex referral
   d. Simple referral
   e. Secondary referral

4. Which of the following illustrates a systems view of a person's healthcare?
   a. John is a 20-year-old schizophrenic who lives with his parents. At times he has been found wandering through the backyards of neighbors "searching for messages that are left for me." His neighbors help John search for the messages and then bring him home.
   b. Dora is a 50-year-old schoolteacher with hyperlipidemia.
   c. Cindy is a 42-year-old woman that was admitted to the hospital yesterday after suffering from an episode of chest pain and diaphoresis. Her cardiac enzymes were slightly elevated and she is scheduled to go for a cardiac catheterization this morning.
   d. Marcus is an 80-year-old widower who lives in an apartment. He receives food from an organization that delivers free meals to people who cannot go out and do not have enough money to buy food every day.
   e. Kara is an 18-year-old with type I diabetes. During the summers she works as a counselor at a camp for children with diabetes.

5. Which of the following was not identified by Koerner as one of the four capacities that are hallmarks of nursing leaders practicing in the community?
   a. Capacity with medication administration
   b. Capacity to create and negotiate partnerships
   c. Capacity to create new order
   d. Capacity for moral courage and integrity

6. Which of the following scenarios encompasses all three discharge planning elements for the patient?

  a. Katie is a 25-year-old woman who is being discharged from the hospital to her home after a motor vehicle accident. The nurse working with her helps her develop goals to increase her activity level at home. They also talk about how Katie can best communicate her needs to her husband who is helping with her rehabilitation. The nurse tells Katie that her first appointment to see a physical therapist has been set up for a week from today.

  b. Katie is a 25-year-old woman who is being discharged from the hospital to her home after a motor vehicle accident. The nurse working with her helps her develop goals to increase her activity level at home. They also facilitate a meeting with Katie and her family to negotiate goals that everyone can agree on. The nurse tells Katie that her first appointment to see a physical therapist has been set up for a week from today.

  c. Katie is a 25-year-old woman who is being discharged from the hospital to her home after a motor vehicle accident. The nurse working with her helps her develop goals to increase her activity level at home. They also facilitate a meeting with Katie and her family to negotiate goals that everyone can agree on. Because Katie is a little overwhelmed right now, the nurse asks her mother if she is able to transport Katie home.

  d. Katie is a 25-year-old woman who is being discharged from the hospital to her home after a motor vehicle accident. The nurse working with her talks to Katie about how she can best communicate her needs to her husband who is helping with her rehabilitation. The nurse tells Katie that her first appointment to see a physical therapist has been set up for a week from today. The nurse collaborates with the pharmacy, the social worker, and the doctor to assure that Katie's medications are ready for her before she goes home.

7. Which of the following are examples of primary healthcare? Select all that apply.

  a. Screening
  b. Health promotion
  c. Protection
  d. Emergency care
  e. Rehabilitation
  f. Treatment

8. Which of the following are components of the case management process? Select all that apply.

  a. Coordinating
  b. Making referrals
  c. Monitoring medical progress
  d. Prescribing medications
  e. Driving a patient to appointments
  f. Filing and completing paperwork

9. Martha Hall is a single 65-year-old woman who has been receiving home nursing care for the past year due to debilitating chronic lower back pain. Twice a week, a nurse comes to her home to help her bathe and care for a surgical wound that is chronically infected. Martha had the opportunity to live in an assisted living facility but chose to live at home instead. Martha is illustrating which of the following national trends on home care? Select all that apply.

  a. Graying of America
  b. Changes in family status
  c. Increased self-care responsibility
  d. Technological advances in medical equipment
  e. Managed care plans
  f. Increased expectations of lay caregivers

10. Darren is a home-health nurse who is working with Laura. Laura has a new colostomy and must learn to care for it. Because Darren wants his patient education to be successful, he knows that he must work collaboratively with Laura and her family. He also knows that there are certain steps he must take. Place the following patient education activities in the order in which they should occur.

  a. Darren asks Laura and her family how much they already know about colostomy care.
  b. Darren notes that Laura wants to be able to change her own colostomy bag by the end of the week.
  c. Darren brings a plastic stoma and a bunch of colostomy bags that Laura and her family can practice on.
  d. Darren watches Laura change her colostomy bag.

CHAPTER 4

Culture and Diversity

SECTION I: LEARNING OBJECTIVES

Upon completion of this chapter, the student will be able to do the following:

1. Discuss characteristics of culture.

2. Define concepts related to culture.

3. Build an understanding of people by viewing human responses in cultural context.

4. Identify patterns of one's own and others' behavior that reflect stereotypical thinking and ethnocentric assumptions.

5. Communicate effectively with people of diverse orientations.

6. Demonstrate an increased awareness of one's own culture and its influence on one's own nursing practice.

7. Conduct an ethnographic interview.

SECTION II: ASSESSING YOUR UNDERSTANDING

Activity A FILL IN THE BLANKS

1. Culture is primarily learned and transmitted via the _____ and other social organizations.

2. Individuals with similar cultural backgrounds may adhere to _____ cultural beliefs or behaviors.

3. _____ _____ have a rich base of cultural knowledge and are able to articulate their knowledge of their culture.

4. Cultural _____ makes people unaware of their own assumptions and subsequently their own cultural biases.

5. Cultural _____ can help restore a sense of control and confidence to patients and their families in times of stress.

6. Persistent gaps in the health status of minorities and non-minorities are referred to as _____ _____.

7. Though often used interchangeably, race refers to _____ characteristics of an individual, whereas ethnic group refers to _____ characteristics.

8. Culturally competent nurses work with patients and use their cultural beliefs to develop an _____ plan of care.

9. Open-ended questions allow patients to use their own _____ to describe their health.

10. The three parts of an ethnographic interview include open-ended questions, _____, and documentation.

Activity B MATCHING

1. *Match the characteristics of culture listed in Column A with their definitions in Column B.*

Column A

___ **1.** Ethnocentric
___ **2.** Dynamic
___ **3.** Stabilizing
___ **4.** Implicit
___ **5.** Unequal sharing

Column B

A. Always changing, typically over long periods of time

B. Learned, accessed, and used by some more than others

C. It has habituated assumptions about the world which are not easily described by its members

D. Using one's own culture as a reference or standard

E. Makes human response predictable

2. *Match the ethnic group in Column A with the commonly held belief in Column B.*

Column A

___ **1.** Chinese
___ **2.** Muslim
___ **3.** Hmong
___ **4.** Southeast Asian
___ **5.** Western

Column B

A. Febrile persons are kept warm with blankets.

B. White is a color associated with death.

C. Gender color coding is common.

D. Autopsy prevents continuation of their society by preventing reunification of body and spirit.

E. Exposure of oneself to a member of the opposite sex is considered highly embarrassing.

Activity C SHORT ANSWER

1. Discuss the importance of cultural diversity.

_____

_____

_____

2. Describe cultural diversity within groups and provide an example.

_____

_____

_____

3. Describe the Tuskegee project and its long-term impact.

_____

_____

_____

4. Define stereotyping and discuss how it can negatively affect a nursing–patient interaction.

_____

_____

_____

5. What does the American Nurses Association (ANA) state about cultural competence?

_____

_____

_____

SECTION III: APPLYING YOUR KNOWLEDGE

Activity D CASE STUDY

Fatima Jattak, a 35-year-old recent Pakistani immigrant, presents at your labor and delivery unit with her husband, Mohammed. She does not speak English. Mohammed, who is also originally from Pakistan, has lived in the United States for several years and speaks fluent English. He offers to serve as an interpreter for his wife during her labor.

1. Discuss why it is important to utilize an interpreter for your interaction with Fatima and her husband.

_____

_____

_____

2. Using the principles of communicating with an interpreter, describe how you would approach your conversation with Fatima.

_____

_____

_____

SECTION IV: PRACTICING FOR NCLEX

Activity E

Answer the following questions.

1. Persistent gaps between the health status of minorities and non-minorities are defined as:
   a. Racism
   b. Ethnocentrism
   c. Health disparities
   d. Cultural relativity

2. The use of one's own culture as a cultural standard is known as:
   a. Ethnocentrism
   b. Ritualism
   c. Culture
   d. Cultural relativity

3. Preconceived and untested beliefs about an individual or group of individuals is:
   a. Racism
   b. Stereotyping
   c. Culturally competent care
   d. Cultural relativity

4. You are caring for Mr. J., a 55-year-old man from Thailand. He has bacterial pneumonia and a temperature of 104°F; yesterday his temperature was 102°F. The physician on call prescribes cool compresses for Mr. J. to help lower his fever. However, Mr. J. insists that you bring him warm blankets because they will help him recover more quickly. You recognize that Mr. J.'s request is an example of:
   a. Cultural ritual
   b. Cultural competence
   c. Cultural stereotyping
   d. Ethnocentrism

5. Culture shock is best defined as:
   a. The acute experience of not understanding the culture in which one is situated.
   b. Using one's own culture as the correct standard for comparison.
   c. Expectations learned over a period of time.
   d. A recognizable and predictable pattern of human behavior.

6. Mr. V. was recently admitted to the Intensive Care Unit following an acute gastroesophageal bleed. His native language is Spanish, and he speaks limited English. When speaking with Mr. V., it is important to remember which of the following? Select all that apply.
   a. Speak directly to the interpreter.
   b. Use interpretive services when communicating patient instructions for discharge.
   c. Use simple sentences.
   d. Rephrase a question if the patient's response does not match the original inquiry.

7. A minority group is defined as a group of people who differ from the majority of persons in their society based on which of the following? Select all that apply.
   a. Race
   b. Religion
   c. Political beliefs
   d. Ethnicity

8. The ANA states that nurses are responsible for delivering culturally competent care for all patients. Culturally competent care accounts for all of the following except:
   a. Individual values
   b. Developmental level
   c. Patient's height
   d. Available technology

9. Mrs. A. is an Alaskan Inuit woman recently admitted to the hospital with a ruptured ovarian cyst. She has expressed that it is very important that her husband be present to receive all medical information. Using the

concepts of culturally competent care, which is the best response?

a. Explain to Mrs. A. that she is required to make all of her own decisions related to her healthcare.

b. Document Mrs. A.'s request in your nursing care plan.

c. Bring Mrs. A.'s husband into the hallway to discuss surgical options for Mrs. A.

d. Explain to Mrs. A. that it is not a good idea to have her husband in the room when discussing such a private matter.

CHAPTER 5

Communication in the Nurse–Patient Relationship

SECTION I: LEARNING OBJECTIVES

Upon completion of this chapter, the student will be able to do the following:

1. Define the four major types of communication.

2. Discuss the elements of the communication process and their relevance to nursing.

3. Describe how language and experience affect the communication process.

4. Explain the nature of the nurse–patient relationship.

5. Distinguish between a professional and a social relationship.

6. Name the elements of an informal nurse–patient contract.

7. Discuss three key ingredients of therapeutic communication.

8. Name two professional self-care safety nets.

9. Identify important assessment areas to address when communicating with patients.

10. Give an example for each type of therapeutic communication technique.

11. Identify three key non-therapeutic responses, explaining how each interferes with therapeutic communication.

12. Describe two special situations that affect communication.

SECTION II: ASSESSING YOUR UNDERSTANDING

Activity A FILL IN THE BLANKS

1. When applying the principles of therapeutic communication to a nurse–patient interaction, it is important to remember that the _____ is the focus of the conversation.

2. A nurse walks into Mr. Z.'s room and introduces herself as his nurse for the evening shift. It is Christmas Eve, and to be festive, she dressed for her shift as an elf. This provides the patient with a/an _____ message about the nursing professional he just encountered.

3. The process of the sender and the receiver using one another's reactions to produce further messages is called _____.

4. Technical _____ often intimidates patients and prevents them from asking questions.

5. The contractual relationship between the nurse and a patient is _____; it is typically verbal and assumed by both parties.

6. When considering elements of therapeutic communication, _____ is the ability to walk in another person's shoes.

7. In the informal nurse–patient contract, the circle of _____ is always respected.

8. When a patient makes a vague statement or complaint, try _____ to enhance a therapeutic nurse–patient interaction.

9. Reviewing a _____ of a conversation can help a nurse to develop his communication skills.

10. When speaking with _____, it is appropriate to play and speak using simple words.

Activity B MATCHING

1. *Match the style of communication in Column A with its definition in Column B.*

Column A

____ 1. Verbal

____ 2. Nonverbal

____ 3. Written

____ 4. Metacommunication

Column B

A. Records the treatment of care and is a primary means of passing along healthcare information.

B. Use of spoken word. Powerful because the specific words and jargon used define the perceptions and realities of people's experiences.

C. Communication about communication or lack thereof. It is anything that is taken into account during an interpreting an interaction.

D. Gestures, facial expressions and posture are all examples.

2. *Match the element of therapeutic communication listed in Column A with its definition in Column B.*

Column A

____ 1. Comfortable sense of self

____ 2. Positive regard

____ 3. Empathy

Column B

A. To unconditionally be able to view a person in a nonjudgmental way.

B. The ability to look at things from another's perspective and to communicate that understanding through verbal and nonverbal communication.

C. Awareness of one's own values, personality, cultural background and style of communication.

Activity C SHORT ANSWER

1. Describe the difference between a congruent relationship and an incongruent relationship among types of communication. Provide an example for each.

_____

_____

_____

2. Who is the key focus in the nurse–patient relationship? Discuss the goals and parameters of this relationship.

_____

_____

_____

3. Discuss two techniques you could utilize to initiate a conversation with a new patient.

_____

_____

_____

4. Explain how silence can be used as a therapeutic communication technique.

_____

_____

_____

5. Discuss special communication strategies that may facilitate a therapeutic communication with an older adult.

_____

_____

_____

SECTION III: APPLYING YOUR KNOWLEDGE

Activity D CASE STUDY

Angie is a 26-year-old patient s/p a dilatation and curettage procedure following a spontaneous miscarriage. This is the first time you have met Angie. As you enter the room, you notice that Angie is staring at the wall and appears sullen and withdrawn.

1. What are some strategies you could use to open your conversation with Angie?

_____

_____

_____

2. Using Table 5-4 as a guide, create a brief process recording of your conversation with Angie.

_____

_____

_____

SECTION IV: PRACTICING FOR NCLEX

Activity E MULTIPLE CHOICE

Answer the following questions.

1. Mrs. Vining has just learned that she has Stage 2 breast cancer. She appears distant and withdrawn. Her shoulders are slumped. She explains "I just never thought this could happen to me". Which answer best describes Mrs. Vining's response?
   a. Incongruent communication
   b. Verbal communication
   c. Congruent communication
   d. Nonverbal communication

2. Which of the following best describes an element of the nurse–patient relationship?
   a. The nurse self-discloses only what is necessary for the patient's benefit.
   b. Conversation for mutual companionship, enjoyment and interaction.
   c. Sharing of life events and activities.
   d. A conversation with the goal of forming a more intimate relationship.

3. Mr. Brandon is a 35-year-old patient with Down syndrome. He is on your unit following heart surgery. He is very weak and has had difficulty with his activities of daily living. Which of the following is an example of his nurse using advocacy as a style of patient communication?
   a. There are starving children all over the world who would love to eat your food.
   b. You have to get up to shower; otherwise you may get a blood clot.
   c. If you don't get up right now to take a walk, you may develop a blood clot. Wouldn't your family be so stressed if you had to stay in the hospital longer?
   d. I know that it has been difficult for you to walk to the bathroom to brush your teeth. How can we make this work for you?

4. Mrs. Miller is a 60-year-old woman s/p a hip replacement. She has had multiple complications following surgery including a skin infection and a blood clot. As a result, she has been a patient on the unit for 6 weeks. You have just returned from vacation and this is your first day caring for Mrs. Miller. One of your colleagues looks at you and describes her as "quite difficult to deal with". You know that all of the following can contribute to difficult behaviors except:
   a. A quiet room
   b. Language barrier
   c. Fatigue
   d. Multiple family members in the room

5. Carl Rogers (1961) studied the process of therapeutic communication. Through his research, the elements of a "helpful" person were described. They include all of the following except which choice?

    a. Empathy

    b. Positive regard

    c. Analysis

    d. Comfortable sense of self

6. Each of the following facilitates a therapeutic nurse–patient relationship except which one?

    a. Closed-ended questions

    b. Rephrasing

    c. Reflection

    d. Active listening

7. Mr. Delmico is a hospice patient that you are visiting in his home. He is explaining the difficulties he is having with his home infusion pump. By making statements such as "I see" and "go on" during your conversation, you are utilizing which therapeutic nurse–patient communication technique.

    a. Restating

    b. Clarification

    c. Reflection

    d. Encouraging elaboration

8. Jimmy is an 18-month-old patient in the Pediatric Intensive Care Unit. He is scheduled to have a subgaleal shunt placed tomorrow, and his mother is quite nervous about the procedure. You feel for the mother and tell her that the surgeon "has done this a million times. Jimmy will be fine". This is an example of what type of non-therapeutic communication?

    a. Rescue feelings

    b. False reassurance

    c. Giving advice

    d. Being moralistic

9. Which of the following are examples of non-professional involvement?

    a. Discussing your recent breakup with your boyfriend with a patient who is also going through a difficult breakup.

    b. Asking a patient if they would like to go out for dinner after they are discharged.

    c. Discussing today's weather forecast.

    d. Asking a patient in hospice care to describe their relationship with various family members.

10. Mrs. Singh recently immigrated to the United States from Mumbai, India. She was just admitted to your unit postoperatively following gallstone removal. She does not speak English. When using the hospital's interpretive services, which of the following are most important?

    a. Speak directly to the patient.

    b. Ensure that family members are present.

    c. Give all of your discharge instructions at once.

    d. Have the interpreter write out all of the information listed in your unit brochure.

CHAPTER 6

Values, Ethics, and Legal Issues

SECTION I: LEARNING OBJECTIVES

Upon completion of this chapter, the student will be able to do the following:

1. Define values, personal values, and professional values.

2. Explain how behaviors relate to values.

3. Apply cultural and developmental perspectives when identifying values.

4. Examine value conflicts and resolutions in nursing care situations.

5. Differentiate law and institutional policies from professional values.

6. Discuss the eight principles of healthcare ethics from the American Nurses Association.

7. Describe a systematic approach for resolving ethical dilemmas.

8. Distinguish among licensure, a standard of care, a crime, and a tort.

9. Define four elements of negligence.

10. Describe legal protections for nurses and cite measures to take.

SECTION II: ASSESSING YOUR UNDERSTANDING

Activity A FILL IN THE BLANKS

1. _____ are abstract ideas that set an individual's standard for decision making.

2. Values are often firmly engrained by _____ _____, but this age group is still willing to accept the values of others that are different from their own.

3. If a person does not develop a sense of _____, their values will reflect the values of others and be externalized rather than internalized.

4. Since there are no absolute guidelines for healthcare decision making, _____ provide a framework for doing so.

5. When a nurse acts on a patient's wishes in order to do good, she is practicing _____.

6. In the U.S. healthcare system, patients are _____ to make decisions about the care that they receive.

7. Keeping patient information _____ is a professional and legal requirement of the nurse.

8. When a nurse develops a treatment plan, it is important that she engage the patient in a discussion to identify _____.

9. When a nurse is accused of _____ it means that she has written something about a patient that is false and injurious to the patient's reputation.

10. Nurses have a _____ to their patients.

11. The doctrine of respondeat superior states that the _____ may be held responsible for the nurses' negligence.

12. Professional _____ cases can be brought against nurses for adverse patient outcomes.

13. To be prosecuted for a crime, a prosecutor must demonstrate _____ intent and a criminal act.

14. The Controlled Substances Act of 1970 states that nurses may administer narcotics to a patient under the direction of an _____ provider.

ACTIVITY B **MATCHING**

1. *Match the age in Column A with Erickson's theory of development in Column B.*

Column A

____ **1.** Infant

____ **2.** Toddler

____ **3.** Preschool

____ **4.** School age

____ **5.** Adolescence

____ **6.** Young adulthood

____ **7.** Middle adulthood

____ **8.** Older adulthood

Column B

A. Loyalty

B. Competence

C. Will

D. Wisdom

E. Love

F. Care

G. Hope

H. Purpose

2. *Match the legal terminology in Column A with its definition in Column B.*

Column A

____ **1.** Living will

____ **2.** Licensure

____ **3.** Standard of care

____ **4.** Tort

____ **5.** Negligence

____ **6.** Malpractice

Column B

A. The legal ability of the nurse to practice in any given state

B. A mistake or failure to be prudent

C. Specifies the type of medical treatment a patient does or does not want to receive should they be incapacitated to make medical decisions

D. Negligence in the practice of a profession

E. Results in a civil trial to assess compensation for the plaintiff

F. The expected level of nursing performance as established by guidelines or authority

ACTIVITY C **SHORT ANSWER**

1. Distinguish between personal values and professional ethics.

_____

_____

_____

2. Describe the difference between beneficence and nonmaleficence.

_____

_____

_____

3. Explain how the concept of justice is practiced in the United States healthcare system.

_____

_____

_____

4. Define licensure and the Nurse Practice Act and discuss their role in nursing practice.

_____

_____

_____

5. Define "Code Status" and discuss why it is important to know the code status of your patient.

_____

_____

_____

SECTION III: APPLYING YOUR KNOWLEDGE

ACTIVITY D CASE STUDY

Ms. Montrose a 65-year-old patient with multiple sclerosis. Two years ago, you cared for Ms. Montrose while she was in the hospital for a pulmonary embolism. On your shift, her condition worsened and Ms. Montrose required 1 minute of CPR and transfer to the ICU. She was a full code status. After her stay in the hospital, Ms. Montrose noted that her right arm was tingling and believes that it was related to the CPR that was done. You are named in a lawsuit in which a patient, Ms. Montrose, is suing the hospital for malpractice.

1. Based on the information given, are you liable for injuries sustained to this patient?

   _____

   _____

   _____

2. Discuss what your legal options are as a registered nurse.

   _____

   _____

   _____

SECTION IV: PRACTICING FOR NCLEX

Activity E MULTIPLE CHOICE

Answer the following questions.

1. Johnny, age 2, is with his mother in clinic today. Johnny continues to grab for the otoscope, then looks sheepishly toward his mother as she tells him "no". According to Kohlberg (1964), Johnny is in which stage of learning?
   a. Conventional
   b. Preconventional
   c. Values
   d. Will

2. Anna is a 2-month-old infant extremely ill from HSV sepsis. Anna's mother and father, Mr. and Mrs. James, have decided to stop additional medical intervention and allow Anna to pass away naturally. Mrs. James does not want her relatives to know that they plan to stop pursuing aggressive medical treatment because it is against their family's religious beliefs to withdraw medical support. What do you tell Mrs. James?
   a. Yes, it is her decision who to inform about the family's medical decision.
   b. Yes, but encourage her to tell her family so that they can provide support.
   c. No, it is wrong to lie to people.
   d. No, you can keep details of her diagnosis from the family, but not the fact that she is dying.

3. Mr. Cunningham is a 40-year-old man admitted s/p repair of a femoral fracture. He discloses that he has a history of an addiction to painkillers and asks that you assist him in adhering to his recovery from this addiction by not administering any narcotics. As you review post-operative orders for Mr. Cunningham, you note that his physician has ordered Codeine 30 mg PO q6 hours for pain. How do you best approach this situation?
   a. Inform the next nurse that the patient does not wish to receive narcotics.
   b. Offer the medication to the patient; if he really doesn't want it, he will tell you.
   c. Ask the physician to remove this order from the patient's chart.
   d. Leave the order in the chart.

4. You are a nurse on the oncology unit and are caring for a patient on hospice care. The patient is weak and is resting. The patient's daughter comes storming onto the unit and demands that you do everything you can to treat her mother. This is an example of what type of values conflict?
   a. Family conflict
   b. Healthcare conflict
   c. Ethical conflict
   d. Individual conflict

5. The nurse administered Acetaminophen (Tylenol) 15 mg/kg to a 2-year-old with a sore throat. After charting the medication, she realized that the patient has a documented allergy to the medication. The patient breaks out in a rash 15 minutes later, his throat swells, and he must be intubated. Which best describes the nurse's actions?

   a. The nurse is guilty of negligence but not malpractice.

   b. The nurse committed a crime and is going to jail.

   c. This was an honest mistake and the nurse is not at fault.

   d. The nurse is guilty of malpractice.

6. You are driving on a back country road when a man flags you down and yells that his wife is having a baby. As a registered nurse you are eager to help. You recall that you are covered under the Good Samaritan Law. This law states which of the following?

   a. That your license is protected if you act in a reasonable manner given the circumstances

   b. That you are required to assist this couple because of your medical knowledge

   c. That your license is at risk and you would face criminal prosecution if an error was made

   d. That you are not allowed to help this couple and instead call 911

CHAPTER 7

Nursing Research and Evidence-Based Care

SECTION I: LEARNING OBJECTIVES

Upon completion of this chapter, the student will be able to do the following:

1. Trace the historical appreciation of nursing research.

2. Explain the contributions of evidence-based research to nursing practice.

3. Discuss the role of evidence-based research in nursing.

4. Review the research process for the beginning professional nursing student.

5. Summarize legal and ethical issues related to nursing research.

SECTION II: ASSESSING YOUR UNDERSTANDING

Activity A FILL IN THE BLANKS

1. _____ research forms a bridge between theory and practice.

2. A systematic investigation designed to test a hypothesis is called _____.

3. Evidence-based practice emphasizes decision making based on the best available evidence and the use of _____ studies to guide decisions.

4. The focus of nursing research must be on generating _____ knowledge to guide nursing practice.

5. _____ research involves the systemic collection and analysis of subjective narrative materials.

6. The PICO model is a mnemonic that helps to formulate good clinical _____ questions.

7. In the problem statement, a relationship is expressed between two or more _____.

8. Privacy of research subjects is protected with anonymity and _____.

Activity B MATCHING

Match the feature of a nursing research method in Column A with the correct research type in Column B.

Column A	Column B
____ 1. The systematic collection of numeric information	A. Quantitative research
____ 2. Requires the researcher to become an instrument	B. Qualitative research
____ 3. Focuses on understanding the whole	
____ 4. The systematic collection of subjective materials	
____ 5. Uses formal protocols to collect data	

Activity C ORDERING

1. Below are historical occurrences that lead to an increased appreciation of nursing research. *Write the correct sequence in the boxes provided below:*

    a. Dr. Allen started the first Canadian nursing research journal.

    b. Publications of nursing research became more common.

    c. Research interest turned to supply and demand for nurses to serve in the military.

    d. The Institute of Medicine urged the federal government to increase the level of funding for nursing research.

    e. Florence Nightingale carefully documented the care of soldiers.

    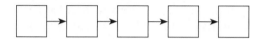

2. Below are the steps of the research process. *Write the correct sequence in the boxes provided below:*

    a. Translation of finding to practice.

    b. Develop a research design and analyze results.

    c. Propose a research question or hypothesis.

    d. Choose a theoretical framework and formulate a problem statement.

    e. Identify a problem area and perform a review of the scientific literature.

    f. Dissemination of the results and communication of findings.

    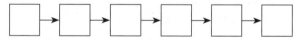

Activity D SHORT ANSWER

1. Why is doing a literature review important for any research project?

    _____

    _____

    _____

2. Why are institutional review boards so important in research?

    _____

    _____

    _____

3. What is the difference between a dependent and an independent variable?

    _____

    _____

    _____

4. How are study results disseminated?

    _____

    _____

    _____

5. What is the goal of evidence-based practice?

    _____

    _____

    _____

SECTION III: APPLYING YOUR KNOWLEDGE

ACTIVITY E CASE STUDY

Answer the following questions, which involve the nurse's role in translating evidence into practice:

Mr. Gage is a 45-year-old patient who has hypertension and hyperlipidemia. Both his biological parents were diagnosed with type II diabetes in their 40s. Mr. Gage has not yet had elevated blood sugar levels when tested but his hemoglobin A1c, a test performed on diabetics to assess blood sugar levels over the last 3 months, was 5.9% which is on the high end of normal. Mr. Gage wants to know what he can do to keep from getting diabetes.

1. What are two examples of a foreground question for this patient and patients like him?

    _____

    _____

    _____

2. What would be a good way to go about finding the most up-to-date information for this patient to answer his question?

    _____

    _____

    _____

    _____

SECTION IV: PRACTICING FOR NCLEX

Activity F **MULTIPLE CHOICE**

Answer the following questions.

1. Which of the following could be considered an example of a qualitative research project?

   a. Kathleen is a BSN student who is looking at the prevalence of alcohol hand sanitizer use on an adult medical floor. She is collecting her data by observing nurses going in and out of rooms and noting how often they use the hand sanitizer and how often they do not.

   b. Jerry is a PhD nursing student who is collecting data on how Somali immigrants perceive the care they receive in one community clinic. He is taping and analyzing interviews with patients that have been in the country and community 2 years or less and who have sought care at least once at this clinic.

   c. Jason is a nurse who is a member of the wound care team on his in-patient floor in the hospital. He is collecting data for a research project that is interested in uptake of information given to patients by nurses. He is giving patients a quiz about the information both before patient education occurs and afterwards.

   d. Marta is on a nursing research team that is interested in the prevalence of anemia in a group of patients suffering from Crohn's disease. She is looking at the serum hemoglobin and ferritin levels of these patients.

2. Which of the following is an example of evidence-based nursing practice?

   a. Dorothea is a nurse working in an obstetric clinic. Because many of her patients experience nausea and vomiting, Dorothea performed a literature review on complementary and alternative medicine treatments. She has chosen to look at studies that have been published in indexes such at PubMed. In her review of the literature she found that ginger was an effective treatment for nausea and was safe during pregnancy. She now recommends ginger to all of her patients.

   b. Jared has been a nurse on the Intensive Care Unit for 10 years. He has noticed that more and more of his patients are getting central line infections during their stay on the floor. Knowing that this can lead to an increased length of stay and worse health outcomes, Jared asks his nurse manager for central line dressing kits which cut down on the number of steps that need to be kept sterile during the process of a dressing change.

   c. Maggie is a nurse practitioner in women's health. She has been a nurse practitioner for 20 years and has successfully treated many women for gonococcal infections with ciprofloxacin. Newer research has found that ciprofloxacin and other fluoroquinolones are not recommended for these patients because of resistance. Maggie continues to prescribe ciprofloxacin because she does not want to change something that works for her patients.

   d. Dora is a nurse on a cardiac floor in the hospital. Dora read yesterday in a nursing journal that people who are 50 and over should be on a daily dose of aspirin. She consults with the prescribing physician about this issue because one of her patients is not currently taking this drug.

3. Which of the following is not a focus of nursing research?

   a. Drug metabolism by Cytochrome P450
   b. Health appraisal
   c. Prevention of trauma
   d. Promotion of recovery
   e. Coordination of healthcare

4. Which of the following is not a criterion for critically evaluating websites when doing a literature review?

   a. Authority
   b. Currency
   c. Objectivity
   d. Coverage
   e. Accessibility

5. The American Nurses Association's Commission on Nursing Education developed guidelines for the investigative function of nurses at different educational levels. Which of the

following is a guideline for a nurse with an associate degree?

a. Assist in collection of data within an established, structured format

b. Reads, interprets, and evaluates research for applicability to nursing practice

c. Identifies nursing problems that need to be investigated and participates in implementation of scientific studies

d. Analyzes and reformulates nursing practice problems so that scientific knowledge and scientific method can be used to find solutions

6. Which of the following is not an example of a problem statement?

a. Is there a relationship between diet soda intake and obesity in adolescent boys?

b. In patients with stage II pressure ulcers, does screening for and treating diagnosed depression decrease healing time?

c. Is it better to tell patients that a medical error has occurred with their care and do an internal investigation or tell them about the error and do an internal investigation?

d. What is it like for teens with cystic fibrosis to experience a lung transplant that fails?

7. Marion is a nurse in a nursing home. She strongly believes that the care she provides be evidence based and tailored to her population. She is constantly looking for ways in which to improve patient outcomes. Recently she has noticed that more and more of the residents she works with have a diagnosis of depression. Marion wants to decrease depression rates. Place the following actions in the order that they should occur following the scientific process of nursing practice.

a. Marion assesses the problem of an increased number of residents with depression.

b. Marion makes a nursing diagnosis.

c. Marion starts a group therapy session once a week for residents to talk about shared experiences.

d. Marion uses anonymous surveys of residents to evaluate depression levels.

CHAPTER 8

Patient Education and Health Promotion

SECTION I: LEARNING OBJECTIVES

Upon completion of this chapter, the student will be able to do the following:

1. Describe important qualities of a teaching–learning relationship.

2. Explain the domains of knowledge and how learning relates to each.

3. Identify four purposes of patient education.

4. Define factors that inhibit and facilitate learning.

5. Discuss important assessment data used to individualize patient teaching.

6. Describe individualized teaching methods and evaluation strategies for patients of different ages or abilities.

7. Give examples of health promotion and disease prevention behaviors.

8. Recognize major factors that affect motivation and health maintenance.

SECTION II: ASSESSING YOUR UNDERSTANDING

Activity A FILL IN THE BLANKS

1. Patient education is a _____ activity that involves both the patient and the healthcare team.

2. Mastering a new skill such as taking a blood pressure is an example of _____ learning.

3. Health promotion activities are meant to increase a patient's level of _____, while disease prevention activities _____ specific diseases.

4. To match a teaching activity with a patient's _____ knowledge, a nurse could ask "what do you know about this medication?".

5. Teaching is best delivered when learning is a high _____ for the patient.

6. The words "compliance" and "noncompliance" have generally been replaced with the term _____, or the extent to which a behavior reflects an agreed upon health plan.

7. The ability to obtain, process, and understand basic health information is known as health _____.

8. The use of dolls to explain a procedure to a child is an example of _____ _____.

9. For women of all ages, the use of a breast _____ is an effective strategy for teaching what a breast lump would feel like.

10. In order to evaluate whether teaching was effective, it is helpful to review the patient _____.

Activity B **MATCHING**

1. Match the nursing activity in Column A with an example in Column B.

Column A

_____ **1.** Disease prevention

_____ **2.** Restoration of health

_____ **3.** Promotion of coping

_____ **4.** Health promotion

Column B

A. Partnering with physical therapy to assist a patient post-stroke walk three times per day

B. Working with your patient to incorporate exercise into their schedule five times per week

C. Teaching a diabetic patient about low-sodium diet

D. Explaining to parents that their child will be intubated following surgery

2. Match the teaching concepts and method in Column A with an example in a newly diagnosed Type 1 Diabetic patient in Column B.

Column A

_____ **1.** Cognitive

_____ **2.** Affective

_____ **3.** Psychomotor

_____ **4.** Repetition

_____ **5.** Individualized

Column B

A. Rescheduling a teaching session so both parents can be present

B. A discussion with the diabetic about the function of insulin in the body

C. A return demonstration of insulin injection

D. Explaining how adherence to an insulin regimen promotes better overall health and will reduce tension within a family

E. Scheduling three sessions with a patient to practice insulin injection

Activity C **SEQUENCING**

1. Place the stages of the *Transtheoretical Model of Change* in the order in which they occur.

a. Preparation

b. Precontemplation

c. Maintenance

d. Action

e. Contemplation

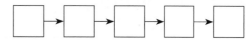

Activity D **SHORT ANSWER**

1. Discuss ways in which teaching can be patient focused.

_____

_____

_____

2. Differentiate between health promotion and disease prevention.

_____

_____

_____

3. Define primary, secondary, and tertiary prevention and provide an example of each.

_____

_____

_____

4. Discuss ways in which consideration of cultural and language needs are important for delivery of healthcare.

_____

_____

_____

5. Describe some important considerations when selecting written material for patient education.

_____

_____

_____

6. Discuss some of the key patient characteristics that should be present to facilitate effective teaching.

_____

_____

_____

SECTION III: APPLYING YOUR KNOWLEDGE

Activity E CASE STUDY

Mr. Morgan is a 65-year-old man with a 40-year pack history of tobacco use. He comes into your clinic today and professes that he is going to quit smoking tomorrow. He informs you that he saw an advertisement for a new smoking cessation medication on television and would like you to ask his nurse practitioner for a prescription.

1. According to the Transtheoretical Model of Change, what stage of change is Mr. Morgan?

_____

_____

_____

2. Write an appropriate NANDA-I nursing diagnosis for Mr. Morgan.

_____

_____

_____

3. List some lifespan considerations you should keep in mind when working with Mr. Morgan.

_____

_____

_____

4. Mr. Morgan's nurse practitioner prescribes this new medication for him. Discuss general strategies of how you might provide Mr. Morgan with information about side effects.

_____

_____

_____

SECTION IV: PRACTICING FOR NCLEX

ACTIVITY F MULTIPLE CHOICE

Answer the following questions.

1. You are working with Mr. Milner, a 55-year-old man who recently underwent a coronary artery bypass graft (CABG). He is taking furosemide and metoprolol following his procedure. Together you and Mr. Milner are developing a plan for a heart healthy diet. During their planning, Mr. Milner states that he really thinks that his diet did not contribute to his heart disease. If he continues to take his medications, he should be fine. According to the *Transtheoretical Model of Change,* what stage of change is Mr. Milner in related to his diet?

a. Contemplation

b. Preparation

c. Precontemplation

d. Maintenance

2. You are working with a panel of diabetic patients. Part of your job description is to provide education to patients about the benefits of healthy food choices. Nurse Adams education has taught a few of her patients the benefit of healthy food choices. This is an example of what type of learning?

a. Affective learning

b. Cognitive learning

c. Psychomotor learning

d. Technical learning

3. Mrs. Bryant is 40 years old. Her family nurse practitioner has prescribed a mammogram as part of Mrs. Bryant's annual examination. Mammograms are an example of which type of preventative healthcare?

a. Primary prevention

b. Tertiary prevention

c. Secondary prevention

d. Health prevention

4. Mrs. Shields is a 46-year-old obese woman diagnosed with hypertension and type 2 diabetes. She tells you that she knows she needs to lose weight. She recently visited her local fitness club, obtained a membership and has signed up for their next water aerobics class. According to the *Transtheoretical Model of*

Change, what stage is Mrs. Shields in relation to her weight loss?

a. Preparation

b. Maintenance

c. Precontemplation

d. Contemplation

5. You are teaching Juan, age 4, about cast care following a tibia-fibula fracture. Which of the following is NOT developmentally appropriate to include in your teaching?

a. Blocking 30 minutes for skill teaching

b. Use of dolls to demonstrate psychomotor skills

c. Ensuring Juan's parents are present

d. Give stickers as a reward for task completion

6. The nurse is working with Ms. Adams, a 26-year-old smoker who is a patient in an outpatient center. Ms. Adams states that she is very committed to quitting smoking to improve her health as well as to provide a good example for her young son. The nurse knows that participating in a smoking cessation support group is a key component to smoking cessation. During discussion, the nurse asks Ms. Adams "on a scale of zero to ten, how likely are you to attend a support group?" Which strategy of motivational interviewing is the nurse using with Ms. Adams?

a. Assessing importance

b. Elicit–provide–elicit

c. Evoking change talk

d. Rating

7. You are working with James, a 15-year-old patient with sickle cell anemia. He was started on a new pain management plan today, and you are evaluating the effectiveness of the plan. Which of the following is NOT appropriate to include in your care?

a. Ask only his parents to be present at the teaching session.

b. Include a note about who was taught this new information in the patient's chart.

c. Ensure James that your conversation is confidential except under extreme circumstances.

d. Answer questions openly and honestly.

8. You are engaged in teaching Zach, a 5-year-old boy that is newly diagnosed with type 1 diabetes. His mother is his primary caregiver and is present with him today. You are preparing to teach insulin injections. Zach's mother informs you that she has a fear of needles. Which of the following are appropriate for a successful teaching session? Select all that apply.

a. Ensure 20 minutes of uninterrupted teaching time.

b. Use a doll so that Zach can practice this skill.

c. Provide Zach's mother with an informational pamphlet about insulin injection.

d. Ask Zach's mother to leave the room because she will be a distraction.

9. You are working with Mrs. Xander, a 60-year-old woman recently diagnosed with Stage 2 ovarian cancer. You would like to provide some health literature to help her educate herself about this new diagnosis. Several of your patients have informed you of internet resources they found particularly helpful. When considering these resources for Mrs. Xander, you know that which of the following are true? Select all that apply.

a. Many websites are above the recommended reading level for patients with low literacy.

b. Sites that target multiple audiences (healthcare providers and patients) provide less individualized information.

c. Lack of stability of web addresses provides confusion and frustration.

d. Websites are always current to provide the most up-to-date information.

10. You are working with Mrs. Jones, age 76, on developing a medication schedule following a new diagnosis of type 2 diabetes. She has difficulty reading the medication labels due to age-related vision changes. Mrs. Jones further confides in you that she has stopped taking the "water pill" because it makes her urinate too frequently. She has stopped taking her ARB because it is "too expensive". Which of the following are appropriate NANDA-I diagnoses for Mrs. Jones? Select all that apply.

a. Ineffective health maintenance related to insufficient resources

b. Deficient knowledge related to cognitive limitations

c. Ineffective therapeutic regimen management related to lack of motivation

d. Ineffective therapeutic regimen management related to side effects of treatment

Caring for the Older Adult

SECTION I: LEARNING OBJECTIVES

Upon completion of this chapter, the student will be able to do the following:

1. Describe the demographics of older adults in North America.

2. Discuss a comprehensive knowledge base that can help nurses display commitment to providing humane and dignified care.

3. Explain functional and physiologic changes that place older adults at greater risk for declines in health and quality of life.

4. Identify health promotion and health maintenance strategies that can give older adults advantages in maintaining optimal health.

SECTION II: ASSESSING YOUR UNDERSTANDING

Activity A FILL IN THE BLANKS

1. The percentage of older adults aged 65 and older is _____ percent of the United States total population.

2. Older adults who live below the poverty level commonly live in large metropolitan areas, rural towns, and the _____ portion of the United States.

3. Older adults tend to experience higher rates of dementia, or irreversible confusion, as well as _____, or acute confusion.

4. The mood disorder _____ often goes unrecognized and is subsequently under diagnosed in the older adult.

5. An overactive detrusor muscle is responsible for _____ incontinence.

6. Skin _____ refers to skin that is intact without any breaks.

7. Good oral health is necessary to meet the _____ needs of the older adult.

8. The prevalence of chronic pain in persons over 60 is _____ the rate of chronic pain in persons younger than 60 years.

9. In _____-focused coping, the individual tries to change the way he thinks about the situation rather than change the situation itself.

10. _____ care is the practice of meeting the needs of an individual at the end of life.

Activity B MATCHING

1. *Match the statistic in Column A with its definition in Column B.*

Column A

___ **1.** 4.1%

___ **2.** 42%

___ **3.** 54.6%

___ **4.** 20.1%

___ **5.** 9.7%

Column B

A. The number of older adults categorized as belonging to a minority population

B. The percentage of noninstitutionalized older adults living with a spouse

C. The percentage of older adults living in institutional settings

D. The percentage of older adults living below the poverty level

E. The percentage of widows living in the United States.

Activity C SHORT ANSWER

1. Why is the use of antipsychotic medication limited in older adults?

2. What are self-care activities and how can dementia or chronic illness impede self-care?

3. Why are falls so common and of such concern in the older adult?

4. Discuss the ways that grief may affect the older adult and how nurses can respond.

5. Describe signs of depression in an older adult.

SECTION III: APPLYING YOUR KNOWLEDGE

Activity D CASE STUDY

Lenora is an 85-year-old widow who lives alone in a single family home. She was recently discharged from the hospital following a fall. She had significant bruising over her left arm and knee but did not break any bones. You are meeting Lenora for the first time to initiate home care services.

1. What questions would you ask Lenora regarding her risk of falls?

2. Why are questions regarding elimination so important?

3. Lenora reveals to you that she has lost interest in taking her daily walk, which she previously loved. What other signs would you look for to indicate that Lenora is suffering from depression?

4. After meeting Lenora, you note that she has not cooked for herself in some time. What other signs may lead you to suspect a cognitive impairment?

_____

_____

_____

SECTION IV: PRACTICING FOR NCLEX

Activity E MULTIPLE CHOICE

Answer the following questions.

1. Patrice is a 77-year-old woman on your unit s/p left knee replacement. She typically stools every morning but has not had a bowel movement in 3 days. You know that which of the following medications places Patrice at increased risk for constipation?

a. Hydromorphone
b. Psyllium
c. Acetaminophen (Tylenol)
d. Furosemide (Lasix)

2. Eleanor is a 78-year-old woman on your rehabilitation unit s/p a cerebrovascular accident (CVA). As you assess her gait, you notice that her left foot is dragging and she is not bending her left knee nor swinging her left arm. How would you best describe what you are visualizing with Eleanor's gait?

a. Spastic
b. Festinating
c. Hemiparesis
d. Ataxic

3. You are performing a home assessment for Miguel, a 90-year-old widower who lives in a third story apartment. As you consider his home environment, you know that what poses the greatest risk of injury-related death or disability for Miguel?

a. Myocardial infarction
b. Falls
c. Dementia
d. Fire

4. Eunice is an 86-year-old female on the medical inpatient unit. She explains that the hospital is quite noisy and that she is having difficulty sleeping. Which of the following is NOT true regarding sleep in the older adult?

a. Sleep medications are usually the first choice in treating sleep disturbance.
b. Stage one sleep increases in the older adult.
c. Deep sleep declines in the older adult.
d. Chronic cardiovascular or respiratory illness can interfere with sleep.

5. Ruth is a 90-year-old woman admitted to your unit s/p CVA. She is A&Ox3 but has limited mobility and hemiparesis of the left side of her body. She is experiencing urinary incontinence. Which of the following is the most appropriate nursing action?

a. Insert a foley catheter to prevent incontinence.
b. Use disposable padding (Chux) to keep the bedding dry.
c. Assist Ruth once per shift to use the commode.
d. Use the Braden scale to assess for pressure ulcers.

6. Amelia is a 78-year-old woman s/p right hip fracture after a fall. She has stopped going to her church over the past few months. She has also asked her neighbor to help her and do her gardening, an activity she previously loved. Amelia tells you "I just don't enjoy gardening like I used to. I am always worried about falling". What would most concern you regarding Amelia?

a. Depression
b. Generalized anxiety disorder
c. Realistic caution
d. Bipolar disorder

7. Victor complains of chronic insomnia. Which medication would you NOT want to administer to Victor?

a. Diuretic in the morning for hypertension
b. Acetaminophen for postoperative pain
c. Nasal decongestant for an upper respiratory infection
d. Beta blocker for blood pressure control

8. Ada, 92-years-old, is admitted to your unit with a community-acquired pneumonia requiring 14 days of intravenous antibiotic treatment. She asks why this happened to her. You know which to be true of immunity in older adults?

   a. Humoral immunity declines

   b. Older adults are more susceptible to pneumonia following respiratory infections.

   c. Nutrition.

   d. Alcoholism

9. James is a 75-year-old African-American man on your inpatient unit following a minor stroke. He expresses to you that he has difficulty finding meaning in life. He is retired from the workforce and recently moved in with his daughter due to financial issues. He does not volunteer or participate in organized activities. You suspect that James may be suffering from depression. Which of the following is a factor of depression in older adults? Select all that apply.

   a. Depression is often underdiagnosed in the older adult.

   b. Patients suffering from strokes and cancer are more likely to report depression.

   c. A recent change in living environment

   d. Older African-American men have the highest rate of suicide.

   e. Currently, older Caucasian males have the highest rate of suicide in the United States.

CHAPTER 10

Nursing Process: Foundation for Practice

SECTION I: LEARNING OBJECTIVES

Upon completion of this chapter, you will be able to do the following:

1. Identify the components of the nursing process.

2. Discuss the requirements for effective use of the nursing process.

3. Explain how critical thinking is used in nursing. Enhance awareness of definitions, behaviors, and standards used in critical thinking. Understand the relationships between knowledge, experience, critical thinking, reflection, clinical reasoning, and nursing judgment.

4. Explore ways to enhance and develop critical thinking skills, especially as they apply to nursing.

SECTION II: ASSESSING YOUR UNDERSTANDING

Activity A FILL IN THE BLANKS

1. The nursing process is a systematic problem-solving approach to provide _____ nursing care.

2. The _____ is the primary source of information for assessment.

3. Diagnostic _____ is the process of gathering and clustering data to propose diagnoses.

4. The _____ is the nurse's label for the problem.

5. The success of a nursing intervention is garnered during the _____ phase.

6. Active listening means paying attention to both _____ cues and spoken responses.

7. The application of theoretical knowledge to an actual patient scenario is referred to as clinical _____.

8. The process of _____ allows nurses to explore their experiences and develop a new appreciation or understanding.

9. The _____ nurse can link theory, practice, and intuition.

10. As a nurse gains more clinical experience, _____ develops.

11. The nursing process is a framework for providing _____ care to individuals, families, or communities.

12. Legally and professionally, the nursing _____ is recognized as the standard method of nursing practice.

13. According to Benner (2000), a nurse who realizes that events, context, and patient situation are as important as the nurses' resources is considered _____.

1. *Match the phase in the nursing process in Column A with an example in Column B.*

Column A

____ **1.** Plan

____ **2.** Assessment

____ **3.** Evaluation

____ **4.** Diagnosis

____ **5.** Implementation

Column B

A. The risk for fluid imbalance secondary to lack of oral fluid intake

B. Ambulation unsuccessful because patient was unable to support his own weight

C. Requested lime gelatin from the nutrition department as requested by the patient

D. The patient will walk three times a day for 10 minutes each time

E. A murmur was auscultated in the pulmonic region

1. Describe the difference between primary and secondary sources of information.

_____

_____

_____

2. Define the nursing process and differentiate between the nurse's and patient's role.

_____

_____

_____

3. Provide examples of the ways in which a nurse can develop critical thinking skills.

_____

_____

_____

4. Discuss the importance of reflection-in-action and reflection-of-action.

_____

_____

_____

5. Describe the five stages of Benner's (2000) model of skill acquisition.

_____

_____

_____

SECTION III: APPLYING YOUR KNOWLEDGE

Activity D CASE STUDY

Mr. Simmons is an 86-year-old man admitted to a hospice care facility with a diagnosis of stage IV lung cancer. His children, grandchildren, and close friends take turns bringing food, reading him the paper, and enjoying his company. You note that during these visits, Mr. Simmons is often quiet and appears relaxed. His wife states that this is the most at peace she has seen Mr. Simmons in a long time. In the evenings when he is alone with staff, he is quite animated, sharing stories about his life's adventures.

1. Using the skill of reflection, try to put yourself in the shoes of Mr. Simmons. Why is his behavior so different during visits with friends and when he is alone? Answers will vary.

   _____

   _____

   _____

2. Provide an example of an assessment from a primary source and from a secondary source.

   _____

   _____

   _____

SECTION IV: PRACTICING FOR NCLEX

Activity E MULTIPLE CHOICE QUESTIONS

Answer the following questions.

1. Benner (2000) has developed a model of skill acquisition outlining the stages of increasing expertise. The practitioner who uses rules to predominantly guide practice would best be described as which of the following?

   a. Advanced beginner

   b. Expert

   c. Novice

   d. Proficient

2. You are sitting with Mrs. Andrews, a 90-year-old patient in a long-term care facility. Mrs. Andrews is describing the challenge of her transition from independent living to assisted living. You are watching Mrs. Andrews' body language as she tenses her body during the conversation. Which of the following best describes the skill you, the nurse, are utilizing?

   a. Listening

   b. Observing

   c. Collaborating

   d. Communicating

3. Nurse Chen is caring for Mrs. B., a 50-year-old post-hysterectomy patient whose care is complicated by a post-operative infection. She is IV on antibiotics. Nurse Chen recalls from a literature review that probiotics are an effective means to prevent thrush in patients receiving antibiotics. This is an example of which phase of the nursing process?

   a. Diagnosis

   b. Implementation

   c. Assessment

   d. Plan

4. You are caring for Mr. M., a 35-year-old man who recently underwent gastric bypass surgery. He is complaining of horrible diarrhea. After a lengthy discussion, you identify that spicy food may be contributing to this problem. You speak with the staff nutritionist to work with the patient to make appropriate food choices. Which of the following best describes your discussion with the patient?

   a. Secondary source information gathering

   b. Primary source information gathering

   c. Team evaluation

   d. Collaborative implementation

5. Nurse White is working on a rehabilitation floor today. She has obtained a pair of crutches for her patient from the physical therapy department. She and her patient set a goal of using the crutches twice daily to ambulate down the hall. However, at the end of the day, the patient was only able to ambulate one time because the crutches were the incorrect height. The patient's inability to ambulate best represents which phase of the nursing process?

   a. Diagnosis

   b. Evaluation

   c. Intervention

   d. Plan

6. A.J. is a 15-year-old man who confides in you that he is considering sexual activity with his girlfriend. He asks you what the best method of birth control is for someone his age. Before answering, you hope to discover more about what A.J. knows about sexual activity and birth control. This is an example of which phase of the nursing process?

   a. Evaluation

   b. Planning

   c. Diagnosis

   d. Assessment

7. You note that the patient you are caring for has had a 20 mm Hg drop in her systolic blood pressure in the last hour. She is slurring her words and cannot tell you what date it is. She has twice asked to speak with her mother, who you know to be deceased. You surmise that the patient is acutely disoriented. You approach an experience nurse to ask for assistance. Your thought process and actions in this scenario can best be described as what?

   a. Clinical experience

   b. Collaboration

   c. Clinical reasoning

   d. Astute nursing

8. Critical thinking relies on the nurse's ability to evaluate a clinical situation. According to the National League of Nurses (2011) which of the following describes the process of evaluation? Select all that apply.

   a. Detect bias

   b. Examine alternatives

   c. Interpret evidence

   d. Revise a plan

CHAPTER 11

Nursing Assessment

SECTION I: LEARNING OBJECTIVES

Upon completion of this chapter, the student will be able to do the following:

1. Describe the assessment phase of the nursing process.

2. Discuss the purpose of assessment in nursing practice.

3. Identify the skills required for nursing assessment.

4. Differentiate the three major activities involved in nursing assessment.

5. Describe the process of data collection.

6. Explain the rationale for data validation.

7. Discuss the frameworks used to organize assessment data.

SECTION II: ASSESSING YOUR UNDERSTANDING

Activity A FILL IN THE BLANKS

1. The first phase of the nursing process is called _____ and is the collection of data for nursing purposes.

2. _____ lays the groundwork for collecting other kinds of assessment data and involves using all senses.

3. _____ consists of asking questions designed to elicit subjective data from the patient or family members.

4. _____ is the visual examination of the patient that is done in a methodical and deliberate manner.

5. The technique of listening to body sounds with a stethoscope placed on the body surface to amplify normal and abnormal sounds is called _____.

6. _____ data are observable, perceptible, and measurable.

7. Past and current health records are considered _____ sources.

8. _____ serve as guides during the nursing interview and physical examination.

9. A(n) _____ assessment is performed when the patient enters a healthcare facility, receives care from a home health agency, or is seen for the first time in an outpatient clinic.

10. _____ is the specialized use of touch for data collection.

Activity B MATCHING

1. Match the type of nursing assessment method in Column A with the correct aim in Column B.

Column A

____ **1.** Time-lapse reassessment

____ **2.** Problem-focus assessment

____ **3.** Emergency assessment

____ **4.** Admission assessment

Column B

A. Identification of a life-threatening situation

B. Comparison of patient's current status to baseline obtained previously

C. Initial identification of normal function, functional status, and collection of data concerning actual or potential dysfunction

D. Status determination of a specific problem identified during previous assessment

2. Match the method of validating data in Column A with the correct example in Column B.

Column A

____ **1.** Comparing cues to normal function

____ **2.** Referring to textbooks, journals, and research reports

____ **3.** Checking consistency cues

____ **4.** Clarifying the patient's statements

____ **5.** Seeking consensus with colleagues about inferences

Column B

A. A patient states that she has a history of sarcoidosis. The nurse looks this disease up in a medical journal in order to find out more about the disease and what to look for.

B. A patient states that they feel shaky, "just like when my sugars are low." The nurse checks the patient's blood glucose and finds that it is 45, well below normal.

C. The nurse knows that babies usually are able to pull themselves to a sitting position by the age of 12 months so they are not worried that Toby is not doing this at the age of 10 months.

D. A patient states that her stomach hurts. The nurse asks her to point to the area that hurts and she points to her lower right abdominal area or quadrant.

E. A nurse performs an assessment of a patient with a red spot on their right heel. Due to the fact that the area is non-blanchable and the patient is immobile much of the time, the nurse comes to the conclusion that this person has a stage II pressure ulcer. He then looks at previous assessments and finds that the last nurse came to the same conclusion.

Activity C ORDERING

1. Below are examples of the four phases of an interview. *Write the correct sequence in the boxes provided below.*

a. The nurse reviews as much information as possible about the patient.

b. The nurse and the patient review the goals attained and the nurse encourages the patient to express their feelings.

c. The nurse and the patient work toward achieving a set goal.

d. The nurse establishes rapport with the patient, introduces themselves and their role, and attempts to alleviate any anxiety.

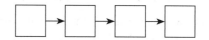

Activity D SHORT ANSWER

1. Why are setting and environment important to consider when performing an assessment?

_____

_____

_____

2. Why is smell an important assessment tool?

_____

_____

_____

3. In what way does the nursing history help the nurse?

_____

_____

_____

4. Describe the type of information that can be gathered from secondary sources.

_____

_____

_____

5. Why is it important to validate information that is gathered in an assessment?

_____

_____

_____

SECTION III: APPLYING YOUR KNOWLEDGE

Activity E CASE STUDY

Answer the following questions, which involve the nurse's role in assessing a patient.

Natalia is a 33-year-old woman who is being admitted to the hospital for a thyroidectomy after being diagnosed with thyroid cancer 2 days ago. You are the nurse who is going to admit her.

1. Describe the process of performing your assessment of this patient.

_____

_____

_____

2. Which framework, or frameworks, will you use to organize your data collection?

_____

_____

_____

SECTION IV: PRACTICING FOR NCLEX

Activity F MULTIPLE CHOICE

Answer the following questions.

1. The assessment phase of the nursing process has to be well organized to prevent omission of pertinent information. Which of the following is an advantage of using the functional health framework?

   a. Patient strengths and assets can be identified.

   b. It provides a guide so that the nurse can systematically examine every part of the body.

   c. It focuses on the patient's major anatomic systems.

   d. It allows the nurse to collect data about the past and present condition of each organ or body system.

2. Which of the following action is taken during the maintenance phase of an interview?

   a. Assess your own feelings or reactions to previous patients that might interfere with the nurse–patient relationship.

   b. Keep focused on the task or goals to ensure that needed data are obtained and goals are achieved.

   c. Review goal or task attainment.

   d. Observe the patient's behavior, and listen attentively.

   e. Establish a verbal contract with the patient, incorporating the goals of the interview.

3. An assessment involves gathering pieces of information about a patient's health status. Which of the following pieces of information is subjective?

   a. Patient has a temperature of 102 °F.

   b. Patient has leukoplakia on her oral mucosa.

   c. Patient has generalized myalgia or muscle pain.

   d. Patient is alert and oriented to person and place but not time or situation.

   e. Patient has ptosis, a drooping of the eyelid, on his right side.

4. Which of the following defines the physical exam technique of auscultation?

   a. The technique of listening to body sounds with a stethoscope placed on the body surface to amplify normal and abnormal sounds.

   b. A visual examination of the patient that is done in a methodical and deliberate manner.

   c. The specialized use of touch for data collection.

   d. A technique in which one or both hands are used to strike the body surface in a precise manner to produce a sound.

   e. Systematic data collection method that uses the four senses to detect health problems.

5. Which of the following is an example of a time-lapse reassessment?

   a. Daren is a nurse in a hospital that happens to walk by a room and notices a patient down on the floor. Daren immediately assesses the patient for airway, breathing, and circulation. Once the presence of these three is established, Daren calls for help and begins a quick neurological exam.

   b. Joan is a nurse who is just coming on to her shift. She has received patient reports from the nursing leaving the floor. To start off her day, she goes into each of her patient's rooms and performs a focused physical assessment based on each individual's diagnosis.

   c. Bob is a nurse in a long-term skilled nursing facility. Noreen is a new patient. Bob wants to gather information from Noreen, which include her health status and any problematic health patterns, and to get a baseline for Noreen's overall functioning.

   d. Natalia is a visiting nurse who has an appointment with Donald, an 85-year-old man with mobility issues. Natalia has worked with Donald in the past on the ways in which he can prevent falls. Today she wants to assess how he is doing with the fall prevention strategies they practiced before.

6. Which of the following techniques facilitate communication during an interview? Select all that apply.

   a. Use broad opening statements

   b. Share observations

   c. Use silence

   d. Use reassuring clichés

   e. Give approval

CHAPTER 12

Nursing Diagnosis

SECTION I: LEARNING OBJECTIVES

Upon completion of this chapter, the student will be able to do the following:

1. Define diagnosis in relation to the nursing process.

2. Describe the components of a nursing diagnosis.

3. Discuss the significance of nursing diagnosis for nursing practice.

4. Differentiate between nursing diagnosis and collaborative problems.

5. Identify the clinical skills needed to make nursing diagnoses.

6. Formulate nursing diagnoses for a patient situation.

7. Discuss the categorization of nursing diagnoses by functional health patterns.

SECTION II: ASSESSING YOUR UNDERSTANDING

Activity A FILL IN THE BLANKS

1. Nursing diagnosis is the _____ of collected patient data.

2. A medical diagnosis describes a _____ of specific organ systems, whereas a nursing diagnosis describes a patient's _____ to a disease process.

3. Actions that require both a physician prescription and a nursing prescription are called _____ health problems.

4. _____ are pieces of information collected during the nurse's assessment.

5. Cluster _____ requires that you look at the whole clinical picture and attach meaning to the cluster.

6. A _____ might help a nurse with limited experience form a nursing diagnosis.

7. In a nursing diagnosis, cues are documented following statements such as _____.

8. Nursing diagnoses increase the _____ of the nursing intervention for each patient.

Activity B MATCHING

1. Match the medical diagnosis in Column A with a potentially paired nursing diagnosis in Column B.

Column A

___ **1.** Uncomplicated seizure

___ **2.** Femoral fracture

___ **3.** Dementia

___ **4.** Respiratory distress syndrome

___ **5.** Rotavirus

Column B

A. Impaired walking

B. Diarrhea

C. Risk for falls

D. Wandering

E. Ineffective airway clearance

2. Match the component of the nursing diagnosis in Column A with an example in Column B.

Column A

___ **1.** Descriptors

___ **2.** Definition

___ **3.** Defining characteristics

___ **4.** Related factors

___ **5.** Risk factors

Column B

A. Body temperature above normal range

B. A reddened area on a patient's sacrum

C. Associated with increased intracranial pressure

D. Deficient or decreased

E. Old age

Activity C ORDERING

1. Place the following events of the nursing diagnosis phase in the order in which they occur:

a. Formulates the nursing diagnosis statement

b. Identifies patterns

c. Validates diagnosis

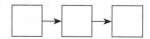

Activity D SHORT ANSWER

1. Describe the legal ramifications of nursing diagnoses.

_____

_____

_____

2. What is the purpose of clustering clues?

_____

_____

_____

3. Discuss the importance of interpreting clustered cues.

_____

_____

_____

4. Describe the four types of nursing diagnoses.

_____

_____

_____

5. Discuss the difference between a nursing diagnosis and a collaborative diagnosis.

_____

_____

_____

SECTION III: APPLYING YOUR KNOWLEDGE

Activity E CASE STUDY

Mrs. Abrams is a 22 year-old new mother to baby Sophia, age 2 hours. Sophia was born with an undiagnosed cleft lip and palate. When you approach Mrs. Abrams, she is crying. She confides "I was so excited about breastfeeding and now it can never happen". Her husband, Mr. Abrams, is quietly sitting in the corner.

1. Considering the family as your patient, develop three actual nursing diagnoses based on the information provided.

_____

_____

_____

2. Develop three risk diagnoses based on the information provided in this example.

_____

_____

_____

SECTION IV: PRACTICING FOR NCLEX

Activity F MULTIPLE CHOICE

Answer the following questions.

1. Which of the following is the best example of a nursing diagnosis?

   a. Gastroesophageal reflux related to low stomach pH as evidenced by foul breath, burning sensation in throat.

   b. Ineffective airway clearance as evidenced by patient not speaking.

   c. Ineffective breastfeeding related to latching as evidenced by nonsustained suckling at the breast.

   d. Cellulitis related to infection as evidenced by warm, reddened skin.

2. Elise is a 57 year-old woman who is caring for her 84-year-old mother-in-law. Which of the following statements would lead you to make a nursing diagnosis of caregiver role strain?

   a. I just don't have time to take a shower.

   b. I feel great but wish that I could get more sleep.

   c. My mother-in-law and I go for a walk daily.

   d. My mother-in-law makes dinner on Tuesday's and I cannot stand her cooking.

3. Can a nurse develop a nursing diagnosis when there is not enough evidence to support the presence of a problem, but the nurse would like to gather more evidence?

   a. Yes, this defines a risk diagnosis.

   b. No, a nursing diagnosis describes an existing problem.

   c. No, the nurse must have all of the evidence before formulating the diagnosis.

   d. Yes, this defines a possible nursing diagnosis.

4. You are treating a patient with congestive heart failure. He informs you that he is having difficulty walking up the stairs in his home. He is frustrated because he used to be a runner, and now he can barely walk to the store. Which of the following is an accurate actual nursing diagnosis for this patient?

   a. Activity intolerance related to congestive heart failure as evidenced by inability to walk up and down stairs.

   b. Activity intolerance as evidenced by inability to walk up and down stairs and inability to walk to the store.

   c. Impaired coping related to new diagnosis of congestive heart failure.

   d. Risk for impaired coping related to congestive heart failure.

5. A nurse makes a nursing diagnosis of constipation after a patient tells her he did not defecate on his last trip to the bathroom. She has no other information on the patient's defecation history. This is an example of which of the following?

   a. Inconsistent cues

   b. Premature closure

   c. Clustering of cues

   d. Cluster interpretation

6. "Acute pain related to instillation of peritoneal dialysate as evidenced by patient wincing and grimacing during procedure, patient description of experience as 'stabbing'" is an example of what type of nursing diagnosis.

   a. Actual diagnosis

   b. Risk diagnosis

   c. Wellness diagnosis

   d. Potential diagnosis

7. Which of the following is an accurately phrased risk diagnosis?

   a. Risk for impaired coping as evidenced by patient crying.

   b. Risk for fluid volume excess related to increased oral intake as evidenced by consuming 3 L of soda.

   c. Risk for pain after surgery.

   d. Risk for falls related to altered mobility.

8. A nursing diagnosis has which of the following parts? Select all that apply.

   a. Risk factors

   b. Defining characteristics

   c. Related factors

   d. Chief complaint

   e. Descriptors

   f. Definition

CHAPTER 13

Outcome Identification and Planning

SECTION I: LEARNING OBJECTIVES

Upon completion of this chapter, the student will be able to do the following:

1. Define outcome identification and planning.

2. Explain the purposes of outcome identification and planning.

3. Discuss the Nursing Outcome Classification and the Nursing Intervention Classification projects.

4. Describe the components of the patient plan of care.

5. Formulate a patient plan of care for a patient given a nursing assessment database.

6. Use a functional health approach to plan patient care.

SECTION II: ASSESSING YOUR UNDERSTANDING

Activity A FILL IN THE BLANKS

1. The Nursing _____ Classification system has 385 outcomes for individuals, families, communities, or caregivers.

2. The top priority for outcome planning is always _____ problems.

3. A short-term nursing outcome is typically fulfilled within one _____.

4. Nursing interventions are any _____ that the nurse performs to enhance patient outcomes.

5. The nursing plan of care uses scientific rationales from nursing literature to illustrate the nurse's _____ process.

6. All nursing diagnoses should be listed in order of _____ for patient care.

7. The focus of the clinical plan of care is the _____.

8. The critical path is based on evidence-based research and the most _____ practice pattern for a particular diagnosis.

9. The critical path is used by the _____ care team.

10. Deviation from the critical path is known as a _____.

Activity B MATCHING

1. *Match the terminology in Column A with its definition in Column B.*

Column A

_____ **1.** Individual plan of care

_____ **2.** Standardized plan of care

_____ **3.** Patient outcome criteria

_____ **4.** Nursing intervention

_____ **5.** Scientific rationale

Column B

A. The plans are written by a group of nursing experts for a patient population with a specific medical diagnosis.

B. Specific, measurable, realistic statements that can be evaluated to judge goal attainment.

C. Provides justification for carrying out the intervention.

D. Created by the RN. The nursing diagnoses are listed, along with specific goals and interventions to resolve the problem.

E. Nursing orders that are specific to the stated goal.

Activity C SHORT ANSWER

1. What is the purpose of outcome identification?

_____

_____

_____

2. List the five components of outcomes criteria.

_____

_____

_____

3. Discuss why the plan of care is so important in the nursing profession.

_____

_____

_____

4. Describe who develops a critical path, how a critical path is used, and why it is so important.

_____

_____

_____

5. What is "variance" from the critical path?

_____

_____

_____

SECTION III: APPLYING YOUR KNOWLEDGE

Activity D CASE STUDY

Fawn is a 46-year-old woman recovering from surgical cholelithectomy. She is two hours post-op. She is currently on bed rest and is NPO.

1. How might a critical path be used in this case?

_____

_____

_____

2. Provide one nursing intervention for the patient at this time and the rationale for that intervention.

_____

_____

_____

3. A licensed provider orders that the patient resume feedings as tolerated. Restate this as a nursing outcome criterion.

_____

_____

_____

SECTION IV: PRACTICING FOR NCLEX

Activity E MULTIPLE CHOICE

Answer the following questions.

1. Jamal is a 16-year-old patient admitted to the medical unit 1 hour ago for sickle cell crisis. His vital signs are as follows: T: 36.8 sublingual, HR: 95, RR: 20, BP: 130/65. He rates his pain as a 9/10. You are talking with the medical resident on service to discuss patient orders. What order are you likely to request first for Jamal?

   a. Narcotic pain medication to treat pain

   b. Septic workup due to BP and HR elevation

   c. Isolation for suspected respiratory illness

   d. Tylenol to treat pain and fever

2. You are caring for Isabel, a 45-year-old ventilator-dependent quadriplegic. You are in the process of placing IV access when the ventilator alarms occlusion. You assess Isabel and she appears mildly uncomfortable but is not in acute distress. What is your first priority in your nursing outcome planning?

   a. Continue to place IV

   b. Ask Isabel to cough and clear her tracheostomy tube

   c. Assess tracheostomy for patency

   d. Call respiratory therapy for help

3. Consider the following statement: "The patient <u>ambulated</u> with the assistance of a cane without incident during his physical therapy session." Which part of the outcome criteria does the underlined portion represent?

   a. Verb (action)

   b. Who

   c. Condition

   d. Criteria

4. Cameron is a 5 year old recently diagnosed with type I diabetes. You are in charge of her discharge teaching plan. You know that site rotation is important for long-term self-care. The statement "will properly identify three areas on her body to inject insulin" represents which of the following?

   a. Scientific rationale

   b. Nursing diagnosis

   c. Nursing intervention

   d. Outcome criteria

5. You are caring for Collin, a 30-year-old man s/p repair of a left femur fracture. He is currently immobilized and on strict bed rest. You enter Collin's room every 2 hours to help him change positions because doing so will help to prevent pressure ulcers. The "help to prevent pressure ulcers" portion of this statement is best described as which of the following?

   a. Rationale

   b. Outcome criteria

   c. Nursing intervention

   d. Nursing diagnosis

6. Georgia is a 56-year-old woman on your inpatient unit 2 hours s/p gallbladder surgery. She is just waking up from anesthesia, and asks you how long it will take until she can go home. You respond that most patients are discharged within 2 days. Your answer is most likely based on which of the following pieces of information?

   a. The individualized plan of care

   b. The scientific rationale

   c. The agencies critical path

   d. The patient outcomes and interventions

7. Eric is a 35-year-old construction worker who fractured his right clavicle on the job. He is on your rehabilitation unit working to regain full function of his right arm. Which of the following represents the best documentation of the evaluation of Eric?

   a. Patient will perform ROM three times per day.

   b. Actively abducts right arm from 0 to 90 degrees, passive ROM from 90 to 180 degrees.

   c. Able to abduct from 0 to 90 degrees without assistance. Will continue to perform ROM three times per day.

   d. Active ROM only twice today, but patient states goal of three times per day tomorrow.

8. Amira is on your surgical unit s/p resection of an intestinal tumor. She is alert and oriented x3. Based on assessment of the patient, a medical order to "ambulate with assistance" is written in the chart. This will be her first time ambulating. Which of the following best represents a nursing outcome?

   a. The patient will ambulate with the assistance of a walker without falling within the next 4 hours.

   b. Physical therapy will be consulted to assist the patient with ambulation.

   c. The patient will ambulate to the restroom three times this shift.

   d. The patient will ambulate with the assistance of a walker sometime today.

9. Which of the following represent appropriate nursing interventions for a patient who is on bed rest s/p surgical intervention? Select all that apply.

   a. Deep breathing using an incentive spirometer every hour

   b. Change of position every 2 hours

   c. Ambulation when patient feels better

   d. Acetaminophen (Tylenol) every 6 hours for treatment of pain

10. You are caring for Samantha who is on your medical unit s/p pneumonia. She has a medical order to "resume oral feeding as tolerated". Which of the following are appropriate nursing interventions related to this medical order? Select all that apply.

   a. Allow Samantha to order her favorite foods from the hospital menu

   b. Auscultate for bowel sounds

   c. Begin feedings with clear broth

   d. Consult with dietitian regarding appropriate foods

11. Elijah is 9 months old admitted to your unit s/p non-accidental trauma. He suffered a left clavicular fracture and fracture of the left femur. He also has a concurrent diagnosis of a stage 2 pressure ulcer. He is alert and oriented x3 and taking food and milk by mouth. Which of the following are appropriate outcome criteria for Elijah? Select all that apply.

   a. Elijah will ambulate to the bathroom two times per day.

   b. Elijah will have complete resolution of pressure ulcer by discharge.

   c. Elijah will assist with turning every 2 hours.

   d. Elijah will feed self under direct supervision five times per day.

12. You are developing a plan of care for a newly admitted patient to your nursing unit. You know that which of the following are important to include in this plan of care? Select all that apply.

   a. Promoting patient participation

   b. Planning care that is realistic and measurable

   c. Allowing for involvement of support people

   d. Providing standardized care

Implementation and Evaluation

SECTION I: LEARNING OBJECTIVES

Upon completion of this chapter, the student will be able to do the following:

1. Define implementation and evaluation.

2. Discuss the purposes of implementation and evaluation.

3. Describe clinical skills needed to implement the plan of care.

4. Explain methods for revising or modifying the plan of care.

5. Describe activities the nurse carries out during the evaluation phase of the nursing process.

6. Discuss quality assurance monitors used in nursing settings.

SECTION II: ASSESSING YOUR UNDERSTANDING

Activity A FILL IN THE BLANKS

1. During the _____ phase actual nursing care is provided.

2. The _____ skills used during implementation include problem solving, decision making, and teaching.

3. Setting _____ does not allow for skipping interventions; it only dictates the order in which interventions are performed.

4. When a nurse performs interventions, he may _____ tasks but remains accountable for supervision of the tasks performed.

5. Team conferences and team rounds are used to discuss a _____ health plan.

6. Interpersonal interventions include _____, supportive, and psychosocial interventions.

7. _____ interventions have the important role of helping patients' preserve function.

8. Evaluation is the nurses' judgment of the _____ of nursing care.

9. In order to properly evaluate a nursing intervention, the nurse must have knowledge of the normal patient _____.

10. The layout of a hospital and nurse–patient ratio are areas of concern in _____ evaluation.

11. Avoid _____ words in professional nursing documentation such as "good" or "inadequate"; such words may have different meaning to different people.

12. Once a nursing diagnosis is resolved, it may be _____ from the plan of care.

Activity B MATCHING

1. *Match the implementation skill or activity in Column A with its definition in Column B.*

Column A

____ **1.** Intellectual skill

____ **2.** Interpersonal skill

____ **3.** Technical skill

____ **4.** Reassessment

____ **5.** Priority setting

Column B

A. Verbal and nonverbal communication

B. Use of equipment, machines, and devices

C. Ranking of nursing diagnoses and patient problems in order of importance

D. Looking for changes in a patient's condition

E. Problem solving, decision making, and teaching

2. *Match the nursing intervention in Column A with its definition in Column B.*

Column A

____ **1.** Psychomotor interventions

____ **2.** Supportive interventions

____ **3.** Surveillance interventions

____ **4.** Coordinating interventions

____ **5.** Educational interventions

Column B

A. Focus on using good communication skills and caring behavior

B. Applying the basic principles of learning and teaching

C. Detecting changes from baseline data and abnormal responses

D. Interventions that require technical expertise

E. Serving as a patients advocate or coordination of care

Activity C SHORT ANSWER

1. Describe the implementation activity of reassessment.

_____

_____

_____

2. Discuss how nurses use education as an intervention.

_____

_____

_____

3. Why are supervisory interventions important?

_____

_____

_____

4. List and differentiate between the three types of interpersonal interventions.

_____

_____

_____

5. Why is evaluation such an important piece of the nursing process?

_____

_____

_____

6. List and describe the types of evaluation skills used by nurses.

_____

_____

_____

7. Discuss how the American Nurses Association (ANA) and the Joint Commission participate in quality improvement.

_____

_____

_____

SECTION III: APPLYING YOUR KNOWLEDGE

Activity D **CASE STUDY**

Mr. P. is a 46-year-old man admitted to your unit at 1 PM following the removal of an intestinal mass. He is ordered to have nothing by mouth (NPO) and to total parenteral nutrition (TPN) initiated. You know that TPN orders take time to process and that the TPN solution will likely not be available until after you leave your shift at 7:30 PM. He currently has a Jackson Pratt (JP) drain in his abdomen which is draining serosanguineous fluid and needs to be emptied every 2 hours. He has an intermittent IV infusion device in his right hand.

1. Based on the information provided and your assessment of Mr. P., develop two risk diagnoses for Mr. P. How would you prioritize these diagnoses?

   _____

   _____

   _____

2. Based on your risk diagnoses, discuss one technical implementation activity and one intellectual implementation activity that you could use to assist Mr. P.

   _____

   _____

   _____

SECTION IV: PRACTICING FOR NCLEX

Activity E **MULTIPLE CHOICE**

Answer the following questions.

1. Priority setting is based on the information obtained during reassessment. Priority setting is used to rank nursing diagnoses. Each of the following contributes to priority setting except which of the following?
   a. Finances of the patient
   b. The patient's condition
   c. Time and resources
   d. Feedback from the family

2. You are a nurse in the Burn Intensive Care Unit (BICU) and are caring for a 3-year-old boy who was burned with scalding hot water. He has burns covering 75 percent of his body. His condition is critical but stable. At 10 AM, you reassess the patient and find that he is agitated and pulling at his endotracheal tube. Which of the following would be your top nursing priority?
   a. Providing medication for agitation
   b. Repositioning to prevent pressure ulcers
   c. Ensuring that the endotracheal tube is secure
   d. Dressing change to prevent infection

3. You are caring for Mr. M., a 48-year-old man with congestive heart failure. Your nurse manager informs you that Mr. M. was enrolled in a clinical trial to assess whether a 10-minute walk, three times per day, leads to expedited discharge. What type of evaluation best describes what the researchers are examining?
   a. Process evaluation
   b. Structure evaluation
   c. Outcome evaluation
   d. Cost-effectiveness evaluation

4. You are caring for Mr. H., a 35-year-old man who is hospitalized following a motorcycle accident. He has a traumatic brain injury. You are working with Mr. H. on self-care behaviors. The following would help you to assess the success of your nursing interventions except which of the following?
   a. Check with the patient to ensure personal goals are met.
   b. Model self-care behaviors for the patient.
   c. Collect data on number of self-care activities performed that day.
   d. Ask patient to discuss his goals for the day at the start of your shift.

5. You are working with Ms. V. today. Ms. V. is having a difficult time accepting her new diagnosis of type II diabetes. You pull up a chair next to Ms. V.'s bed and hold her hand while listening to her story. What type of nursing intervention are you engaging in?
   a. Supportive intervention
   b. Psychosocial intervention
   c. Coordinating intervention
   d. Supervisory intervention

6. Mr. J. is a 56-year-old man s/p admission for a myocardial infarction and coronary artery bypass graft. He is preparing to go home tomorrow. Mr. J. expresses that he feels unprepared to cook heart healthy foods. You sit with Mr. J. and review the heart healthy nutrition plan, asking him to identify which foods would be appropriate for him to eat. What type of nursing intervention are you engaging in?

   a. Supervisory intervention

   b. Educational intervention

   c. Coordinating intervention

   d. Supportive intervention

7. Nurse Mayweather is auscultating lung sounds. She notes crackles in the LLL which were not present at the start of the shift. Nurse Mayweather is engaged in what type of nursing intervention?

   a. Educational intervention

   b. Psychomotor intervention

   c. Maintenance intervention

   d. Surveillance intervention

8. Nurse Sanchez is a community health nurse in a largely Hispanic community. She has noticed that a large percentage of her patients with type II diabetes struggle to find food choices that are a compatible with the cooking style of their culture. Nurse Sanchez decides to organize a cooking class to demonstrate to patients with type II diabetes how to prepare culturally appropriate foods. Nurse Sanchez actions could be labeled as what type of nursing intervention? Select all that apply.

   a. Educational intervention

   b. Psychosocial intervention

   c. Supervisory intervention

   d. Supportive intervention

9. The purpose of the nursing intervention classification (NIC) is which of the following? Select all that apply.

   a. Creation of a standardized language

   b. Assistance to determine the cost of service nurses provide

   c. Demonstration of the impact of nurses

   d. To create busy work for the nursing professional

CHAPTER 15

Documentation and Communication in the Healthcare Team

SECTION I: LEARNING OBJECTIVES

Upon completion of this chapter, the student will be able to do the following:

1. Describe the importance of timely, accurate communication in healthcare.

2. Describe the purposes of the patient record.

3. List key principles of charting.

4. Discuss the relevance of electronic records in documentation.

5. Properly record nursing progress notes by SOAP, PIE, FOCUS, or narrative format.

6. Identify flow sheets, plans of care, and critical pathways used in patient records.

7. Identify critical components for safe patient handoff.

8. Describe communication tools (such as SBAR, TeamSTEPPS) that improve organization of communication.

9. Discuss the importance of confidentiality and the RN's legal responsibility in documenting and reporting.

SECTION II: ASSESSING YOUR UNDERSTANDING

Activity A FILL IN THE BLANKS

1. Written or typed communication, or _____, serves as a permanent record of patient information and care.

2. _____ takes place when two or more people share information about patient care, either face to face, or by audiotape or voice mail, or by telephone.

3. _____ means keeping patient information private.

4. _____ charting is when a nurse waits until the end of their shift to chart on their patients which can lead to errors in documentation.

5. _____ are tables that have vertical and horizontal columns that allow nurses to document routine assessments and procedures.

6. A _____ occurs when the patient does not proceed along a clinical pathway as planned.

7. _____, or transfer of care for a patient from one health provider to another.

8. Physicians order _____ when a specialist or health team member must provide an expert opinion or specialized care for a patient.

9. An _____ is any unusual happening, such as a fall, medication error, malfunctions in equipment, or injury to a patient, visitor, or employee, that occurs during the performance of healthcare activities.

10. An _____ is a review of records which is used for quality assurance as well as reimbursement purposes.

Activity B MATCHING

1. *Match the documentation type listed in Column A with the correct description in Column B.*

Column A

___ **1.** PIE

___ **2.** SOAP

___ **3.** FOCUS

___ **4.** Narrative

___ **5.** Charting by exception

Column B

A. Data, action, response

B. Problem, interventions, evaluations

C. Standard met, you can sign or check off; if standards are not met, you can write a narrative or note

D. Subjective data, objective data, assessment, and plan

E. Information provided in written sentences or phrase, usually time sequenced

Activity C ORDERING

1. In order to promote clear and concise communication, the SBAR template for communication was developed. Following this template, write the following statements in the correct sequence in the boxes provided below:

a. Marta is a 80-year old woman who was admitted to the floor yesterday after total hip replacement. Past medical history includes hypertension and osteoarthritis.

b. I would recommend ordering a pain medication for breakthrough pain. I will recheck BP half an hour after administering pain medications.

c. Blood pressure elevation secondary to elevated pain.

d. Marta's BP is 210/93, HR is 102, pain is 8/10 on the pain scale.

Activity D SHORT ANSWER

1. Why it is important to document as care occurs?

_____

_____

_____

2. What is a nursing discharge summary?

_____

_____

_____

3. How is home care documented for Medicare and Medicaid patients?

_____

_____

_____

4. Describe the resident assessment instrument and what it is used for.

_____

_____

_____

5. What is a care plan conference?

_____

_____

_____

SECTION III: APPLYING YOUR KNOWLEDGE

Activity E CASE STUDY

Answer the following questions, which involve the nurse's role in assessing a patient:

You are a nurse taking care of Jan, a 38-year-old woman, who was admitted to the hospital for pyelonephritis (a kidney infection). She has been receiving IV fluids as well as IV antibiotics for 2 days. She states that her pain is mild, a 1/10 on the pain scale. It is located in her lower back. She is hungry and would like to order a meal. She denies any burning with urination currently although she did have this for about 2 weeks prior to coming into the hospital. She noticed some blood in her urine two days ago but none currently. Her vital signs are as follows: BP 122/63, HR 58, Temp 102.8, O₂ saturation 99%.

1. What is a possible SOAP note for this patient?

_____

_____

_____

2. From your assessment, you decide to call and communicate Jan's status to her primary provider. What could a possible SBAR report look like?

_____

_____

_____

SECTION IV: PRACTICING FOR NCLEX

Activity F MULTIPLE CHOICE

Answer the following questions.

1. Which of the following is not a purpose of the medical record?
   a. Legal document
   b. Reimbursement
   c. Contract
   d. Care planning

2. Which of the following is an example of using medical records for quality assurance purposes?
   a. Records are randomly selected to determine whether certain standards of care were met and documented.
   b. The nurse considers all data on the patient record when developing goals, outcome criteria, interventions, and evaluation criteria for and with patients.
   c. Data are gathered from groups of records to determine significant similarities in disease presentation, to identify contributing factors, or to determine the effectiveness of therapies.
   d. The medical record is used, by a student, to learn how a disease might present itself in certain patients.

3. Which of the following is not typically found in the patient care summary or kardex?
   a. Code status
   b. Respiratory assessment
   c. Activity status
   d. IV therapy

4. You are a nurse taking care of a 49-year-old man who was admitted for acute pancreatitis. He was admitted yesterday and has been on IV fluids, has been kept NPO (nothing by mouth), and has been given IV pain medications since. During your nursing assessment he tells you that his pain is a 4/10 on the pain scale. It starts out in his epigastric area and radiates to his back. He also has been nauseous this morning. Your facility charts by exception. You finish filling out the flow sheet and have to write a progress note. Which of the following is an example of writing a progress note that represents charting by exception for this patient?
   a. Forty-nine-year-old man, 125 mL/h of normal saline, NPO, pain 4/10 on pain scale with 2 mg IV dilaudid every 4 hours
   b. 4/10 pain on pain scale, epigastric radiating to back; also complains of nausea
   c. NPO, 4/10 pain, epigastric radiating to back, nausea
   d. 4/10 pain located in epigastric area and radiating to back with nausea; on IV fluids

5. Which of the following is a note that includes all elements of a SOAP note?

    a. Patient complains of nausea, one episode of nausea yesterday. Also with diarrhea. Mucous membranes are moist, good turgor. BP 130/85, HR 92. Nausea and vomiting of unknown etiology. Will give an antiemetic, will reassess.

    b. Patient complains of nausea, vomiting, and diarrhea × 3 days. States that she can't recall any sick contacts, denies any recent travel. Mucous membranes moist, BP 130/85, HR 92. Will give an antiemetic and reassess.

    c. Patient complains of nausea and vomiting × 3 days. Vital signs stable. Most likely due to gastroenteritis.

    d. Patient with nausea, vomiting, diarrhea, most likely secondary to gastroenteritis. Will give an antiemetic and reassess in half an hour.

6. In order to improve communication within the healthcare system, tools were created to standardize the process and assist with clarity and conciseness. SBAR is one such tool. In this tool, which of the following does R stand for?

    a. Reinforcing data

    b. Response

    c. Recommendation

    d. Report

7. Which of the following charting formats permit documentation on any significant topic, not just patient problems?

    a. CBE

    b. SOAP

    c. PIE

    d. FOCUS

8. Which of the following is a correct abbreviation to use in documentation?

    a. PO

    b. Sub q

    c. Per os

    d. BT

9. You are a nurse taking care of a 15-year-old man with cystic fibrosis. You are at the start of your shift and you go in to his room to introduce yourself and do a safety check. You notice that he is receiving a IV fluids with potassium. When you double check to see if this is what he is supposed to be on, you notice that these fluids were supposed to have been stopped 32 hours ago. Which of the following should you not do in this situation?

    a. Fill out an incident report

    b. Attach a copy of the incident report to the chart

    c. Stop the infusion and document the time

    d. Report error to primary provider

10. Which of the following is not true regarding a medication administration record (MAR)?

    a. If the patient refuses the dose you don't have to document this on the MAR.

    b. The MAR distinguishes between routine and "as needed" medications.

    c. The MAR identifies routine times for medication administration.

    d. When using an electronic MAR, the nurse has to log off so that the next person using the computer does not sign off a medication under their name by mistake.

11. You are a nurse taking care of a 66-year-old man post knee surgery. You are following a clinical pathway that guides the care of this patient after this specific procedure. He is 2 day post his operation and the clinical pathway states that you should advance his diet. You enter his room to discuss this order and find him vomiting in his wastebasket. What is a change in patient care that deviates from the clinical pathway called?

    a. Never events

    b. Variance

    c. Audit

    d. Deviation

12. Which of the following are high-risk errors made in documentation? Select all that apply.

    a. Inadequate admission assessment

    b. Failure to document completely

    c. Charting in advance

    d. Batch charting

    e. Falsifying patient records

13. Which of the following are principles of documentation? Select all that apply.

    a. Subjective

    b. Confidentiality

    c. Accuracy

    d. Objective

    e. Timely

CHAPTER 16

Health Assessment

SECTION I: LEARNING OBJECTIVES

Upon completion of this chapter, the student will be able to do the following:

1. Organize a nursing assessment.

2. Discuss preparation of the patient and the environment to foster data collection.

3. Differentiate between subjective and objective data.

4. Discuss methods to obtain subjective information during the patient interview.

5. Describe the techniques of inspection, palpation, percussion, and auscultation used in the physical assessment.

6. Describe methods to obtain objective data during the physical examination.

7. Individualize the nursing assessment based on lifespan considerations.

SECTION II: ASSESSING YOUR UNDERSTANDING

Activity A FILL IN THE BLANKS

1. _____ data are those symptoms, feelings, perceptions, preferences, values, and information that only the patient can state and validate.

2. Data sources such as another healthcare provider and clinical notes are labeled _____.

3. Assessment of nutrition includes dietary habits and _____ needs.

4. The way in which a person reacts and adapts to stress is called _____ behavior.

5. Sexual _____ is a complex integration of physiologic, psychological, and social aspects of human nature.

6. The degree to which sound propagates is called _____.

7. With _____ aphasia, patients are unable to understand simple directions.

8. An involuntary, rhythmic oscillation of the eyes noted during the evaluation of extraocular movements is called _____.

9. The area that is located in the second intercostal space, right sternal border of the precordium is called the _____ area.

10. _____ data can be directly observed or measured, such as vital signs or appearance.

11. Objective data concerning the patient's cognitive abilities are obtained through the _____ examination.

Activity B MATCHING

1. *Match the words used to describe skin in Column A with the correct definition in Column B.*

Column A

___ **1.** Cyanosis

___ **2.** Pallor

___ **3.** Jaundice

___ **4.** Erythema

___ **5.** Turgor

Column B

A. A change in the color of the skin to gray, blue, or purple due to hypoxia

B. Redness of the skin, usually from irritation or inflammation

C. A yellow tone to the skin, observed in liver disease

D. Used to describe how quickly skin returns to position after being pinched and released

E. A change in the color of the skin so that it appears pale.

2. *Match the words used to describe breath sounds in Column A with the correct definition in Column B.*

Column A

___ **1.** Vesicular

___ **2.** Bronchial

___ **3.** Bronchovesicular

Column B

A. Loud, high pitched, sound, which is normal if heard over the trachea

B. Soft and breezy, with inspiration lasting longer than expiration, that is normally heard over the lungs

C. A breezy, lower pitched sounds normally heard over the bifurcation of the main bronchi or posteriorly behind the scapulae

Activity C ORDERING

1. You are a nurse on an inpatient medical floor. You are just coming on to your shift and have gotten report on your patients from the nurse who is leaving. Your plan is to first perform an assessment of each of your patients. The first patient you start with is a 34-year-old woman named Dorothea who was admitted early this morning for pain in her right calf that is thought to be a deep vein thrombosis. In order to be thorough, in what order should you perform your assessment of this patient. *Write the correct sequence in the boxes provided below.*

a. You palpate the right calf to assess for temperature and moisture.

b. You observe the patient for any signs of pain such as grimacing or guarding.

c. You obtain the patient's vital signs.

d. You inspect the skin for color.

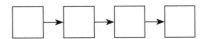

Activity D SHORT ANSWER

1. Why is performing a complete assessment important?

_____

_____

_____

2. In what type of environment should the patient assessment be performed?

_____

_____

_____

3. Why is it important to acknowledge one's own cultural beliefs as a nurse?

_____

_____

_____

4. Why is it important to assess a patient's sexuality?

_____

_____

_____

5. What are the lifespan considerations of assessing the school-age child and adolescent?

_____

_____

_____

Activity E CROSSWORD

Use the clues to complete the crossword puzzle.

Across

2. A curvature of a portion of the spine to the side laterally. The measure of vibration that is heard as pitch during auscultation.
4. What a nurse uses to make specific observations of physical features and behavior.
5. Used to make specific observations of physical features and behaviors.
6. Fluid which is accumulated in tissue, causing an indentation when pressed on for 5 seconds.

Down

1. This is used to determine whether a structure is air-filled, fluid-filled, or solid.
3. An instrument used during a physical assessment, which collects and transmits sound.

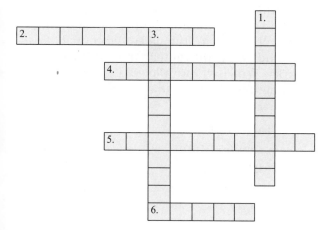

SECTION III: APPLYING YOUR KNOWLEDGE

Activity F CASE STUDY

Answer the following questions, which involve the nurse's role in assessing a patient.

Jordana is a 16-year-old woman who is being hospitalized for increasing shortness of breath. Jordana had cystic fibrosis and so has been in and out of the hospital her entire life. She is currently on a transplant list for new lungs. She knows that if she is diagnosed with an infection during this hospital stay she will be put farther down on the transplant list. Her mom is currently in her room and is visibly upset. Jordana is trying to comfort her.

1. Jordana most likely plays many roles. What roles could those be and why is assessing for them be important?

_____

_____

_____

2. What would your objective assessment of this patient's respiratory status look like?

_____

_____

_____

SECTION IV: PRACTICING FOR NCLEX

Activity G MULTIPLE CHOICE

Answer the following questions.

1. Your patient has been complaining of persistent headaches. Which of the following is an example of subjective data? Choose one.
   a. Temperature is 104.1°F.
   b. The patient appears lethargic.
   c. Pain is a 4 out of 10 on a pain scale.
   d. The patient is alert and oriented to person, place, and time.
   e. Heart rate is 100 bpm.

2. Palpation is the use of hands and fingers to gather information through touch. Different parts of the hand are more suitable for different tactile sensations. Which part of the hand is best for sensing temperature?

   a. The dorsum

   b. The palm

   c. The fingertips

   d. The knuckles

3. A nurse is assessing a new patient's level of activity and exercise. Which of the following should be addressed with every patient? Choose one.

   a. Whether they have anemia.

   b. Whether they have a program of regular physical activity.

   c. Whether they have proper dietary habits.

   d. Whether they have home maintenance skills.

4. You are evaluating a patient's orientation after they were brought into the ER following a car accident. Which of the following is indicated by "Oriented x3"? Choose one.

   a. Oriented person, situation, and time.

   b. Oriented to hospital, person, and date.

   c. Oriented to person, place, and time.

   d. Oriented to person, place, and situation.

5. Your patient, Mrs. Rodrigquez, has requested a translator so that she can understand the questions that you are asking her during the patient interview. You know which of the following is important when working with a patient translator?

   a. That talking directly to the translator facilitates the transfer of information.

   b. That talking loudly helps the translator and the patient understand the information better.

   c. That it is always okay to not use a translator if a family member can do it.

   d. That translators may need additional explanations of medical terms.

6. Cranial nerve function is important for normal sensory functioning. Which cranial nerve is important for the sense of smell? Choose one.

   a. Cranial nerve I

   b. Cranial nerve II

   c. Cranial nerve III

   d. Cranial nerve IV

7. The Glasgow Coma Scale is a standardized assessment tool for a person's level of consciousness. Which of the following patients would this scale not be appropriate for?

   a. Dana is in the Intensive Care Unit for acute pancreatitis and is asking for pain medications.

   b. Thomas is in the Intensive Care Unit after having a stroke yesterday.

   c. Jordan is recovering from brain surgery for repair of an aneurysm.

   d. Sonya has a brain tumor and is in the hospital because of respiratory depression.

8. It is important to ask several questions about a person's pain experience during the patient interview. Which of the following topics are important to address when assessing pain? Select all that apply.

   a. Aggravating factors

   b. Functional goal

   b. Duration

   c. Quality

   e. Location

   f. Intensity

9. During an assessment of the pupils, a beam of light is directed through the pupil and into the retina which stimulated the cranial nerve III and causes the muscles of the iris to constrict. Which of the following are evaluated by doing this? Select all that apply.

   a. Size

   b. Visual acuity

   c. Accommodation

   d. Reaction to light

   e. Internal structures

   f. Shape

CHAPTER 17

Vital Signs

SECTION I: LEARNING OBJECTIVES

Upon completion of this chapter, the student will be able to do the following:

1. Describe the procedures used to assess the vital signs: temperature, pulse, respirations, and blood pressure.

2. Describe factors that can influence each vital sign.

3. Identify equipment routinely used to assess vital signs.

4. Identify rationales for each route of temperature assessment.

5. Identify the location of commonly assessed pulse sites.

6. Describe how to assess orthostatic hypotension.

7. Recognize normal vital sign values among various age groups.

SECTION II: ASSESSING YOUR UNDERSTANDING

Activity A FILL IN THE BLANKS

1. The state of normal body temperature in a patient is termed _____.

2. Adult pulse rates above 100 beats per minute are called _____.

3. _____ is an abnormally slow respiratory rate, usually below 12 breaths per minute.

4. The absence of respirations, _____, is often described by the length of time in which no respirations occur.

5. Cardiac output is the product of _____ volume and heart rate.

6. An _____ gap is the absence of Korotkoff sounds between phases I and II.

7. _____ is the condition in which blood pressure is chronically elevated.

8. _____ is blood pressure below 100/60 mm Hg.

9. An abnormally slow pulse rate is called _____.

10. _____ refers to normal respiratory rhythm and depth.

Activity B MATCHING

1. *Match the common sites where arteries can be palpated for find a pulse in Column A with the correct description of where they can be found normally in Column B.*

Column A

____ **1.** Pedal

____ **2.** Carotid

____ **3.** Femoral

____ **4.** Popliteal

____ **5.** Radial

____ **6.** Apical

Column B

A. Beneath the sternomastoid muscle which runs from below the ear to the clavicle and sternum

B. At the level of the fifth intercostal space, midclavicular line

C. On the thumb side of the inner aspect of the wrist

D. In the anterior, medial aspect of the thigh, just below the inguinal ligament, about halfway between the anterior superior iliac spine and the symphysis pubis

E. Behind the knee in the lateral aspect of the hollow area at the back of the knee joint.

F. On the dorsal aspect of the foot, lateral to the tendon that runs from the great toe toward the ankle

2. *In order to properly take a manual blood pressure it is important to know what you are listening for as the bladder deflates. Match the Korotkoff phases in Column A with the correct description of what is being heard in Column B.*

Column A

____ **1.** Phase I

____ **2.** Phase II

____ **3.** Phase III

____ **4.** Phase IV

____ **5.** Phase V

Column B

A. Marked by crisper, more intense sounds; clear intense tapping

B. Absence of sound

C. Initiated by the onset of faint, clear tapping sounds of gradually increasing intensity

D. Sound has a swishing quality

E. Characterized by muffled, blowing sounds

Activity C ORDERING

1. In order to correctly obtain a blood pressure, a proper cuff size should be used, the cuff should be placed appropriately, and certain steps should be followed. *Write the correct sequence of steps in the boxes provided below.*

a. Clean stethoscope and palpate for the brachial artery.

b. Perform hand hygiene, identify the patient, and allow for privacy.

c. Wrap a deflated cuff snuggly around upper arm in the appropriate fashion.

d. While palpating the brachial or radial artery, inflate cough until pulse disappears then slowly release valve noting when pulse reappears.

e. Wait 1 to 2 minutes then, while listening over the brachial artery with a stethoscope, inflate cuff and allow it to slowly release.

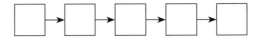

Activity D SHORT ANSWER

1. How does age affect body temperature?

_____

_____

_____

2. What types of medications affect respirations and how do they affect them?

_____

_____

_____

3. Why is it important to perform part of the respiratory assessment without the patient being aware that you are doing so?

_____

_____

_____

4. Describe what resistance is in relation to blood pressure.

_____

_____

_____

5. What is orthostatic hypotension and what are the symptoms?

_____

_____

_____

SECTION III: APPLYING YOUR KNOWLEDGE

Activity E **CASE STUDY**

Answer the following questions, which involve the nurse's role in assessing a patient for fluid, electrolyte, and acid–base imbalance.

Josie is a three-and-a-half-year-old girl who is seen in her primary care office for breathing problems. Josie takes albuterol for asthma. She started experiencing cold symptoms 2 days ago with fever, chills, and breathing problems. You hear audible wheezing. You are the nurse who is taking her vital signs which are as follows: Temperature 99 °F, Pulse 140, Respirations 34, and Blood Pressure 110/80.

1. What are some of the factors, which could be causing a pulse of 140?

_____

_____

_____

2. How would you go about decreasing the fear Josie might have of getting her vital signs taken in the first place?

_____

_____

_____

SECTION IV: PRACTICING FOR NCLEX

Activity F **MULTIPLE CHOICE**

Answer the following questions.

1. Which of the following is not true of respiration?
   a. Inspiration is a passive process.
   b. Normal tidal volume is 500 mL/minute.
   c. External respiration is the process of taking oxygen into and eliminating carbon dioxide from the body.
   d. During inspiration, the pressure in the airway becomes negative and air flows inward.

2. It is very important to assess for the quality of someone's respirations as well as describe what you hear with auscultation. Which of the following describes stridor?
   a. High-pitched musical sound
   b. Respirations that require excessive effort
   c. Discontinuous popping sounds
   d. A harsh inspiratory sound that may be compared to crowing

3. Which of the following describes diastolic blood pressure?
   a. During ventricular relaxation, blood pressure is due to elastic recoil of the vessels.
   b. The blood pressure measured during ventricular contraction.
   c. The pressure is highest when the ventricles of the heart eject blood into the aorta and pulmonary arteries.
   d. The flow of blood produced by contractions of the heart and the resistance to blood flow through the vessels.

4. Which of the following piece of equipment is no longer used for temperature measurement?
   a. Electronic thermometers
   b. Glass mercury thermometers
   c. Tympanic membrane thermometers
   d. Paper thermometers

5. Which of the following is not a characteristic used to describe the pulse?
   a. Frequency
   b. Quality
   c. Depth
   d. Rhythm

6. Which of the following is true regarding the autonomic nervous system and its affect on the rate of a person's pulse?
   a. Sympathetic nervous system activation occurs in response to a variety of stimuli including changes in intravascular volume.
   b. Stimulation of the parasympathetic nervous system results in an increase in the pulse rate.
   c. Stimulation of the sympathetic nervous system results in a decrease in the pulse rate.
   d. The sympathetic nervous system is the dominant activation during resting states.

7. Which of the following is not used to describe the quality of a person's pulse?
   a. Full
   b. Galloping
   c. Bounding
   d. Thready

8. The body loses heat continually through several different processes. Which of the following is an example of how heat is lost through evaporation?
   a. Diaphoresis
   b. Conduction
   c. Convection
   d. Radiation

9. Which of the following is not known to cause false blood pressure readings?
   a. Having the patients legs crossed at the knee
   b. Smoking
   c. Eating
   d. Being in a warm environment

10. Which of the following is true regarding the different sites for assessing body temperature? Select all that apply.
    a. Temperatures should not be taken orally in infants.
    b. Rectal temperatures should not be taken on anyone who is neutropenic.
    c. Tympanic temperature readings closely reflect core body temperature.
    d. Temporal artery thermometer readings may be affected by perspiration or air blowing over the face.

CHAPTER 18

Asepsis and Infection Control

SECTION I: LEARNING OBJECTIVES

Upon completion of this chapter, the student will be able to do the following:

1. Identify the six components of the chain of infection.

2. Identify ways that infection may occur.

3. Describe factors that increase the risk of infection in various settings.

4. Discuss the role of healthcare personnel and health agencies in infection control.

5. Identify ways that caregivers can increase their protection against infectious exposure.

6. Explain ways that caregivers can decrease the transmission of infection to patients.

7. Differentiate between medical and surgical asepsis.

8. Demonstrate good hand hygiene technique and identify key occasions and reasons for incorporating it as an integral part of practice.

9. Describe appropriate situations for using cleaning, disinfection, and sterilization.

10. Describe proper use of barriers also known as personal protective equipment (PPE).

11. Discuss the two-tier system of isolation.

12. Identify age-related and cultural considerations in preventing the transmission of infectious diseases.

SECTION II: ASSESSING YOUR UNDERSTANDING

Activity A FILL IN THE BLANKS

1. Pervasive infection by bacteria that is transported in the blood is known as _____.

2. Some bacteria secrete _____ into the host which typically results in serious illness.

3. The three factors associated with healthcare-associated infections are _____, therapeutic regimen, and patient resistance.

4. For infection control, all healthcare personnel should receive an annual _____ vaccine.

5. Hand hygiene consists of either washing with soap and water or using a _____ sanitizer.

6. A chemical or antibiotic that kills bacteria is called _____.

7. Negative flow rooms are required for a diagnosis of _____.

8. It is imperative that physicians and nurses discard all _____ after completing a procedure.

9. Insertion of a urinary catheter and a central line dressing change require the use of _____ asepsis.

10. Ear infections and upper respiratory infections are most common among the _____ age group.

MATCHING

Match the term listed in column A with its definition in Column B.

Column A

____ **1.** Disinfectant

____ **2.** Antiseptic

____ **3.** Bactericidal

____ **4.** Bacteriostatic

____ **5.** Sterilization

Column B

A. Inhibits replication of bacteria

B. Chemical used to cleanse living objects

C. The complete destruction of all living organisms including spores

D. Kills all bacteria

E. Chemical used to cleanse lifeless objects

SEQUENCING

Place the events in the chain of infection in the order in which they occur.

a. A susceptible host

b. The source

c. The portal of entry

d. Infectious agent

e. The portal of exit

f. The mode of transmission

SHORT ANSWER

1. Explain why an infection with the fungus *Candida albicans* is considered opportunistic.

_____

_____

_____

2. List the four strategies of the CDC in preventing the spread of antibiotic-resistant organisms.

_____

_____

_____

3. What can nurses do to protect themselves from needlesticks?

_____

_____

_____

4. What is the difference between medical asepsis and surgical asepsis?

_____

_____

_____

5. Discuss some factors that may contribute to poor hand hygiene.

_____

_____

_____

6. Explain what is meant by "standard" precautions.

_____

_____

_____

SECTION III: APPLYING YOUR KNOWLEDGE

CASE STUDY

Vanessa is a 28-year-old nurse on your pediatric medical unit. She is 4 months pregnant. As you examine the assignment board, you note that Vanessa was assigned a patient with an undiagnosed rash. The child's parents do not believe in vaccination and subsequently the child has not received any of his childhood immunizations.

1. You are the charge nurse. What is your most appropriate action regarding Vanessa? Provide a rationale for your decision.

_____

_____

_____

2. What type of precautions would be appropriate to use when caring for this patient?

_____

_____

_____

3. You now need to place an IV in this patient. How would you do so?

_____

_____

_____

SECTION IV: PRACTICING FOR NCLEX

Activity F MULTIPLE CHOICE

Answer the following questions.

1. Anisa is a 12 year old hospitalized with pneumonia. You receive her culture and sensitivity report on her tracheal aspirate. Anisa is infected with a strain of *Streptococcus pneumoniae,* which is particularly prone to cause infections, also referred to as what?
   a. Virulent
   b. Pathogenic
   c. Specific
   d. Source

2. Aleah is an employee on the medical unit at the local children's hospital. You are an occupational health nurse educating Aleah on various routes of exposure. You know that as a hospital employee, Aleah is most susceptible to infection by what mode of transmission?
   a. Contact
   b. Vehicle
   c. Droplet
   d. Airborne

3. You are a nurse caring for Judy, a 55-year-old post-operative patient. She returns to the ICU after surgery intubated and mechanically ventilated with a Salem sump nasogastric tube, a Foley catheter, and a PICC line in place. Based on your knowledge of the most common hospital-acquired infections, which apparatus is most important to remove first?
   a. Urinary catheter
   b. PICC line
   c. Salem sump nasogastric tube
   d. Endotracheal tube

4. You are working with Elsie, a 55-year-old woman diagnosed with human immunodeficiency virus (HIV). You also have another patient today who has an upper respiratory infection. What is the most important thing you can do to prevent Elsie from acquiring this infection?
   a. Wear gloves every time you touch Elsie.
   b. Wear a mask and gown in Elsie's room.
   c. Avoid direct contact with Elsie.
   d. Perform hand hygiene before and after entering Elsie's room.

5. Which of the following is NOT appropriate regarding the use of gowns as PPE?
   a. Use of paper or cloth gowns is appropriate.
   b. Don a gown when splashing is a possibility.
   c. Use one gown per person per shift.
   d. Use a gown each time you enter the room.

6. Which of the following patients would require a negative flow room?
   a. A 21-year-old man with latent tuberculosis who is post-op following repair of a femoral fracture
   b. A 4-year-old boy with meningitis
   c. An 81-year-old man with active tuberculosis and a productive cough
   d. A 3-year-old with influenza A and a productive cough

7. Anita is a nurse working with you on the medical unit. She comes to you and informs you that she just cut herself with a scalpel that was left on a procedure tray. Without knowing anything about the patient's or Anita's history, you know that Anita is most at risk for which infectious disease?

   a. Hepatitis B

   b. Hepatitis C

   c. HIV

   d. Methicillin-resistant *Staphylococcus aureus* (MRSA).

8. Senna is a 34-year-old woman pregnant with her first child. You notice on her lab results that she is not immune to rubella. When is it most imperative that Senna protect herself from a rubella infection?

   a. First trimester

   b. Second trimester

   c. Third trimester

   d. Immediately postpartum

9. You are working as a new graduate nurse in a long-term care facility. You are frequently required to perform surgical asepsis procedures for your job. Which of the following

would NOT be appropriate? Select all that apply.

   a. Nails that are cut to ½ inch beyond the nail bed

   b. Artificial nails with dark purple nail polish

   c. Artificial nails with intact, clear nail polish

   d. Nails that are chewed down to the nail bed

10. You are working with Anna, a new graduate nurse. She states that she was exposed to a patient's blood and that she was not wearing any PPE. Which of the following would be considered significant blood exposures by occupational health? Select all that apply.

    a. Hepatitis B

    b. Hepatitis C

    c. Tuberculosis

    d. HIV

11. You are about to enter the room of a patient with a strain of influenza A. You prepare to don your PPE. Which of the following would be appropriate? Select all that apply.

    a. Gloves

    b. Gown

    c. Mask with face shield

    d. Respirator

CHAPTER 19

Medication Administration

SECTION I: LEARNING OBJECTIVES

Upon completion of this chapter, the student will be able to do the following:

1. Describe essential components of a medication order.

2. Discuss pharmacokinetic principles of drug action.

3. List the six rights of proper medication administration.

4. Calculate proper drug dosage using different systems of drug measurement.

5. Discuss the importance of designing systems within healthcare institutions for medication administration that emphasize patient safety.

6. Discuss important assessment data to obtain from the patient during the initial interview and before medication administration.

7. Develop an individualized teaching plan to improve patient knowledge of medications.

8. Incorporate evaluation of medication effectiveness and documentation into safe medication administration practices.

9. Describe recommended guidelines and procedures for medication administration by each route.

SECTION II: ASSESSING YOUR UNDERSTANDING

Activity A FILL IN THE BLANKS

1. A _____ name is the name given to a medication by the United States Adopted Names Council and is the drug's official name thereafter.

2. The _____ name is used by the pharmaceutical company for a 17-year period in which it has the exclusive rights to make and sell the drug.

3. A _____ is a legal order for the preparation and administration of a medication.

4. _____ is the process by which a drug moves through the body and is eventually eliminated.

5. _____ is the process of removing the drug or its metabolites from the body.

6. A medication's desired and intentional effects are called its _____ effects.

7. A severe allergic reaction, called an _____ reaction, requires immediate medical intervention because it can be fatal.

8. Drug _____ is when a drug precipitates from solutions, or is chemically inactivated, if mixed with another medication.

9. Drugs known to cause birth defects are called _____.

10. _____ injections are given into the dermis which is the layer of tissue located beneath the skin's surface.

11. _____ injections are given into the layer of fat located below the dermis and above the muscle tissue.

12. _____ injections are given into the muscle layer beneath the dermis and the subcutaneous tissue.

13. _____ substances are drugs that are considered to have either limited medical use or high potential for abuse or addiction.

14. _____ refers to the physiologic and biochemical effects of a drug on the body.

Activity B MATCHING

1. *Match the oral preparation of a given medication in Column A with the correct description in Column B.*

Column A	Column B
____ **1.** Elixir	**A.** Gelatinous container to hold powder or liquid medicine
____ **2.** Emulsion	
____ **3.** Suspension	**B.** Liquid preparation of medication with alcohol base
____ **4.** Capsule	
	C. Suspension within an oil base
	D. Medication in liquid, which must be shaken before administration because it separates

2. *Match the drug class in Column A with the correct action in Column B.*

Column A	Column B
____ **1.** Antihypertensives	**A.** Decrease nausea
____ **2.** Antiemetics	**B.** Increase urine production and elimination
____ **3.** Diuretics	
____ **4.** Corticosteroids	**C.** Decrease blood pressure
____ **5.** Bronchodilators	**D.** Open airways
	E. Decrease inflammation

Activity C CROSSWORD

Across

2. The process of chemically changing the drug in the body.
4. The process by which the medication is delivered to the target cells and tissue.
6. The name given to a medication that is based on its molecular structure.

Down

1. The process by which a medication enters the bloodstream.
3. Medications which are designed to be absorbed through the skin for systemic effects.
5. St. John's wort or Echinacea.

Activity D SHORT ANSWER

1. What are the dangers of nonprescription medications?

_____

_____

_____

2. Why is it important to ask a person if they are taking any herbal medications?

_____

_____

_____

3. What are patient rights in regard to medication administration?

_____

_____

_____

4. What is medication reconciliation and why is it important?

_____

_____

_____

5. Why is it important to assess a person before giving them their medications?

_____

_____

_____

SECTION III: APPLYING YOUR KNOWLEDGE

Activity E CASE STUDY

Answer the following questions, which involve the nurse's role in medication administration.

Tara is a 55-year-old woman who is in the hospital for diabetic ketoacidosis. Her blood sugars have been stabilized and she will be going home on subcutaneous insulin which is new for her. She also takes lisinopril for hypertension and atorvastatin for hypercholesterolemia. Her medication administration record while in the hospital states that she is to take the following:

Lispro insulin sliding scale, subcutaneous AC and HS (before meals and before bedtime)

Insulin Sliding Scale*	Blood Glucose Level	Units of Short-Acting (i.e., Lispro) Insulin to be Given
	150–200	1 unit
	200–250	2 units
	250–300	4 units
	>300	Recheck BG and notify provider

*A sliding scale order for insulin administration changes from patient to patient. This is not an actual order and should not be memorized.

Lisinopril 10 mg PO once a day
Atorvastatin 20 mg PO once a day

You are a nurse caring for Tara:

1. What are you going to assess before administering these medications?

_____

_____

_____

2. What are you going to include in your patient teaching regarding these medications?

_____

_____

_____

SECTION IV: PRACTICING FOR NCLEX

Activity F MULTIPLE CHOICE

Answer the following questions.

1. Which of the following contains all the components of a valid order?
   a. John Smith, Coumadin, once a day, by mouth
   b. John Smith, Atenolol 50 mg, twice a day, by mouth
   c. John Smith, Lovenox 120 mcg, subcutaneously, periumbilical
   d. John Smith, 70 units, BID, SL

2. The National Formulary is a list of medications, which are regulated by the US government. It describes medications based on certain categories. Which of the following category does the National Formulary not describe?
   a. Source
   b. Physical properties
   c. Purity
   d. Side effects

3. Which of the following is a drug class that strengthens cardiac contraction?
   a. Inotropes
   b. Antiarrhythmics
   c. Anticoagulants
   d. Diuretics

4. You are a nurse taking care of a patient who asks you if she can have some acetaminophen to help with her headache. You check to see if there is an order for acetaminophen and notice that she is able to have 650 mg every 4 hours for pain. What type of order is this considered?

   a. Standing order

   b. PRN order

   c. One-time order

   d. STAT order

5. Which of the following is not true regarding Nurse Practice Acts?

   a. They were established to describe legitimate nursing function.

   b. They vary among states.

   c. They define the boundaries of your functions as a nurse.

   d. They describe what medications nurses can prescribe.

6. Which of the following is a sign of a severe allergic reaction to a medication?

   a. Angioedema

   b. Hives

   c. Pruritus

   d. Rhinitis

7. You are a nurse taking care of George, a 56-year-old man with end-stage liver disease. You have a prescription to give 20 g of lactulose every 6 hours to treat his hepatic encephalopathy. On hand, you have containers of lactulose which have 30 g in 45 mL. How many milliliters are you going to administer every 6 hours to George?

   a. 15 mL

   b. 22.5 mL

   c. 67.5 mL

   d. 30 mL

8. Which of the following describes buccal medication administration?

   a. Placing a medication under the tongue and allowing it to dissolve

   b. Placing a medication underneath the upper lip or in the side of the mouth

   c. Placing a medication through a nasogastric tube

   d. Placing a medication, which is designed to be absorbed through the skin for systemic effects, on the skin

9. Which of the following medications are dropped into the ear to treat ear infections or to soften and remove ear wax?

   a. Otic

   b. Ophthalmic

   c. Parenteral

   d. Nasal

10. Which of the following medication interaction illustrates a synergism?

    a. Jane takes a Tylenol PM to help her sleep. She also takes an oxycodone for pain related to recent hip surgery, which makes her even more drowsy.

    b. Jane is taking doxycycline, an antibiotic, for rosacea. She takes this with her morning vitamins, which includes calcium carbonate. She has not noticed a change in her symptoms.

    c. Jane is taking metoprolol for her blood pressure and metformin for her diabetes. Her provider has told her that these are same to take together.

    d. Jane was told not to take tretinoin topical, Retin A, if she is pregnant because it may be teratogenic.

11. Which of the following would be considered a "right" of drug administration Select all that apply.

    a. Right drug

    b. Right documentation

    c. Right class

    d. Right dose

    e. Right patient

CHAPTER 20

Intravenous Therapy

SECTION I: LEARNING OBJECTIVES

Upon completion of this chapter, the student will be able to do the following:

1. Explain the purpose of intravenous infusion therapy.

2. Identify the two major types of solutions administered intravenously.

3. List equipment necessary to administer peripheral and central intravenous therapy.

4. State guidelines for site selection in peripherally inserted venipuncture.

5. Outline the nurse's role in initiating, monitoring, maintaining, and discontinuing intravenous therapy.

6. Describe differences in the nursing care and maintenance of central venous catheters and peripheral catheters.

7. Discuss the purpose of total parenteral nutrition (TPN) and monitoring considerations.

8. Discuss indications for blood component therapy and safe transfusion practices.

9. Describe potential complications of intravenous therapy, total parenteral nutrition, and blood transfusions.

10. Identify principles of patient and family education associated with intravenous therapy.

SECTION II: ASSESSING YOUR UNDERSTANDING

Activity A FILL IN THE BLANKS

1. Crystalloids are fluids that are clear, whereas _____ are fluids that contain proteins or starch molecules.

2. The _____ veins are usually the quickest and easiest to access for IV placement.

3. As the gauge (number) on the IV catheter increases, the size of the lumen _____.

4. The peripherally inserted central catheter (PICC) is inserted peripherally but delivers fluid into a _____ vein.

5. A needleless connector should be wiped for _____ seconds prior to access to prevent infection.

6. One way to prevent phlebitis is to rotate the peripheral IV site every _____ hours.

7. Pain in the chest, shoulder or back in a patient with an IV may be indicative of a _____ embolism.

8. Assess a peripheral IV site at least once every _____.

9. When performing tubing and/or IV change use strict _____ technique.

10. TPN must be administered through a _____ IV.

Activity B MATCHING

1. *Match the complication listed in Column A with its sign/symptom in Column B.*

Column A

_____ **1.** Air embolism
_____ **2.** Phlebitis
_____ **3.** Septic shock
_____ **4.** Extravasation

Column B

A. Headache, tightness in chest, changes in BP

B. Pain in chest, shoulder, or back; dyspnea, hypotension

C. Pain, swelling, and discoloration at the site

D. Redness and warmth along cannulated vein; burning pain; vein feels cordlike

Activity C SHORT ANSWER

1. What is the difference between isotonic and hypotonic solutions? Provide an example of when you would use each.

_____

_____

_____

2. Describe the five-step central catheter bundle (CCB) used to prevent catheter-associated blood stream infections (CABSI).

_____

_____

_____

3. What is the difference between infiltration and extravasation?

_____

_____

_____

4. Discuss special considerations when placing a peripheral IV in the infant.

_____

_____

_____

5. Describe the difference between type A, B, AB, and O blood.

_____

_____

_____

6. Describe some common blood transfusion reactions.

_____

_____

_____

SECTION III: APPLYING YOUR KNOWLEDGE

Activity D CASE STUDY

You are a home healthcare nurse visiting Selma, an 86-year-old woman who is on daily home antibiotic therapy for 2 weeks to treat an infected pressure ulcer. She had a PICC placed 3 days ago for treatment. Her daughter calls and asks if you can come early today because she is worried that her mother may have an infection.

1. Describe the steps that a home care nurse should take when administering nutrition or medications in the home.

_____

_____

_____

2. Why would a PICC line be an appropriate choice for this patient?

_____

_____

_____

3. What signs might Selma exhibit that would make you suspicious of a CABSI?

_____

_____

_____

4. You decide to infuse the antibiotic through Selma's PICC line. The volume to be infused is 200 mL over 1 hour. Your tubing has a drop factor of 10 drops/mL. Calculate the drops per minute.

_____

_____

_____

SECTION IV: PRACTICING FOR NCLEX

Activity E **CASE STUDY**

Answer the following questions.

1. You are working the night shift in the ER when an ambulance arrives carrying a man s/p motor vehicle accident (MVA). His initial BP is 100/56 and you note that he is bleeding heavily from a laceration on the forehead. Fifteen minutes later, you reassess your patient and find that his BP is 95/58. What IV fluid would you expect to be ordered?

a. 0.45% NS

b. 0.9% NS

c. 3% NS

d. D_5 ¼ NS

2. Alex is a 15 year old diagnosed with ALL. You draw his morning labs and note a hematocrit of 28, WBC of 10, platelets 68. Which of the following would you expect that a licensed practitioner would order?

a. Packed red blood cells

b. White blood cells

c. Platelets

d. a & c.

3. You are placing an IV in a newly admitted 30-year-old man. What size catheter (lumen size and length, respectively) is most appropriate?

a. 20 gauge, 1 inch

b. 14 gauge, 1 inch

c. 18 gauge, 2 inches

d. 24 gauge, 2 inches

4. Elaine is a 28-year-old woman pregnant with multiples. She is diagnosed with hyperemesis gravidarum (excessive vomiting during pregnancy). She is unable to keep enteral fluids down. A licensed practitioner orders home IV therapy for 2 weeks. What type of IV access is most appropriate for Elaine?

a. An implanted access port

b. A peripheral IV

c. A PICC

d. A tunneled catheter

5. Which of the following patients would most likely require placement of an implantable port?

a. A 58-year-old woman with stage 3 breast cancer requiring weekly chemotherapy.

b. An 18-year-old man s/p gunshot wound in the ICU requiring multiple blood transfusions.

c. A 12-year-old girl with sickle cell anemia requiring frequent pain medication administration.

d. A 45-year-old man with a history of colon cancer that is currently in remission.

6. You are the nurse on a medical unit when the medical assistant approaches you and informs you that Mrs. G.'s IV dressing is curling at the edges and appears wet. What is your best approach to this situation?

a. Assess the dressing and redress it if the dressing is not intact.

b. Assess the dressing and delegate the dressing change to the medical assistant if the dressing is not intact.

c. Reinforce the dressing with a tegaderm.

d. Leave the dressing change for the next shift.

7. You are placing an IV on Collin for parenteral nutrition. He asks you why he needs a second IV. You explain that you need to change the IV site every 72 hours to prevent what complication?

a. Air embolism

b. Infiltration

c. Infection

d. Phlebitis

8. You are the nurse caring for Amira, a 6-year-old patient on the hematology–oncology floor. During a packed red blood cell transfusion, Amira complains of pain at her peripheral IV site. You assess the sight and notice that the site is purple. What is your best course of action?

   a. Call the physician and notify them of a transfusion reaction.

   b. Stop the transfusion and aline lock the peripheral IV.

   c. Stop the transfusion and discontinue the peripheral IV.

   d. Continue the transfusion and note your findings in the chart.

9. You are preparing a packed red blood cell transfusion for your patient. You check the patient's blood type in the electronic medical record (EMR) and not that it he is blood type B. What does this mean?

   a. The patient has anti-A antibodies.

   b. The patient has anti-B antibodies.

   c. The patient has both anti-A and anti-B antibodies.

   d. None of the above.

10. You are infusing ampicillin IV for Mr. B. The medication is diluted in 100 mL of NS and is to infuse over 1 hour. You have tubing with a drop factor of 20 drops/mL. What is the drip rate of this infusion?

    a. 16 drops/minute

    b. 33 drops/minute

    c. 5 drops/minute

    d. 20 drops/minute

11. You are infusing 0.9% NS to a hypovolemic patient s/p an MVA. You are ordered to infuse 1,000 mL of fluid over 1 hour. Your tube has a drop factor of 5 drops/mL. What is the drip rate of your infusion?

    a. 17 drops/minute

    b. 100 drops/minute

    c. 167 drops/minute

    d. 83 drops/minute

12. Which of the following would cause your IV drip rate to increase? Select all that apply.

    a. Increase the height of the IV pole

    b. Raise the patient's arm

    c. Changing the tubing to unclog an air vent

    d. Unkink the IV tubing

13. You are placing a peripheral IV in Charlie, a 2 year old being treated with IV antibiotics for pneumonia. Which of the following principles are appropriate when placing an IV on a child this age? Select all that apply.

    a. Select a site near a joint space such as the AC fossa.

    b. Explain the procedure to the patient.

    c. Perform the procedure in a separate room.

    d. Decorate the IV with stickers and smiley faces.

Perioperative Nursing

SECTION I: LEARNING OBJECTIVES

Upon completion of this chapter, the student will be able to do the following:

1. Describe the three phases of perioperative patient management.

2. Discuss the effects of surgery on health and function.

3. Identify lifespan considerations for the patient undergoing a surgical procedure.

4. Describe appropriate perioperative patient teaching.

5. Discuss emotional support, safety, and asepsis during the intraoperative phase.

6. Identify appropriate nursing assessments in the recovery facility and during the postoperative period.

7. List common postoperative complications and appropriate nursing interventions to prevent or treat each postoperative complication.

8. Develop an appropriate discharge plan for the surgical patient.

SECTION II: ASSESSING YOUR UNDERSTANDING

Activity A FILL IN THE BLANKS

1. The _____ phase of patient care may be short (<1 day) or long (months) depending on the diagnosis and procedure.

2. Patients who undergo procedures using a minimally invasive technology called a _____ are often sent home the same day.

3. Leg exercises, _____ hose and sequential compression devices (SCDs) help maintain peripheral circulation and promote venous return to the heart.

4. A paralytic _____ is a condition in which a portion of the bowel becomes temporarily paralyzed.

5. _____ is often referred to as the fifth vital sign.

6. An appropriate nursing intervention for the surgical patient is to help them identify how they have handled _____ in the past.

7. Teaching about the surgical procedure is best done in the _____ period.

8. Concerns about Hepatitis B and human immunodeficiency virus have led to _____ blood donations for elective procedures.

9. A bowel preparation is often ordered prior to _____ surgery.

10. Completing the preoperative _____ is a quick way to show that all patient preparation activities have been accomplished and safety measures have been taken.

11. The _____ nurse is responsible for managing patient care in the operating room.

12. A _____ is used prior to the start of surgery to ensure that the team is on the same page.

13. Intravenous administration of anxiolytics and narcotics without general anesthesia is known as _____ sedation.

14. Enteral feedings are often held in the postoperative period until _____ returns.

15. The patient is expected to void within _____ hours of surgery.

16. In order to maintain _____, keep all items within the sterile field.

17. Intraoperative and postoperative glucose levels are typically kept less than _____ mg/dL.

Activity B MATCHING

1. *Match the developmental stage in Column A with the appropriate perioperative nursing intervention Column B.*

Column A

___ **1.** Newborn

___ **2.** Toddler

___ **3.** School-age

___ **4.** Adolescent

___ **5.** Older adult

Column B

A. When possible, allow visual and hearing aids until after anesthesia is administered; use positioning aids for those with altered mobility

B. Use of a treatment room; teach using demonstration doll; provide tasks such as holding anesthesia mask

C. Holding and rocking; distraction during procedures; maintain a calm, minimal sensory environment

D. Offer privacy; provide extensive teaching; offer tasks such as holding anesthesia masks

E. Remove clothing and apply grounding pad after anesthesia is administered; allow parents to hold while anesthesia is administered; use of treatment room

Activity C SHORT ANSWER

1. Describe ways to prevent atelectasis in a post-surgical patient.

_____

_____

_____

2. Why is a comorbid diagnosis of diabetes mellitus of concern in surgical candidates?

_____

_____

_____

3. Define malignant hyperthermia and describe postoperative signs of this disorder.

_____

_____

_____

4. Describe some cultural considerations that may arise during the perioperative period.

_____

_____

_____

5. Describe the process of informed consent.

_____

_____

_____

SECTION III: APPLYING YOUR KNOWLEDGE

Activity D CASE STUDY

You are caring for Juan, an 8-year-old who will undergo a tonsillectomy and adenoidectomy (T&A) later today. He is present in the preoperative center with his mother and father. You are the preoperative nurse in charge of his care.

1. Describe some developmentally appropriate tasks that you could perform for Juan.

_____

_____

_____

2. Describe the process of informed consent for a dependent minor.

_____

_____

_____

3. List some tasks that may be included on your preoperative checklist.

_____

_____

_____

4. Write an appropriate psychosocial nursing diagnosis for Juan or his family.

_____

_____

_____

SECTION IV: PRACTICING FOR NCLEX

Activity E **MULTIPLE CHOICE**

Answer the following questions.

1. Avery is a 15-year-old patient with acute lymphoblastic leukemia (ALL). Avery is a practicing Jehovah's Witness and has asked not to receive blood products. You know that the prognosis for ALL is very good but patients often require blood products during treatment. Which of the following is the most appropriate action?

  a. Tell Avery that her request is not appropriate.

  b. Document Avery's request in her medical record.

  c. Request an ethics consultation.

  d. Tell Avery that her request will be upheld.

2. Paul is a 42-year-old patient s/p liver biopsy. He is extubated but remains NPO and on strict bed rest. He does not have a Foley catheter in place. It has been 4 hours since Paul last voided. When asked he informs you that he does not feel that he needs to go. What is your next course of action?

  a. Reposition in bed to position Paul in a manner that will encourage micturition.

  b. Call the physician to obtain an order for Foley catheter placement.

  c. Call the physician to obtain an order for straight catheterization.

  d. Return in 6 hours to recheck.

3. Ames is an 87-year-old man who underwent a hip replacement today. He is telling you that his parents, who are deceased, are coming to visit him today. He continues to tell you that he needs to cut the lawn and run errands. Last time you entered the room, he was trying to climb over the bed rail. Which term best describes Ames' condition?

  a. Dementia

  b. Delirium

  c. Narcotic overuse

  d. Boredom

4. A 2-year-old toddler just underwent a T&A surgery You are the post-anesthesia care unit (PACU) nurse caring for him. What is the best course of action regarding the developmental care of this child?

  a. Give the child a new teddy bear.

  b. Extubate the child as soon as possible.

  c. Administer Acetaminophen (Tylenol) before the child wakes.

  d. Allow the parents into the PACU before the child wakes.

5. You are taking a history on Kumar who informs you that he has an allergy to adhesive tape. When you ask Kumar to describe his reaction to the tape, he describes it as "blotchy and reddened". What type of allergic reaction is this?

  a. Type I

  b. Type II

  c. Type III

  d. Type IV

6. You are caring for Samuel, a 4 year old undergoing a laparoscopy for a ruptured appendix. His blood pressure is unstable and his abdomen is dusky in appearance. Which of the following best describes the use of informed consent in this case?
   a. Informed consent will be waived because the procedure is emergent.
   b. The surgeon may sit with the family while the patient is prepped for surgery as long as the procedure is not delayed.
   c. The surgeon will meet with Samuel and his parents prior to surgery, explain the procedure, and answer any questions they may have.
   d. Informed consent should be obtained when the surgeon meets with the family after the procedure.

7. Amanda is undergoing a knee replacement tomorrow morning. She is ordered nothing by mouth (NPO) prior to surgery. She asks you how long she can drink water prior to the procedure. Based on your knowledge of standard protocols, which of the following is your best response?
   a. 2 hours
   b. 4 hours
   c. 6 hours
   d. 12 hours

8. Anya is a 2 year old who is undergoing a surgical repair of a fractured radius and ulna. Which of the following is developmentally appropriate care for Anya?
   a. Take Anya into the operating room 2 hours before the surgery.
   b. Place an IV after Anya has received a rectal anxiolytic.
   c. Tell Anya's parents they can meet you in her inpatient room.
   d. Allow Anya to bring all of her stuffed animals into the OR.

9. You are the circulating nurse caring for Thomas, a 45-year-old man undergoing left knee arthroscopic exploratory surgery. What task ensures that the team is on the same page and will perform the procedure on the right patient and at the right site?
   a. Operative site marking
   b. Preoperative checklist
   c. Procedural pause (time-out)
   d. Informed consent

10. You are the circulating nurse caring for Ezekiel, a 72-year-old man undergoing removal of a liver tumor. His wife is waiting in the family waiting area. Which of the following are appropriate actions in the intraoperative period? Select all that apply.
    a. Provide emotional support immediately before the surgery.
    b. Explain in detail what is happening to Ezekiel's wife during the surgery.
    c. Notify Ezekiel's wife when the procedure is over.
    d. Bring Ezekiel's wife back to be with him as soon as possible.

11. Patients with a latex allergy may have intolerance to which of the following items? Select all that apply.
    a. Balloons
    b. Condoms
    c. Underwear
    d. Gloves

12. Peyton is a 4-month-old patient on your unit following repair of a cleft lip/palate. She has just awake from anesthesia and is crying. Which of the following would be an appropriate first intervention? Select all that apply.
    a. Administer 0.1 mg/kg morphine IV.
    b. Hold Peyton in a rocking chair.
    c. Offer a pacifier.
    d. Distract Peyton with a stuffed toy.

Safety

SECTION I: LEARNING OBJECTIVES

Upon completion of this chapter, the student will be able to do the following:

1. Identify national organizations that focus on safety concerns of patients and healthcare workers.

2. Recognize the importance of safety in the home and healthcare environments.

3. Relate special safety considerations to specific developmental stages.

4. Identify factors that affect safety and common manifestations of altered safety.

5. Identify safety risks through assessment.

6. Discuss nursing interventions to promote safe homes and healthcare environments.

7. Individualize a teaching plan for individuals with identified safety risks.

SECTION II: ASSESSING YOUR UNDERSTANDING

Activity A FILL IN THE BLANKS

1. Safety is the _____ priority in Maslow's hierarchy of needs.

2. The science of _____ focuses on body positioning during work maneuvers.

3. Safety errors that result in death or serious injury must be reported as a _____ event.

4. Each hospital must have a _____ plan in which bioterrorism is addressed.

5. The Institute of Medicine (2000) defines patient safety as the _____ of adverse outcomes stemming from the processes of healthcare.

6. _____ are the age group at highest risk for poisoning.

7. Cigarette smoke and _____ are known causes of lung cancer.

8. A _____ provides an excellent time to assess skin integrity in the inpatient setting.

9. To prevent back injury, a _____ team is often called to assist with the movement of a patient.

10. A _____ is a physical or chemical devise used to prevent a patient from moving.

Activity B MATCHING

1. *Match the organization in Column A with their role or goal in Column B.*

Column A

___ **1.** Joint Commission

___ **2.** Occupational Safety and Health Administration (OSHA)

___ **3.** Quality and Safety Education for Nurses

___ **4.** Center for Disease Control

___ **5.** Institute of Medicine

Column B

A. Collects and publishes epidemiologic data related to safety

B. Publishes annual patient safety goals for healthcare facilities' compliance

C. Establishes regulations for safety in the physical work environment, such as air quality, ergonomics, prevention of infection transmission from used and uncapped needles and prevention of exposure to toxic substances

D. Authored the 2000 report *To Err is Human*

E. Provide a framework for the knowledge, skills and attitudes necessary for future nurses

Activity C SEQUENCING

Properly order the sequence of events for managing a fire in a healthcare setting.

a. Pull the alarm, call code red and alert personnel

b. Extinguish the fire

c. Remove patient from immediate danger

d. Close all doors and windows

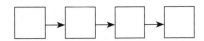

Activity D SHORT ANSWER

1. Discuss some safety concerns for the toddler age group.

_____

_____

_____

2. Discuss some aging-related factors that place older adults at increased risk for burns.

_____

_____

_____

3. List some safety concerns present in the hospital environment.

_____

_____

_____

4. What diagnostic tests provide clues to patient safety?

_____

_____

_____

5. What are some ways that nurses promote safety on an adult inpatient unit?

_____

_____

_____

SECTION III: APPLYING YOUR KNOWLEDGE

Activity E CASE STUDY

You are performing an in home assessment for Anita and Juan, a married couple with two children, Genevieve age 2 years and Sean age 6 years. Anita's mother, Luisa, age 80, also lives with the family. Luisa was diagnosed with Parkinson's disease several years ago. You are asked to help the family provide a safe environment for everyone in the home.

1. What particular concerns do you have regarding Luisa's safety?

_____

_____

_____

2. What particular concerns do you have regarding the safety of Genevieve and Sean?

_____

_____

_____

3. What modifications can Anita and Juan make to their home to increase safety?

_____

_____

_____

4. Luisa is admitted to the hospital for a respiratory infection. What can you do to protect her from falls?

_____

_____

_____

SECTION IV: PRACTICING FOR NCLEX

Activity F MULTIPLE CHOICE

Answer the following questions.

1. You are a school nurse at the local elementary school. A mother arrives to pick up her 6-year-old son and has her 2-year-old daughter in tow. Based on your developmental knowledge of toddlers, which of the following behaviors would most concern you?
   a. The 2 year old leaning against the screen of a window in a classroom.
   b. The 2 year old and 6 year old each holding the mother's hand.
   c. The 2 year old helping mom to open the front door of the school.
   d. The 6 year old riding a bike on the playground with his friend.

2. You are caring for an 18 month-old boy s/p a tracheostomy. He is recovering well and wanting to be more active. You select a toy from the playroom for him to play with. Which toy is most developmentally appropriate?
   a. A beaded bracelet
   b. Dominos.
   c. A rocking horse
   d. Marbles

3. Axel is a 14-year-old man in your clinic for his well-child exam. When you ask his mother if she has any questions for the practitioner, she states "he sleeps so much. I am worried about how lazy he is". Which of the following do you know to be true about sleep in adolescents?
   a. Trying to balance too many activities can result in sleep deprivation.
   b. Increased sleep is the result of boredom.
   c. Adolescents require less sleep than adults; this is clearly an underlying medical concern.
   d. Increased sleep guarantees adolescents will behave in a safe manner.

4. Which of the following is the most common cause of unintentional injury death in the United States?
   a. Automobile accidents
   b. Falls
   c. Poisoning
   d. Fires

5. Anita is a 40-year-old woman admitted to the hospital s/p surgical repair of a radius/ulnar fracture. During your initial assessment, you notice bruising on her inner thigh and the back of her neck in different stages of healing. You also notice several small, circular burns on Anita's forearm. Anita works as a chef at a local restaurant and tells you that her work environment is quite small; she is always bumping into things. What is your most appropriate action?
   a. Notify OSHA of unsafe work conditions.
   b. Provide Anita with a pamphlet on workplace safety.
   c. Offer to provide Anita with some burn cream for her arm.
   d. Ask Anita if she is being abused and notify the proper authority.

6. Owen is a 15-year-old patient who is waking up post-operatively. He became combative and tried to strangle one of the nurses. A support team was called and 4-point restraints were emergently applied. How soon does a licensed provider need to assess the patient and place the restraint order?

   a. 15 minutes

   b. 4 hours

   c. 1 hour

   d. 30 minutes

7. Unintentional injuries are a major cause of disability and death in the United States. For adults, where do unintentional injuries fall on the list of leading causes of death?

   a. Fifth

   b. Tenth

   c. First

   d. Eighth

8. You are volunteering in a free community health clinic at the local YMCA. One of the services offered is vehicle restraint checks for children. Which of the following principles apply to infant and child restraints? Select all that apply.

   a. Infants should be rear-facing up to the age of 2 years.

   b. Booster seats should be used until the child is 4'9".

   c. Children over 30 lbs. only need a lap and shoulder belt.

   d. Infants should remain in the infant seat until the age of 2 years.

9. Ava is a 5-year-old girl admitted to the ICU s/p head trauma from a bike accident. She is awake but confused, and continues to pull at her IV tubing and catheter. A restraint is ordered. Which of the following might be appropriate for Ava? Select all that apply.

   a. Four-point soft restraints

   b. Isolation

   c. A sedating medication

   d. 4 side rails up

Hygiene and Self-Care

SECTION I: LEARNING OBJECTIVES

Upon completion of this chapter, the student will be able to do the following:

1. Discuss the importance of self-care and hygiene in health and illness.

2. Describe the effects of health and illness on the ability to perform self-care.

3. Discuss important subjective and objective areas of assessment when identifying self-care deficits and individualizing a plan for self-care.

4. Demonstrate basic hygiene skills such as bathing, shampooing hair, perineal care, foot care, back massage, toileting, and bed making.

5. Demonstrate proper care of eyes, ears, and teeth, including aids such as dentures, eyeglasses, contact lenses, and hearing aids.

6. List beneficial patient teaching for each of the four areas of self-care.

SECTION II: ASSESSING YOUR UNDERSTANDING

Activity A FILL IN THE BLANKS

1. _____ refers to a person's ability to perform primary care functions without the help of others.

2. _____ is the observance of health rules relating to activities such as bathing, feeding, toileting, and dressing oneself.

3. Cavities in the tooth enamel are caused by deposits of _____, a substance primarily composed of bacteria and saliva that forms on teeth.

4. _____ is when the oral mucosa of an older adult becomes drier as saliva production lessens.

5. Mouth odor is called _____.

6. Infestation with lice is called _____.

7. Hair loss is also called _____.

8. Difficulty swallowing, or _____, may occur as a result of disease or trauma to cranial nerves.

9. _____ is another word for urination.

10. A bedside _____ is a portable chair with a toilet seat and a waste receptacle beneath that can be emptied.

11. A _____ is a plastic receptacle into which the penis can be placed to facilitate urinating without spilling.

12. The _____ is a large protuberant abdominal skin fold which provides a dark, moist environment where fungal infection can occur.

13. Lice found on the hair of the head, eyebrows, eyelashes, and beard is known as pediculosis _____.

14. When plaque remains of the teeth, it hardens into _____, which cannot be removed by simple brushing.

Activity B   MATCHING

1. *Match the lifespan stage listed in Column A with the correct self-care activities in Column B.*

Column A

___ **1.** Infant

___ **2.** Toddler

___ **3.** School-age child

___ **4.** Adolescent

Column B

A. Eating patterns are erratic, can drink from a cup and use a spoon

B. Need reminders to bathe, brush teeth, and change clothes regularly

C. Daily bathing and shampooing become important to counteract body odor

D. Begin to develop eye–hand coordination, can hold a spoon and feed themselves

2. *Match the level of self-care listed in Column A with the correct description in Column B.*

Column A

___ **1.** Level 0

___ **2.** Level 1

___ **3.** Level 2

___ **4.** Level 3

___ **5.** Level 4

Column B

A. Patient requires assistance or supervision from another to complete self-care activities

B. Patient uses equipment or devices to perform self-care activities independently

C. Patient requires assistance or supervision from another and uses devices or equipment

D. Patient is completely dependent on another to perform self-care activities

E. Patient is independent in self-care activities

Activity C   ORDERING

1. Providing oral care on an unconscious patient can be more difficult. Certain considerations must be taken so that you don't' cause them harm. Write the correct sequence of steps to providing oral care to a patient who is unconscious in the boxes provided below:

a. Brush teeth and gums with toothpaste.

b. Place patient in a side-lying position.

c. Place towel and emesis basin under the patient's chin.

d. Perform hand hygiene and identify the patient.

e. Use a small bulb syringe to flush water into the oral cavity.

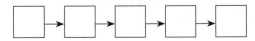

Activity D   SHORT ANSWER

1. What are characteristics of routine self-care?

_____

_____

_____

2. Why is the patient's ability to feed himself or herself so important?

_____

_____

_____

3. Why is it important to assess the feed of an older adult?

_____

_____

_____

4. What are the key things to look for during a physical assessment pertaining to self-care?

_____

_____

_____

5. What could be the focus of health promotion having to do with self-care and hygiene?

_____

_____

_____

SECTION III: APPLYING YOUR KNOWLEDGE

Activity E **CASE STUDY**

Answer the following questions, which involve the nurse's role in assessing a patient.

You are a nurse taking care of Al, an 85-year-old male who is recovering slowly from hip surgery. He has been very week and unable to participate in most of his self-care activities. At this time he is too tired and week to get out of bed or bathe himself.

1. What would be an appropriate nursing diagnosis for this patient and what could be some related factors?

   _____

   _____

   _____

2. How would you assist this person in caring for their dentures if they are not able to do it?

   _____

   _____

   _____

SECTION IV: PRACTICING FOR NCLEX

Activity F **MULTIPLE CHOICE**

Answer the following questions.

1. Self-care refers to a person's ability to perform primary care functions, in four areas, without the help of others. Which of the following is not one of these areas?

   a. Bathing

   b. Toileting

   c. Feeding

   d. Driving

2. Skylar is a 45-year-old woman with multiple sclerosis. She is able to perform most functions of self-care but recently she has been having problems with balance which has made it hard to get dressed. Which of the following factors is affecting Skylar's ability to perform self-care?

   a. Cognitive

   b. Neuromuscular

c. Sensory

d. Motivation

3. Walt is an 80-year-old man in a skilled nursing facility. He has recently become incontinent of urine. He is very angry by this change and has been expressing this anger toward anyone who is helping to care for him. When you walk in his room to perform an initial assessment of him, as his nurse, he states, "Get away from me. I can get to the restroom on my own. You don't know what I need." Which of the following responses would be the most therapeutic for the patient in this situation?

   a. "Walt, it sounds as if you are angry."

   b. "Walt, remember that you are having problems with getting to the bathroom in time. Can I help you?"

   c. "Walt, if you try to get to the bathroom by yourself you might fall."

   d. "Walt, go ahead and go to bathroom. Let me know if you need anything."

4. A nurse is taking care of a patient with schizophrenia who only recently started taking her medications again. When she is off of her medications she often forgets to bathe and does not wear clothing that is appropriate for the weather. In order to assess her normal pattern of self-care while on her medications, which of the following questions would be most appropriate to ask her?

   a. Do you want to bathe regularly?

   b. What are your expectations about bathing at this time?

   c. Are you not able to bathe yourself?

   d. What kind of soap do you like to use?

5. Stella is a 43-year-old woman who is undergoing chemotherapy for ovarian cancer which has metastasized. She has been experiencing increase nausea and vomiting associated with her treatment. Self-care activities have been very hard for her to complete. Which of the following is an internal resource that Stella has to help her attain her self-care goals?

   a. She has hot water to bathe in.

   b. She has good mobility around her home.

   c. She has motivation to participate in self-care.

   d. She has family and friends who help her with self-care.

6. A nurse is taking care of an elderly woman with good mobility but who is unable to stand for long periods of time secondary to muscle weakness. Which of the following methods for bathing would be most appropriate for this patient?

   a. Stand-up shower

   b. Sit-down shower with shower chair

   c. Bed bath

   d. Towel or bag bath

7. Lois is a 35-year-old woman who is 1 day postpartum. She is complaining of moderate perineal pain after delivery and would like to clean the area. Which of the following methods of bathing is most appropriate for Lois?

   a. Sitz bath

   b. Sit-down shower chair

   c. Bag bath

   d. Partial bath at a washbasin

8. There are many problems that can occur on the feet which, if found, need to be assessed further. Which of the following common foot problem is a cone-shaped lesion, which is usually found on the fourth or fifth toe over a toe joint?

   a. Callus

   b. Corn

   c. Plantar wart

   d. Bunion

9. Which of the following patients is most at risk for foot difficulties?

   a. 80-year-old man with coronary artery disease

   b. 45-year-old woman with type II diabetes

   c. 91-year-old man with renal insufficiency

   d. 34-year-old woman who is paraplegic.

10. You are a nurse taking care of a 68-year-old woman who was admitted for pneumonia. She is feeling very week and tired. She has soiled linens. Which of the following would be the most appropriate action for her at this time?

    a. Give her a bed bath and change the linens.

    b. Change the linens with her in the bed.

    c. Cover the soiled area and wait until she has more energy to change the linens.

    d. Don't do anything at this time and wait until she has rested to change the linens.

11. You are going to bathe a bed-bound patient. What do you do first?

    a. Close the door or bed curtains.

    b. Perform hand hygiene.

    c. Raise bed to high position.

    d. Lay a towel across the patient's chest.

12. You are a nurse taking care of a patient who needs a bed bath. Which of the following actions can you delegate to a nursing assistant?

    a. Skin assessment during bed bath

    b. Back massage

    c. Wound care

    d. Assessment of sensation in lower extremities

13. Which of the following are recommendations that should be given to a patient with poor circulation in order to prevent problems with their feet? Select all that apply.

    a. Inspect feet daily.

    b. Avoid crossing your feet.

    c. Cut thick toenails with a sharp razor or knife.

    d. Walk barefoot whenever possible.

    e. Soak feet in warm water once a day.

CHAPTER 24

Mobility

SECTION I: LEARNING OBJECTIVES

Upon completion of this chapter, the student will be able to do the following:

1. Explain normal functions of the musculoskeletal system and characteristics of normal movement.

2. Identify factors, including lifespan considerations, that can affect or alter mobility.

3. Describe the impact of immobility on physiologic and psychological functioning.

4. Discuss appropriate subjective and objective data to collect to assess mobility status.

5. Demonstrate nursing interventions such as positioning, ambulating, transferring, providing range of motion, and using assistive devices.

6. Plan strategies to avoid musculoskeletal injury to the nurse and patient during patient care.

7. Develop appropriate community-based nursing interventions for preventing and managing mobility problems.

SECTION II: ASSESSING YOUR UNDERSTANDING

Activity A FILL IN THE BLANKS

1. The diaphysis is the medical term for the shaft of the bone, while the _____ is the medical term for the end of the bone.

2. When flexor muscles contract, extensor muscles _____.

3. When assisting with patient movement, use of the large muscle groups in the _____ will help to prevent injury.

4. Exercise is considered _____ when the heart rate is elevated enough to provide cardiovascular conditioning.

5. Adequate calcium, _____, and Vitamin D are necessary for bone health.

6. The _____ provides the blood supply and innervations to the bone.

7. _____ is the degeneration of the articular surface of a weight-bearing joint.

8. A _____ is the shortening of a muscle with associated fibrotic changes.

9. Muscle _____ is a major risk of prolonged immobility.

10. _____ contractures are the most common type of contracture.

Activity B **MATCHING**

1. *Match the joint movement in Column A with its definition in Column B.*

Column A	Column B
___ **1.** Adduction	**A.** Turning a body part to face upward
___ **2.** Flexion	**B.** Decreasing the angle between two bones
___ **3.** Supination	
___ **4.** Inversion	**C.** Moving a body part away from midline
___ **5.** Abduction	**D.** Turning a body part to face downward
___ **6.** Pronation	**E.** Turning the feet inward so the toes point midline
	F. Moving the body part toward the midline

2. *Match the gait described in Column A with its description in Column B.*

Column A	Column B
___ **1.** Ataxic gait	**A.** One leg drags or is swung around to propel it forward
___ **2.** Spastic gait	
___ **3.** Waddling gait	**B.** Unsteadiness and staggering
___ **4.** Hemiplegic gait	**C.** Stiff in appearance; toes appear to "catch"
___ **5.** Festinating gait	**D.** Walking on the toes as if being pushed
	E. Feet are wide apart and everted

Activity C **SEQUENCING**

1. Provide the order in which infant motor development occurs.

  a. Crawling
  b. Standing
  c. Stepping reflex
  d. Pulling self up
  e. Rolling over
  f. Head control

☐ → ☐ → ☐ → ☐ → ☐ → ☐

Activity D **SHORT ANSWER**

1. How is balance maintained?

_____

_____

2. What steps can a nurse take to plan for patient ambulation or movement in the inpatient setting?

_____

_____

_____

3. Describe the phases of a normal gait. What would you look for in your assessment?

_____

_____

_____

4. Discuss some risk factors of prolonged immobility.

_____

_____

_____

5. Why are immobile patients at increased risk for urinary tract infections?

_____

_____

_____

SECTION III: APPLYING YOUR KNOWLEDGE

Activity E **CASE STUDY**

Peter is a 35-year-old man who was in a motorcycle accident several weeks ago. His leg was crushed and required amputation below the knee. Peter is now a patient on your rehabilitation unit. He tells you that he does not want to participate in physical therapy today, he would rather stay in bed.

1. What might be contributing to Peter's current desire to stay in bed?

   _____

   _____

   _____

2. Discuss two physical risks of prolonged immobility (answers will vary).

   _____

   _____

   _____

3. Compose two NANDA nursing diagnoses for Peter.

   _____

   _____

   _____

4. What nursing activities should be done to promote mobility in Peter?

   _____

   _____

   _____

SECTION IV: PRACTICING FOR NCLEX

Activity F MULTIPLE CHOICE

Answer the following questions.

1. Jim is a 21-year-old college football player. As a part of his workout regimen, Jim often engages in squats and lateral arm holds. These are examples of what type of exercise?
   a. Isotonic
   b. Aerobic
   c. Isometric
   d. Anaerobic

2. You are working with James, a 45-year-old man who is interested in starting an exercise program. You inform James that exercise has all of the following benefits except which?
   a. Decreases appetite
   b. Prevents constipation
   c. Improves sleep quality
   d. Enhances mood

3. Ezra is an active, healthy 2-year-old child. His mother asks you what she can expect developmentally from Ezra over the next few years. What is your best response?
   a. Ezra will refine both gross and fine motor skills but longitudinal growth will slow.
   b. Ezra will continue to grow rapidly, but gross and fine motor skill acquisition will slow.
   c. Ezra will regress in fine and gross motor skill development.
   d. Ezra will continue to grow rapidly and will refine both gross and fine motor skills.

4. Jane is a 65-year-old woman that has come in for her annual physical exam. She has asked you what to expect in terms of aging. You tell her that the following are normal signs of aging with the exception of which one?
   a. Osteoporosis
   b. Flattening of the lumbar spine causing the head to tilt forward
   c. Slowed reaction time
   d. Decrease in flexibility

5. Mr. Conway is admitted to your unit following an amputation of the left leg below the knee. You are responsible for developing his nursing plan of care. This plan of care should include all of the following except which?
   a. Encourage ROM at least every 8 hours
   b. Elevate the stump to prevent pressure ulcers
   c. Involve physical therapy in the plan of care
   d. Teach patient to use a trapeze for transfers

6. Susan is a 45-year-old woman admitted to your unit after undergoing a hysterectomy. She has been immobile for 2 days. Susan has a 20 pack year history of smoking. She also takes oral estrogen to manage her hot flashes. As you assess Susan, you notice that her left leg is dark purple and measures 2 inches larger than her right leg. What is Susan most at risk for?
   a. Pulmonary embolism
   b. Arterial insufficiency
   c. Pressure ulcer
   d. Surgical wound infection

7. Eloise is an 85-year-old Caucasian woman. She walks 1 mile every morning and every evening. She continues to smoke, but has cut back to half a pack per day. Eloise had a total oophorectomy at age 45 secondary to stage I ovarian cancer. She is currently not on any medications. Which of the following is not a primary risk factor for osteoporosis for this patient?

   a. Oophorectomy at age 45

   b. Smoking

   c. Caucasian race

   d. Sedentary lifestyle

8. You are conducting a home assessment of a 90-year-old male patient with a history of several minor strokes that have left him with a hemiplegic gate. You are particularly concerned about falls. What activities would help to prevent falls for this patient? Select all that apply.

   a. Removal of clutter on the floor

   b. Place a nightlight in the bathroom and the hallways

   c. Move bedroom to the ground floor

   d. Install hardwood floors

9. Frank is a clerical assistant for an inpatient hospital unit. He spends most of his day at a desk. Which of the following would you advise Frank to do to minimize damage to his musculoskeletal system? Select all that apply.

   a. Hold his breath only when lifting heavy objects

   b. Adjust the height of the work area

   c. Face the direction of the activity he is performing

   d. Use a wide stance and lift with the large leg muscles

10. Which structures are primarily responsible for voluntary movement? Select all that apply.

    a. Cerebral cortex

    b. Pyramidal tract

    c. Cerebellum

    d. Hypothalamus

11. Alexis is a recent paraplegic following an MVA. She is a patient on your rehabilitation unit and has several daily appointments with physical therapy and occupational therapy. Which of the following would be most appropriate to do to ensure safe transfers? Select all that apply.

    a. Transfer Alexis by yourself.

    b. Use a transfer belt when moving Alexis to a wheelchair.

    c. Teach Alexis to use the trapeze for transfer and upper body exercise.

    d. Use the under-axilla lift technique to transfer Alexis to a wheelchair.

12. Lucille is a 90-year-old widower who lives alone in her home. You know that older patients are at increased risk for falls. What other factors contribute to increased risk for falls in patients? Select all that apply.

    a. Ataxic gait

    b. History of a fall 5 years ago

    c. Diuretics

    d. Installed carpeting

25

Respiratory Function

SECTION I: LEARNING OBJECTIVES

Upon completion of this chapter, the student will be able to do the following:

1. Identify factors that can interfere with effective oxygenation of body tissues.

2. Describe common manifestations of altered respiratory function.

3. Discuss lifespan-related changes and problems in respiratory function.

4. Describe important elements in the respiratory assessment.

5. List three appropriate nursing diagnoses and outcomes for the patient with altered respiratory function.

6. Describe nursing measures to ensure a patent airway.

7. Discuss safe administration of oxygen using different modes of delivery.

8. Identify home care considerations for the respiratory patient.

SECTION II: ASSESSING YOUR UNDERSTANDING

Activity A FILL IN THE BLANKS

1. The bronchi continue to branch in treelike fashion into _____, which connect the larger conducting airways with the lung parenchyma.

2. The gas-exchanging portion of the lung is made up of millions of tiny air sacs called _____.

3. _____ is the physical process of moving air into and out of the lungs so gas exchange can take place.

4. A hallmark of common allergic asthma, _____ is when airways narrow and air exchange is limited.

5. Blood-filled respiratory secretions are called _____.

6. Very slow breathing can cause _____, low oxygen levels in the blood.

7. Abnormally high carbon dioxide in the blood is called _____.

8. A $PaCO_2$ above 45 mm Hg indicates _____, in which breathing rate and depth are insufficient to clear carbon dioxide adequately from the blood.

9. The _____ is an artificial airway consisting of a plastic tube surgically implanted just below the larynx into the trachea.

10. _____ occurs when stiffer lungs as well as their alveoli collapse.

11. _____ refers to normal respiratory rhythm and depth.

Activity B MATCHING

1. *Match the breathe sounds heard on auscultation in Column A with the correct description in Column B.*

Column A	Column B
____ **1.** Normal breathing	**A.** A low-pitched, rumbling sound
____ **2.** Crackles	**B.** Severe, continuous, high-pitched sound heard on inspiration
____ **3.** Course crackles	
____ **4.** Wheezes	
____ **5.** Stridor	**C.** Soft, rustling sound, inspiration is notable while expiration is quiet
____ **6.** Pleural friction rub	
	D. Continuous, high-pitched, musical sound
	E. A dry rubbing or grating sound
	F. Discontinuous sounds heard on inspiration

Activity C CROSSWORD

Across

1. The subjective felling of labored breathing and breathlessness.

4. The process by which oxygen and carbon dioxide move between the alveoli and the blood, from an area of greater concentration or pressure to an area of lower concentration or pressure.

Down

2. A respiratory illness that often led to patients experiencing pain with deep breathing because each breath increases pressure on pain receptors that are already compressed and irritated by swollen, inflamed tissue.

3. A bluish skin discoloration caused by a desaturation of oxygen on the hemoglobin in the blood.

5. The vibration of air movement through the chest wall, which is assessed with palpation.

Activity D ORDERING

1. Ventilation is the physical process of moving air into and out of the lungs. It starts with inspiration and ends with expiration but there are a series of steps within each of these that allow for gas exchange to take place. *Write the correct sequence of steps in the boxes provided below.*

a. The diaphragm and intercostal muscles relax, causing the thorax to return to its smaller resting size.

b. The diaphragm and external intercostal muscles contract.

c. The thorax volume enlarges and a decrease in intrathoracic pressure occurs.

d. The lungs expand and pressure drops in the airways causing a rush of air into the lungs.

e. Pressure in the chest increases, allowing air to flow out of the lungs.

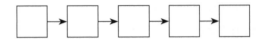

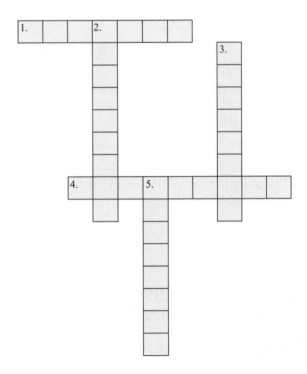

Activity E SHORT ANSWER

1. Briefly describe how oxygen is transported from the lungs to other tissues in the body.

_____

_____

_____

2. How does the upper respiratory tract protect the respiratory system?

_____

_____

_____

3. Why is teaching adolescents about respiratory health so important?

_____

_____

_____

4. How does posture affect someone's ability to breathe deeply?

_____

_____

_____

5. Why is it important to further assess someone's normal breathing pattern even if they report that it is fine?

_____

_____

_____

6. What is incentive spirometry and why should it be incorporated into health promotion teaching with patients?

_____

_____

_____

SECTION III: APPLYING YOUR KNOWLEDGE

Activity F CASE STUDY

Answer the following questions, which involve the nurse's role in assessing a patient for fluid, electrolyte, and acid–base imbalance.

Crystal is a 45-year-old woman who was diagnosed with esophageal cancer. She went for a resection of the cancer yesterday and had a tracheostomy placed. Post operatively she is doing well except that she is very upset that she has a tube.

1. What is a potential nursing goal and matching outcome criteria for this patient?

_____

_____

_____

2. What will your care of the new tracheostomy entail?

_____

_____

_____

SECTION IV: PRACTICING FOR NCLEX

Activity G MULTIPLE CHOICE

Answer the following questions.

1. Martin is a 58-year-old smoker who was admitted to the hospital with worsening shortness of breath over the last 2 days. He states that he is having some chest discomfort. You, as his nurse, ask him further about this in order to characterize whether this may be cardiac related, musculoskeletal related, or respiratory related. Martin states that when he breathes in, he feels as if the air passing into his lungs is burning him. It is also very painful to swallow. Based on what Martin is telling you, which of the following illness do suspect is causing Martins chest discomfort?

   a. Acute bronchitis

   b. Pneumonia

   c. Coronary artery disease

   d. Emphysema

2. Which of the following is a major organ of the upper respiratory tract?

   a. Trachea

   b. Bronchi

   c. Lungs

   d. Pharynx

3. Erin is a 35-year-old woman whom you are taking care of in the emergency department for a cough and hemoptysis for 3 days. Erin states that she has smoked one and a half packs of cigarettes for the last 5 years. In trying to identify risk factors for Erin you calculate her pack-year history to write on the intake form. Which of the following is Erin's pack-year of smoking?

   a. 5

   b. 7.5

   c. 5.5

   d. 7

4. Which of the following is a sign of dyspnea specific to infants?

   a. Panting respirations

   b. A forward-leaning position

   c. Nasal flaring

   d. Increased respiratory rate

5. Katrina is a 24-year-old woman who was admitted to the hospital for an exacerbation of symptoms related to her cystic fibrosis. During your assessment of Katrina, you notice a bluish color around her lips. Which of the following is Katrina exhibiting in this scenario?

   a. Cyanosis

   b. Eupnea

   c. Hypercapnia

   d. Hypoxemia

6. Which of the following is not true regarding the structure of the respiratory system?

   a. The trachea is part of the lower respiratory tract.

   b. The lungs move actively.

   c. Oxygen crosses the epithelium of the alveoli and into the blood stream.

   d. Branches that come off of the bronchi are called bronchioles.

7. Which of the following describes how carbon dioxide levels determine the frequency and depth of ventilation?

   a. Breathing increases when carbon dioxide levels decrease.

   b. An increase in circulating carbon dioxide causes and increase in the release of hydrogen ions, stimulating chemoreceptors in the aortic arch and carotid arteries, causing deeper and more rapid breathing.

   c. A decrease in the partial pressure of oxygen in arterial blood causes an increase in carbon dioxide levels which in turn causes breathing to be slowed and more shallow.

   d. When carbon dioxide levels in the blood increase, chemoreceptors are stimulated, causing deeper and more rapid breathing.

8. Burt is a 55-year-old obese man who complains of excessive daytime sleepiness, morning headaches, and sore throat. His wife states that he snores a lot. Which of the following diseases is Burt most likely suffering from?

   a. Chronic obstructive pulmonary disease

   b. Chronic bronchitis

   c. Sleep apnea

   d. Pneumonia

9. Which of the following diagnostic procedures measure lung size and airway patency, producing graphic representations of lung volumes and flows?

   a. Chest x-ray

   b. Bronchoscopy

   c. Skin tests

   d. Pulmonary function tests

10. Which of the following are characteristics of a normal breathing pattern? Select all that apply.

   a. The average adult moves about a quarter of a liter of air per breath.

   b. Normal breathing occurs at a rate of 12 to 20 breaths per minute in the adult.

   c. Usually a person breathes slightly faster when awake than when asleep.

   d. Exhaling normally takes twice as long as inhaling.

   e. The athlete normally breathes more slowly and deeply while at rest than someone who is less fit.

   f. Normally, each breath is the same size.

CHAPTER 26

Cardiac Function

SECTION I: LEARNING OBJECTIVES

Upon completion of this chapter, the student will be able to do the following:

1. Discuss factors that contribute to normal cardiac output and tissue perfusion.

2. Discuss cardiovascular changes that occur across the lifespan.

3. Describe the causes of altered cardiovascular function.

4. Describe how altered cardiovascular function can affect normal activities.

5. Perform a basic nursing assessment of cardiovascular function.

6. Identify common procedures and diagnostic tests used in the evaluation of the cardiovascular patient.

7. Discuss nursing measures directed at promoting and restoring cardiovascular function.

SECTION II: ASSESSING YOUR UNDERSTANDING

Activity A FILL IN THE BLANKS

1. The adult heart pumps _____ quarts of blood every minute.

2. The heart's ability to generate its own electrical impulse is referred to as _____.

3. Cardiac _____ is the amount of blood pumped through the circulatory system each minute.

4. The equation for cardiac output is CO = heart rate (HR) + _____.

5. A pulse oximeter measures tissue _____, or the flow of oxygen to tissue.

6. Annual blood pressure screening begins at age _____ years.

7. Smoking cessation reduces the risk of cardiovascular disease by _____ %.

8. Metabolic syndrome, or syndrome X, is a cluster of symptoms including diabetes, _____, elevated lipids, central adiposity and atherosclerosis.

9. A HR increase of _____ bpm is expected during light physical activity (i.e., walking).

10. The risk of a dislodged deep vein thrombosis (DVT) is either _____ or _____.

11. A weight gain of _____ lbs in 1 week is a warning sign of worsening heart failure.

12. Antiembolism stockings should be removed for _____ minutes every 8 hours.

13. Patients with heart disease should reduce their _____ intake to less than 2.5 g per day.

14. After nitroglycerin administration, it is most important to assess a patient's _____.

1. *Match the name of the valve or cells in Column A with its location in Column B.*

Column A	Column B
____ **1.** Tricuspid	**A.** Where electrical impulses are initiated
____ **2.** Mitral	
____ **3.** Sinoatrial (SA) node	**B.** Valve between the left atria and ventricle
____ **4.** AV junction	**C.** Valve between the right ventricle and the pulmonary arteries
____ **5.** Pulmonic	
____ **6.** Aortic	
	D. Valve between the left ventricle and the systemic circulation
	E. Where electrical impulses pause allowing the atrium to contract before the ventricles.
	F. Valve between the right atria and ventricle

2. *Match the medical terminology in Column A with the appropriate definition in Column B.*

Column A	Column B
____ **1.** Intermittent claudication	**A.** Limb pain caused by poor blood flow
____ **2.** Angina	**B.** Temporary decreased blood flow to the brain
____ **3.** Transient ischemic attack	**C.** A solid mass that can develop in an artery or vein
____ **4.** Syncope	**D.** Chest pain caused by decreased blood flow
____ **5.** Thrombus	**E.** Temporary loss of consciousness which may signal loss of oxygen to the brain

1. Where are coronary arteries located and what is their function?

_____

_____

_____

2. Map the flow of blood through the heart and systemic circulation, starting in the right atrium.

_____

_____

_____

3. Discuss the gender differences between men and women with regard to heart disease.

_____

_____

_____

4. Why are type "A" and type "D" persons at increased risk for cardiovascular events?

_____

_____

_____

5. What are some signs of decreased blood flow to the brain?

_____

_____

_____

6. Discuss nonpharmacologic patient education pearls for venous stasis prevention.

_____

_____

_____

SECTION III: APPLYING YOUR KNOWLEDGE

Activity D CASE STUDY

Edgar is a 44-year-old Latino police officer. He is married with three children and is the primary income provider for the family. He often picks up overtime shifts, and a 60-hour week is not uncommon. Edgar's wife, Josephina, works part time at the family restaurant two evenings per week, leaving Edgar to care for the children. Edgar lifts weights three times per week at the police station and admits that meals during the day often consist of "convenience" foods. His body mass index is 31. Today he is in the office for an annual physical, his vital signs are as follows: resting HR – 102, RR – 12, BP – 148/92.

1. What are some of Edgar's modifiable risk factors for heart disease.

   _____

   _____

   _____

2. It is suspected that Edgar has signs of heart failure. What labs would you expect to be drawn today?

   _____

   _____

   _____

3. What diagnostic testing procedures may be performed today?

   _____

   _____

   _____

4. What is an appropriate NANDA-I risk diagnosis for Edgar?

   _____

   _____

   _____

5. Edgar suddenly reports that he is experiencing chest pain. What would you do?

   _____

   _____

   _____

SECTION IV: PRACTICING FOR NCLEX

Activity E MULTIPLE CHOICE

Answer the following questions.

1. You are admitting Jacob, a 6-year-old child s/p tonsillectomy, to your surgical unit. You obtain his weight and place EKG and a pulse oximeter on Jacob's left finger. Jacob's HR reads 100 bpm and the pulse oximeter reads 99%. These readings best indicate which of the following?

   a. Adequate tissue perfusion
   b. Diminished stroke volume
   c. High cardiac output
   d. Heart failure

2. Adele is a 3-month-old infant who comes to your ED with her parents. She is working hard to breathe and is diaphoretic. You place her on continuous cardiac monitoring and note a HR of 246 bpm. What does this information tell you about her coronary artery perfusion?

   a. The heart is working harder to fill the coronary arteries.
   b. There is inadequate time for the coronary arteries to fill.
   c. The coronary arteries must be blocked.
   d. HR does not affect the function of the coronary arteries.

3. You are caring for Tyler, a 5-year-old child in the ED for 3 days of vomiting and diarrhea. He has not taken food by mouth for 3 days, but has kept fluids down. You take his BP and it reads 88/45 mm Hg. What is your reaction to this blood pressure?

   a. This BP is indicative of shock.
   b. This BP is normal for his age.
   c. This BP is too high for his age.
   d. This BP is low for his age but does not represent shock.

4. John has used cigarettes for 10 pack years. He is considering a smoking cessation program. You know that persons who quit smoking have the same cardiovascular risk factors as nonsmokers in how many years?

   a. 3 to 4 years.
   b. 1 to 2 years.
   c. 5 to 10 years.
   d. 20 years.

5. You are checking vital signs on Mr. V., a 47-year-old man in the community health center on the local Native American reservation. His blood pressure reading today is 156/82. Mr. V. tells you that, since his wife passed away 2 years ago, he commonly consumes convenience foods. He smokes two packs of cigarettes per day. Which of the following is NOT a modifiable risk factor for Mr. V.'s heart disease?

   a. Cigarette smoking
   b. Hypertension
   c. Native American heritage
   d. Food choices

6. Kimberly is a 35-year-old single woman who was admitted to your unit s/p a DVT. She is on a heparin drip and transitioning to lovenox therapy. As you prepare your patient teaching, it is important to teach Kimberly that all of the following contribute to DVT formation except which?

   a. Oral contraceptives
   b. Alcohol use.
   c. Smoking
   d. Pregnancy

7. John is a 60-year-old man with a 5-year diagnostic history of heart failure. John takes hydrochlorothiazide 25 mg daily to manage symptoms. John tells you that he feels great, but sometimes notices some swelling in his ankles at the end of the day. What lab test would you expect a healthcare provider to order to check for worsening heart failure?

   a. B-type natriuretic peptide (BNP)
   b. Troponin

   c. CK-MB
   d. Complete blood count (CBC).

8. Which of the following contributes to health disparities with relation to blood pressure? Select all that apply.

   a. Less access to fresh foods in urban, poor neighborhoods.
   b. High intake of salty or fried foods.
   c. Sedentary lifestyle secondary to unsafe outdoor space.
   d. Working 40 hours per week.

9. You are advising Mrs. S., a 64-year-old patient that has a family history of heart disease. She has concerns that she is at risk for developing heart disease. Which of the following is true regarding heart disease in women? Select all that apply.

   a. Women are more likely to develop diabetes following a myocardial infarction.
   b. Women are more likely to die following a myocardial infarction.
   c. Women tend to develop heart disease later in life than men.
   d. Women tend to present with chest pain or pressure when suffering from a myocardial infarction.
   e. Women having a myocardial infarction tend to have an atypical presentation such as gastrointestinal symptoms.

10. Elena is a 43-year-old woman admitted to the hospital s/p chest pain and cardiac ischemia. You are reviewing her list of daily medications. You know that which of the following might actually increase Elena's risk for cardiovascular problems? Select all that apply.

    a. Cold medication
    b. Diuretic
    c. Statin
    d. Oral contraceptives

CHAPTER 27

Fluid, Electrolytes, and Acid–Base

SECTION I: LEARNING OBJECTIVES

Upon completion of this chapter, the student will be able to do the following:

1. Describe physiologic factors that affect fluid, electrolyte, and acid–base homeostasis.

2. Discuss common alterations in fluid, electrolyte, and acid–base balance.

3. Explain the impact of age on fluid and electrolyte status.

4. Describe assessment parameters for the patient with potential or actual fluid and electrolyte imbalances.

5. Identify appropriate nursing diagnoses for patients with fluid imbalance.

6. Implement appropriate patient teaching to prevent or manage fluid and electrolyte imbalance.

SECTION II: ASSESSING YOUR UNDERSTANDING

Activity A FILL IN THE BLANKS

1. _____ fluid is a main type of body fluid that is located within cells.

2. _____ fluid is extracellular fluid that is located between the cells.

3. _____ refers to the proportion of dissolved particles in a volume of fluid.

4. Chemical compounds that partially separate in solution are called _____.

5. _____ is the movement of a solvent or solutes from an area of higher solvent or solute concentration.

6. Any substance that can donate free H^+ ions to a solution is called an _____.

7. In a _____ solution, the effective concentration of solute is greater than that of the blood plasma.

8. Stretch receptors, also called _____, are located in major arteries and veins and monitor vascular volume.

Activity B   MATCHING

1. Match the processes of fluid and electrolyte movement in Column A with the correct definition in Column B.

Column A

____ **1.** Diffusion

____ **2.** Osmosis

____ **3.** Active transport

____ **4.** Filtration

Column B

A. The movement of a fluid through a semi-permeable membrane

B. The process, requiring energy, by which ions and other molecules are moved across membranes from an area of lesser concentration to an area of greater concentration

C. The movement of a solvent or solutes from an area of higher solvent or solute concentration to an area of lower solvent or solute concentration

D. The transfer of water and dissolved substances through a permeable membrane from a region of high pressure to a region of low pressure

2. Match the electrolyte in Column A with the correct importance in Column B.

Column A

____ **1.** Phosphorus

____ **2.** Potassium

____ **3.** Calcium

____ **4.** Magnesium

Column B

A. Important in energy metabolism, for the structure of bones and membranes, and synthesis of nucleic acids (RNA and DNA)

B. Important in regulating neuromuscular function and cardiac activity

C. Important for proper cell membrane structure, wound healing, synaptic transmission in nervous tissue, membrane excitability, muscle contractility, and teeth and bone structure

D. Important for normal cardiac, neural, and muscle function and contractility

Activity C   ORDERING

1. The renin–angiotensin–aldosterone system regulates the volume of extracellular fluid within narrow limits by adjusting fluid intake and the urinary excretion of sodium, chloride, and water. *Write the correct sequence in the boxes provided below. The missing words are Renin, Angiotensin, Angiotensin I, Angiotensin II, and Aldosterone.*

a. Converting enzymes in the lungs and other vascular beds convert _____ into _____, a potent vasoconstrictor.

b. Decreased arterial blood pressure, decreased renal blood flow, increased renal sympathetic nerve activity, or low blood sodium levels stimulate _____ release.

c. _____, an enzyme secreted by cells in the kidney, splits _____, produced by the liver and circulating into the blood, into _____.

d. _____ stimulates the secretion of _____ which is produced by the adrenal cortex and both regulate sodium reabsorption in the distal tubules and collecting ducts of the kidney.

e. Chloride and water passively accompany the reabsorbed sodium, resulting in the reabsorption of saline which is extracellular fluid.

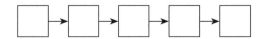

Activity D SHORT ANSWER

1. What are some lifespan considerations for fluid and electrolyte balance in the older?

_____

_____

_____

2. What are the ways in which water and electrolytes can be lost from the body?

_____

_____

_____

3. What things would be important to ask about in order to identify patients at risk for fluid, electrolyte, and acid–base imbalance?

_____

_____

_____

4. When is it important for a nurse to monitor a patient's intake and output?

_____

_____

_____

5. What are changes in the skin and mucous membranes that can indicate a fluid imbalance?

_____

_____

_____

SECTION III: APPLYING YOUR KNOWLEDGE

Activity E CASE STUDY

Answer the following questions, which involve the nurse's role in assessing a patient for fluid, electrolyte, and acid–base imbalance.

John is a 60-year-old man who has a diagnosis of congestive heart failure. He has been admitted to the hospital for increasing shortness of breath and swelling in his legs (edema). You are the nurse taking care of John.

1. Explain the reason for John's fluid imbalance and why he is experiencing shortness of breath and edema?

_____

_____

_____

2. What is a nursing intervention that you could use to help John now and in the future?

_____

_____

_____

SECTION IV: PRACTICING FOR NCLEX

Activity F MULTIPLE CHOICE

Answer the following questions.

1. Because metabolism continually produces acids, maintenance of pH within these incredibly narrow limits depends on two processes, buffering and compensation. Which of the following describes a function of buffering?

a. It helps to prevent large changes in pH by absorbing or releasing H^+ ions.

b. The lungs, under the control of chemoreceptor areas in the brainstem respiratory center, are responsible for controlling the amount of carbon dioxide in the blood.

c. The renal system excretes acids and bases from the body as needed.

d. The kidneys influence the maintenance of the normal acid–base balance by changing the rate of excretion or retention of H^+ and HCO^{3-} ions.

2. Many chronic medical problems adversely affect a person's ability to maintain normal fluid, electrolyte, and acid–base homeostasis. Which of the following describes complications related to liver disease?

a. The secretion of aldosterone and antidiuretic hormone is stimulated due to a lowered blood pressure, which results in extracellular fluid volume and water excess.

b. Increased plasma levels of antidiuretic hormone lead to water excess.

c. There may be an abnormal loss or accumulation of sodium, chloride, potassium, and fluid in the body, resulting in extracellular fluid and water excesses or deficits. Hyperkalemia and hypocalcemia are common and metabolic acidosis occurs in this disease's final stage.

d. A disruption of acid–base balance occurs. A disruption in this organ's ability to excrete carbon dioxide causes the pH of the person's blood to fall.

3. Which of the following is not a primary intracellular electrolyte?

a. Chloride

b. Potassium

c. Phosphate

d. Sulfate

4. Which of the following is a common anion?

a. Magnesium

b. Potassium

c. Chloride

d. Calcium

5. Edema happens when there is which of the following fluid volume imbalance?

a. Extracellular fluid volume deficit

b. Water deficit

c. Water excess

d. Extracellular fluid volume excess

6. Which of the following is not true regarding magnesium?

a. The liver regulates magnesium levels by breaking down the ion when serum levels are low.

b. Normal serum magnesium level ranges from 1.4 to 1.74 mEq/L.

c. Up to 60% of magnesium is in bone.

d. Magnesium is important in regulating neuromuscular function and cardiac activity.

7. Sodium is the most abundant cation in the extracellular fluid. Which of the following is true regarding sodium?

a. Normal serum sodium levels range from 145 to 155.

b. Sodium is regulated by the renin–angiotensin–aldosterone system.

c. If sodium is low, it means that there is not enough water.

d. Sodium is not regulated by natriuretic peptides.

8. Potassium is essential for normal cardiac, neural, and muscle function and contractility of all muscles. Which of the following is false about potassium?

a. Insulin promotes the transfer of potassium from the extracellular fluid into skeletal muscle and liver cells.

b. Aldosterone enhances renal excretion of potassium.

c. A person loses approximately 30 mEq of potassium.

d. Normal serum potassium ranges from 5.5 to 6.0 mEq/L.

9. Which of the following is not true regarding calcium?

a. Approximately 60% of the body's calcium is found within the bones and teeth.

b. Normal total serum calcium levels range between 8.9 and 10.1 mg/dL.

c. Calcium is present in the blood primarily in both ionized and bound protein states.

d. The cell membrane structure depends on calcium.

10. Calcium is important to function in many ways. Calcium is important for which of the following? Select all that apply.

a. Wound healing

b. Regulate vitamin D absorption

c. Respiratory function

d. Synaptic transmission in nervous tissue

e. Membrane excitability

f. Blood clotting

CHAPTER 28

Nutrition

SECTION I: LEARNING OBJECTIVES

Upon completion of this chapter, the student will be able to do the following:

1. Identify essential nutrients and examples of good dietary sources for each.

2. Describe normal digestion, absorption, and metabolism of carbohydrates, fats, and proteins.

3. Discuss nutritional considerations across the lifespan.

4. List factors that can affect dietary patterns.

5. Describe manifestations of altered nutrition.

6. Explain nursing interventions to promote optimal nutrition and health.

7. Discuss nursing responsibilities for interventions used to treat altered nutritional states.

SECTION II: ASSESSING YOUR UNDERSTANDING

Activity A FILL IN THE BLANKS

1. The body cannot synthesize _____ nutrients in adequate amounts and must therefore obtain them through diet.

2. _____-soluble vitamins must be consumed daily to maintain adequate levels in the body.

3. Poor appetite, fatigue, mental depression, apathy, and constipation are all symptoms of Vitamin _____ deficiency.

4. Vitamin _____ is critical for iron absorption.

5. Most of the sodium in the diet comes from consumption of _____ foods.

6. Cretinism is a sign of chronic _____ deficiency in infancy.

7. _____-density lipoprotein cholesterol is also known as "good" cholesterol.

8. The body's _____ metabolic rate is the number of calories needed to carry out activities at rest.

9. By the end of the first year an infant's weight typically _____.

10. Obesity is classified as a body mass index (BMI) of _____ or greater.

11. Foods high in vitamin _____ affect the effectiveness of the drug warfarin (Coumadin).

12. A serum _____ has a 2-day half-life and is considered a very sensitive and specific marker of nutrition status.

Activity B   MATCHING

1. *Match the term listed in Column A with its definition in Column B.*

Column A

_____ **1.** Kilocalorie (kcal)

_____ **2.** Catabolism

_____ **3.** Carbohydrates

_____ **4.** Protein

_____ **5.** Vitamins

Column B

A. The process of breaking down body stores

B. Organic compounds that are essential to the body in small quantities for growth, development, maintenance, and reproduction

C. The amount of energy needed to raise 1 kg of water 1 °C

D. Vital for growth and repair of all body systems

E. Simple and complex sugars

Activity C   SHORT ANSWER

1. Discuss some differences between fat-soluble and water-soluble vitamins.

_____

_____

_____

2. Describe the characteristics of iron-deficiency anemia. Who is at highest risk?

_____

_____

_____

3. List some of the recommendations from the USDA's website choosemyplate.gov.

_____

_____

_____

4. Describe the difference between refined and enriched grains.

_____

_____

_____

5. Discuss the increased nutritional needs of a woman during pregnancy.

_____

_____

_____

6. What are some nursing strategies to promote healthy nutrition in the hospital setting?

_____

_____

_____

SECTION III: APPLYING YOUR KNOWLEDGE

Activity D   CASE STUDY

Ava is a 78-year-old woman who lives alone in a single family home. Her daughter Betty lives in a nearby suburb and visits every other Sunday. Betty calls you because she has noticed that her mother is losing weight and appears to be frail. She asks if you have any advice to help her mother to gain weight.

1. What are some factors that contribute to nutritional status in the older adult?

_____

_____

_____

2. Discuss any special micronutrient needs that Ava would have.

_____

_____

_____

3. Ava is 5'2". How would you approximate her ideal body weight (IBW)?

_____

_____

_____

4. You weigh Ava and calculate her BMI to be 17.5. What does this place Ava at risk for?

_____

_____

_____

SECTION IV: PRACTICING FOR NCLEX

Activity E   **MULTIPLE CHOICE**

Answer the following questions.

1. You are working with Jim, a 54 year old with a history of constipation. Jim asks if there is anything he could add to his diet to ease defecation. Your best response would be what?

   a. Carbohydrates

   b. Fiber

   c. Protein

   d. Alcohol

2. Maria is a 45-year-old patient on your inpatient unit. She has just resumed eating a normal diet. You check a blood sugar with her morning labs and the result is 98 mg/dL. How would you interpret this blood glucose?

   a. Normal

   b. Mildly elevated

   c. Severely elevated

   d. Low

3. You are a nurse in a rural health center when you meet Matthew, age 4. You notice as he enters the clinic that his legs appear to be bowed. When he smiles, you also note that his dentition is quite malformed for a child his age. What vitamin deficiency would you most suspect?

   a. Vitamin A

   b. Vitamin B

   c. Vitamin C

   d. Vitamin D

4. Alexis is a 16-year-old adolescent who informs you that she became a vegetarian 1 year ago. Lately she complains that she is fatigued and has trouble concentrating. A quick blood test ordered by her licensed provider informs you that she has pernicious anemia. This is a deficiency of what vitamin?

   a. Vitamin C

   b. Vitamin B12

   c. Folic acid

   d. Vitamin A

5. Janine is a 28-year-old woman patient in your outpatient clinic with a chief complaint of fatigue. Her physician has prescribed her ferrous sulfate 325 mg to treat iron-deficiency anemia. You are teaching Janine about medication administration. What food would be best consumed with her ferrous sulfate?

   a. A glass of milk

   b. A piece of bread

   c. A glass of orange juice

   d. A can of soda pop

6. All of the following factors increase the basal metabolic rate EXCEPT which?

   a. Fever

   b. Stress

   c. Growth

   d. Exercise

7. Annika is 6 weeks pregnant and is in your clinic for her first prenatal exam. She asks you how her nutritional needs have changed now that she is pregnant. Which of the following is your best response?

   a. You are now eating for two. Enjoy!

   b. You should double your caloric intake to sustain the pregnancy.

   c. You will need additional nutrients such as calcium, folic acid, and protein.

   d. Food choices during pregnancy have little impact on your baby.

8. You are working with James, a 45-year-old construction worker. You obtain his height and weight and calculate that his BMI is 28. How would you best classify James?

   a. Underweight

   b. IBW

   c. Overweight

   d. Obese

9. Selma is a 66-year-old woman with atrial fibrillation for which she is on warfarin (Coumadin) therapy. She asks you if she has any dietary restrictions. Which of the following foods would Selma need to monitor her intake of?

   a. Bananas

   b. Spinach

   c. Mangos

   d. Broccoli

10. You are working with Charlotte, a 46-year-old woman who is working to lose weight. Based on recommendations from the USDA regarding diet modification, which of the following is NOT appropriate advice for Charlotte?

    a. Eat a variety of foods that you enjoy, but less quantity.

    b. Drink nonfat or 1% mild.

    c. Drink juice for majority of fluid intake.

    d. Make fruits and vegetables at least half of your intake.

11. Jimmy is a 6 year old that you are caring for on an inpatient unit for treatment of intestinal malabsorption syndrome. Which of the following might be signs of calcium deficiency? Select all that apply.

    a. Bowed legs

    b. Enlarged skull

    c. Pale mucous membranes

    d. Hypertension

12. You are working with Jim, a 54-year-old obese man who is interested in losing weight. He asks you why trans fats are so bad for you. Your best response includes which of the following? Select all that apply.

    a. Trans fats raise HDL levels

    b. Trans fats lower HDL levels

    c. Trans fats raise LDL levels

    d. Trans fats raise cholesterol levels

13. You are working with Jane, a 35-year-old woman who is interested in losing weight. Based on current recommendations from the USDA and what you know about a typical U.S. diet, which of the following are appropriate recommendations for healthy weight loss? Select all that apply.

    a. Cut carbohydrates to 45% of intake

    b. Increase the number of complex carbohydrates

    c. Decrease the number of calories ingested

    d. Increase physical activity

CHAPTER 29

Skin Integrity and Wound Healing

SECTION I: LEARNING OBJECTIVES

Upon completion of this chapter, the student will be able to do the following:

1. Describe the structure and function of the integumentary system.

2. Identify factors affecting integumentary function and the manifestations of impaired function.

3. Identify the components of nursing assessment of skin integrity.

4. Describe normal wound healing.

5. Describe the scientific principles of moist wound healing.

6. Discuss nursing interventions to promote skin integrity.

7. Explain the scientific principles in the application of heat and cold to injured areas.

8. Describe the categories and function of wound dressings and how to select the appropriate dressing for wound healing.

SECTION II: ASSESSING YOUR UNDERSTANDING

Activity A FILL IN THE BLANKS

1. An _____ is a type of acute wound created intentionally as part of surgical treatment.

2. _____ tissue appears wrinkled and is lighter in appearance than healthy tissue.

3. An inflammation of the skin, most often producing epidermal and dermal damage or irritation, possibly accompanied by pain, itching, redness, and blisters is called _____.

4. An _____results when skin rubs against a hard surface and skin scrapes away the epithelial layer.

5. _____ occurs when two surfaces rub together.

6. In a full-thickness wound, the proliferation phase begins with the development of _____ tissue, which appears beefy, red, and granular, and consists of a matrix of collagen embedded with macrophages, fibroblasts, and capillary buds.

7. A _____ is a localized collection of blood.

8. _____ is a total or partial disruption in wound edges.

9. A _____ is an abnormal tube-like passageway that forms between two organs or from one organ to outside the body.

Activity B MATCHING

In Column A with the correct description in Column B.

Column A

_____ **1.** Stage I

_____ **2.** Stage II

_____ **3.** Stage III

_____ **4.** Stage IV

_____ **5.** Unstageable

_____ **6.** Suspected deep tissue injury

Column B

A. Full-thickness tissue loss, subcutaneous fat may be visible but bone, tendon, or muscle is not

B. Full-thickness tissue loss in which the base of the ulcer is covered by slough and/or eschar

C. Purple or maroon localized area of discolored intact skin or blood-filled blister due to damage of underlying soft tissue from pressure and/or shear

D. Intact skin with non-blanchable redness of a localized area, usually over a bony prominence

E. Full-thickness tissue loss with exposed bone, tendon, or muscle

F. Partial-thickness loss of dermis presenting as a shallow open ulcer with a red-pink wound bad, without slough

Activity C ORDERING

1. Wounds heal through a systemic four-phase process. Write the correct sequence of phases in the boxes provided below.

   a. Proliferative

   b. Maturation

   c. Inflammatory

   d. Hemostasis

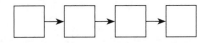

Activity D SHORT ANSWER

1. In what way is newborn skin different from that of other age groups?

_____

_____

_____

2. Why is good nutrition important for skin health?

_____

_____

_____

3. Describe what shear force is and how it puts someone at risk for developing a pressure ulcer.

_____

_____

_____

4. Why may wound healing be decreased in obese patients?

_____

_____

_____

5. What should be included in health promotion to address skin care in patients?

_____

_____

_____

SECTION III: APPLYING YOUR KNOWLEDGE

Activity E CASE STUDY

Answer the following questions, which involve the nurse's role in assessing a patient.

Soriah is a 37-year-old woman who is seen in the clinic for severe psoriasis. She has been experiencing severe pruritus and has scratched so much that she has caused excoriations and, in one area, a superimposed infection has caused an abscess. This abscess is fairly deep and is draining quite a bit of purulent drainage. After seeing her primary care provider, she is sent to you for wound care and patient teaching.

1. What can you, as the nurse, do to help with Soriah's symptoms?

   _____

   _____

   _____

2. What type of wound care would you provide for Soriah and why?

   _____

   _____

   _____

SECTION IV: PRACTICING FOR NCLEX

Activity F MULTIPLE CHOICE

Answer the following questions.

1. Which of the following is true about the dermis?
   a. It is responsible for producing the proteins collagen and elastin.
   b. It is the outermost layer.
   c. It is responsible for producing keratin.
   d. It is the thickest skin layer.
   e. It contains melanocytes which produce melanin.

2. Which of the following is not considered a skin appendage?
   a. Hair
   b. Connective tissue

   c. Sebaceous gland
   d. Eccrine sweat glands

3. You are evaluating a patient who was admitted with second-degree burns. Which of the following describes a second-degree burn?
   a. Usually moist with blisters, they may be pink, red, pale ivory, or light yellow-brown
   b. Superficial, may be pinkish or red with no blistering
   c. May vary from brown or black to cherry red or pearly white, bullae may be present
   d. Also called a superficial partial-thickness burn, can appear dry and leathery

4. Which of the following describes the third phase of the wound healing process called proliferative?
   a. The onset of vasoconstriction, platelet aggregation, and clot formation.
   b. Is marked by vasodilation and phagocytosis as the body works to clean the wound.
   c. Epidermal cells, which appear pink, reproduce and migrate across the surface of the wound in a process called epithelialization.
   d. The number of fibroblasts decreases, collagen synthesis stabilized and collagen fibrils become increasingly organized, resulting in greater tensile strength of the wound.

5. You are treating a patient who has a wound with full-thickness tissue loss and edges that do not readily approximate. You know that the open wound will gradually fill with granulation tissue. What type of wound healing describes this?
   a. Primary intention
   b. Maturation
   c. Secondary intention
   d. Tertiary intention

6. The nurse is assessing a patient's surgical wound after abdominal surgery and sees that the viscera is protruding through the abdominal wound opening. Which term best describes this complication?
   a. Fistula
   b. Dehiscence
   c. Hemorrhage
   d. Evisceration

7. Which of the following is not a protective function of the skin?

   a. Sebum gives the skin an acidic pH, which retards the growth of microorganisms.

   b. Keratin protects against the sun's ultraviolet rays.

   c. Microorganisms that inhibit the growth of pathogens are present on the skin.

   d. It contains cells such as macrophages that protect it.

8. Adequate blood flow to the skin is necessary for healthy, viable tissue. Adequate skin perfusion requires four factors. Which of the following is not one of these factors?

   a. Local capillary pressure must be lower than external pressure.

   b. The heart must be able to pump adequately.

   c. The volume of circulating blood must be sufficient.

   d. Arteries and veins must be patent and functioning well.

9. Which of the following is part of the graded criteria for predicting pressure ulcers using the Braden Scale? Select all that apply.

   a. Sensory perception

   b. Nutrition

   c. Age

   d. Ability

   e. Friction

10. A nurse is assessing a patient's surgical wound and sees drainage that is pale pink-yellow, thin, and contains plasma and red cells is called what? Which of the following describes this type of drainage?

    a. Serous

    b. Purulent

    c. Serosanguineous

    d. Sanguineous

Infection Prevention and Management

SECTION I: LEARNING OBJECTIVES

Upon completion of this chapter, the student will be able to do the following:

1. Name the major components of the body's normal resistance to infection and the role of each.

2. Differentiate between cellular and humoral immunity and between active and passive immunity.

3. Identify possible risk factors for infection or infectious diseases.

4. Name four common healthcare-associated infections (HAIs).

5. Recognize common manifestations of infection.

6. Identify common diagnostic and laboratory tests used to identify or confirm an infectious process.

7. Describe major consequences of an infectious process.

8. Describe nursing measures that strengthen defense mechanisms against infection.

9. Children who receive adequate nutrition have fully operational immune systems by age _____ months.

10. Normal flora that cause disease under the right conditions are said to be _____.

SECTION II: ASSESSING YOUR UNDERSTANDING

Activity A FILL IN THE BLANKS

1. The first line of defense against invading organisms is intact _____ and mucous membranes.

2. Five signs of local inflammation are erythema, _____, edema, pain, and tissue impairment.

3. The thymus begins to shrink during _____ which leads to a decline in cell-mediated and humoral immunity.

4. A _____ invades a cell and uses its metabolic processes to replicate itself.

5. Stress causes the release of cortisol which can lead to _____ and impaired immune system function.

6. The _____ period is the time between exposure to the organism and the time when the organism is shed through body secretions.

7. "Traveler's diarrhea" is a colloquial term used to describe diarrhea following ingestion of endemic _____ or _____ in the drinking water.

8. Patient's with a lactate level greater than _____ mmol/L should be treated with the Severe Sepsis Resuscitation Protocol, regardless of blood pressure.

9. The minimum inhibitory complex (MIC) allows healthcare providers to determine which _____ is effective in treating a specific infection.

10. When IV contrast is used for an imaging study, it is important that the nurse monitor the patient for an _____ reaction.

ACTIVITY B MATCHING

1. Match the term in Column A with its definition in Column B.

Column A

_____ 1. Leukocytes

_____ 2. Fever

_____ 3. T lymphocytes

_____ 4. B lymphocytes

Column B

A. The hypothalamus response to pyrogens released by macrophages

B. Critical in fighting fungi and protozoa

C. When activated, these cells attack and destroy microbes

D. Produce antibodies in response to a wide range of bacteria and viruses

2. Match the medical terminology in Column A with its associated value in Column B.

Column A

_____ 1. Normal white blood cell (WBC) count

_____ 2. Normal lymphocyte level

_____ 3. Normal immature granulocytes (bands)

_____ 4. Normal lactate level

_____ 5. Normal eosinophil level

Column B

A. <10%

B. 50–70%

C. 0.3–2.6 mmol/L

D. 0–3%

E. 5,000–10,000 cells/mm^3

ACTIVITY C SEQUENCING

1. Place the stages of the communicable period, or the time frame in which a disease can be passed from one to another, in the order in which they occur.

    a. Convalescence

    b. Prodromal

    c. Incubation

    d. Acute

Activity D SHORT ANSWER

1. Differentiate between active and passive immunity and provide an example of each.

    _____

    _____

    _____

2. Discuss age-related changes that lead to a decline in immune system function in older adults.

    _____

    _____

    _____

3. What is the difference between incubation and prodromal phases of the communicable period?

    _____

    _____

    _____

4. List some important questions to ask when collecting a history on a patient with an acute illness.

    _____

    _____

    _____

5. Why is it important to maintain sterility during collection of culture samples?

    _____

    _____

    _____

6. Discuss some nonpharmacologic nursing interventions that are helpful during an acute illness.

_____

_____

_____

SECTION III: APPLYING YOUR KNOWLEDGE

Activity E   **CASE STUDY**

Alex is a 75-year-old man on your unit following a knee replacement. He is post-op day 4. Today Alex complains of pain at the site of the incision. On exam, you note that the incision is erythematous and edematous. There is thick yellow pus draining from the site. His vital signs are as follows: Temperature 36.7 °C, HR 77, RR 12, BP 110/70.

1. Write an appropriate NANDA-I nursing diagnosis for Alex.

_____

_____

_____

2. List specific lab values and vital sign changes that would indicate an infection? How might Alex's age affect these values?

_____

_____

_____

3. The attending physician on the unit orders a wound culture of Alex's surgical site. Describe how you would collect this.

_____

_____

_____

4. What nursing interventions can help Alex from developing further complications or a secondary infection?

_____

_____

_____

SECTION IV: PRACTICING FOR NCLEX

Activity F   **MULTIPLE CHOICE**

Answer the following questions.

1. You are caring for Jane, age 4 months, following surgical repair of a tracheal-esophageal fistula. When collecting her vital signs, you note her rectal temperature to be 39.5 °C. You know what to be true of fever in young children?

a. Young children who have temperatures this high will almost always have febrile seizures.

b. Young children rarely mount a fever to an invading organism; this must be an error.

c. Young children typically mount a fever after a surgical procedure and it should go away.

d. Young children often have a vigorous immune response to infection and thus high fevers.

2. You are caring for Mr. Porter, a 66-year-old man admitted to your unit s/p left hip replacement. He has been out of surgery for 3 days. On your initial assessment, Mr. Porter has a heart rate of 96 bpm and a respiratory rate of 32. He is diaphoretic. On a scale from 1 to 10, Mr. Porter describes his pain as a 7 and points to the left side of his chest. What is the most likely cause of Mr. Porter's distress?

a. Pneumonia

b. Myocardial infarction

c. Referred post-operative pain

d. Urinary tract infection

3. Nurse James is working with an 82-year-old man following gallbladder surgery. He is NPO and has IV access in his hand. He also has a Foley catheter in place. He is able to ambulate with the aid of a walker. All of the following lower this patient's immunity except which?

a. Ambulation

b. Foley catheter

c. IV access

d. Surgical incision

4. You are a nurse in a preoperative surgical unit. As a standard of care, all patients are swabbed for methicillin-resistant *Staphylococcus aureus* (MRSA). Prior to his surgery, you note that Mr. C.'s results have come back positive. He asks you what this means. What is your best response?

   a. These results indicate that you are infected with MRSA.

   b. These results indicate that you are contaminated with MRSA.

   c. Two positive tests are required before results can be confirmed.

   d. These results indicate that you are colonized with MRSA.

5. Mrs. V. is a 38-year-old woman in your clinic today with an acute illness. As you collect Mrs. Vinings' vital signs, you note that her oral temperature is 38.6 °C. What do you report to the physician?

   a. Mrs. V. has a low-grade fever.

   b. Mrs. V. has a high-grade fever.

   c. Mrs. V. is hyperpyrexic.

   d. Mrs. V. drank some hot coffee on the way in.

6. Mr. Dent is a 20-year-old man seen in your clinic today for purulent penile discharge. He discloses that he has had five sexual partners in the past month. Mr. Dent states that he always uses a condom. Which of the following is the most appropriate NANDA-I nursing diagnosis for Mr. Dent?

   a. The risk for infection related to increased exposure to pathogens.

   b. The risk for infection related to promiscuous sexual practices.

   c. Knowledge deficit related to improper use of barrier method.

   d. Knowledge deficit related to route of disease transmission.

7. You are caring for Peter, age 4 years, who is being treated for osteomyelitis in his left femur. He is on a 28-day course of IV vancomycin to be administered daily at 1300. Today is day 3 of treatment, and the pharmacist asks you to draw a peak vancomycin level. What would be the most appropriate time to draw this blood?

   a. 1500

   b. 1200

   c. 2000

   d. Wait until day 5 of treatment

8. You are working with Pam, age 15, in your community health clinic. It is early October, and Pam is worried that she will become ill and miss school, stating "I am always getting sick this time of year". What health promotion activities are appropriate to include in your teaching today? Select all that apply.

   a. Proper hand-washing techniques

   b. Instructions to shower daily with Hibiclens

   c. Administration of influenza immunization

   d. Information on sleep hygiene

9. Which of the following are critical to the functioning of a healthy immune system? Select all that apply.

   a. Thymus

   b. Spleen

   c. Tonsils

   d. Liver

10. You are working with Mrs. P. a 50-year-old woman s/p liver transplant. She is on multiple immunosuppressive drug therapies, is intubated, and is NPO with parenteral nutrition running through a central line. Which of the following would raise your suspicion that Mrs. P. is developing septicemia? Select all that apply.

   a. A HR of 80 bpm

   b. Increased urine output

   c. A temperature of 39.5 °C

   d. A WBC count of 15,000 with 12% bands

CHAPTER 31

Urinary Elimination

SECTION I: LEARNING OBJECTIVES

Upon completion of this chapter, the student will be able to do the following:

1. Describe the structure and function of the urinary system.

2. Outline the process of micturition.

3. List and describe alterations in normal voiding patterns.

4. Recognize age-related differences in urinary elimination.

5. Describe factors that can alter urinary function.

6. Discuss nursing assessment of urinary function.

7. Identify nursing diagnoses related to urinary elimination.

8. Describe nursing interventions to promote normal urinary elimination.

9. Discuss interventions for altered urinary function.

10. Develop appropriate collaborative and community-based nursing interventions to manage problems with voiding.

SECTION II: ASSESSING YOUR UNDERSTANDING

Activity A FILL IN THE BLANKS

1. The body of the bladder is composed of three layers of smooth muscle, collective called the _____ muscle.

2. _____ is the process of excreting urine from the body.

3. Water excretion is called _____.

4. _____ is distention of the kidney pelvis with urine secondary to the increased resistance caused by obstruction to normal urine flow.

5. _____ is an infection of the bladder.

6. _____ is the formation and excretion of excessive amounts of urine in the absence of a concurrent increase in fluid intake.

7. The sudden, involuntary loss of small amounts of urine that accompanies a sudden increase in intra-abdominal pressure is called _____ incontinence.

8. The involuntary voiding, with no underlying pathophysiologic origin, after the age at which bladder control is usually achieved is called _____.

9. A _____ is the protrusion or herniation of the bladder into the vaginal canal, which can produce symptoms of stress incontinence, frequency, dribbling, and inability to empty the bladder completely.

Activity B   MATCHING

1. *Match the structures of the urinary tract in Column A with the correct function in Column B.*

Column A

____ **1.** Kidneys

____ **2.** Urethra

____ **3.** Ureter

____ **4.** Bladder

Column B

A. Acts as a passageway for urine from the kidneys to the bladder

B. Has a functional unit called a nephron which forms urine and helps to maintain fluid and electrolyte imbalance

C. Acts as a storage compartment for urine

D. An exit passageway for urine, it is controlled by a band of muscles that allow for voluntary control of urination

Activity C   ORDERING

1. The kidneys regulate the volume and composition of the body's extracellular fluid. They perform this function by selectively retaining wanted water and other substances and excreting unwanted water and other substances in urine. This happens in a sequence of processes. *Write the correct sequence in the boxes provided below.*

a. The renal arteries bring blood into the kidneys.

b. Varying amounts of H^+ and K^+ ions, as well as ammonia, creatinine, uric acid, and other metabolites are secreted.

c. The tubule actively and passively reabsorbs substances that the body wants to retain such as electrolytes and varying amounts of water.

d. The glomerulus filters blood into a glomerular filtrate.

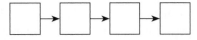

2. In order to properly apply an external catheter, it is important to follow certain steps. Write the correct sequence of steps in the boxes provided below.

a. Put on disposable gloves, wash the penis and pubic area.

b. Apply self-adhesive sheath or skin protector.

c. Explain the procedure to the patient, raise the bed, and assist patient to a supine position.

d. Grasp penis in nondominant hand and apply sheath.

e. Wash hands, identify the patient, and provide for privacy of the patient.

f. Attach drainage bag and perform hand hygiene.

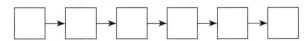

Activity D   SHORT ANSWER

1. How does loss of body fluid affect urination?

_____

_____

_____

2. What are some ways that a nurse can increase normal pattern identification in patients with urinary issues?

_____

_____

_____

3. What things would be important to ask about for risk identification in patients with urinary issues?

_____

_____

_____

4. Why is it important to assess for both fluid intake and output?

_____

_____

_____

5. Describe the risks associated with catheterization and how to prevent them.

_____

_____

_____

SECTION III: APPLYING YOUR KNOWLEDGE

Activity E CASE STUDY

Answer the following questions, which involve the nurse's role in assessing a patient.

Tony is a 19-year-old man who has been a paraplegic since the age of 12. Until recently, he has had an indwelling urinary catheter but has suffered from multiple urinary tract infections and trauma to his urethra. In order to hopefully decrease the incidence of infection and to allow his urethra to heal, a suprapubic catheter was placed. He will be going home later today.

1. What does nursing assessment of Tony's suprapubic catheter entail?

_____

_____

_____

2. What are some home care considerations for Tony?

_____

_____

_____

SECTION IV: PRACTICING FOR NCLEX

Activity F MULTIPLE CHOICE

Answer the following questions.

1. Which of the following does not illustrate a normal lifespan variant regarding urination?
   a. Natalia is 8 years old. She is continent during the day but is incontinent two times during the night.
   b. Norris is a 3 and a half years old. He is showing interest in being ready for toilet training by showing that he can undress himself and by being able to stay dry for 2 hours at a time.
   c. Charles is a 5 hours old. His urine appears pink tinged.
   d. Dana is 10 years old. She has been voiding straw-colored urine six or seven times a day.

2. Which of the following is true regarding the normal urination?
   a. Catheterized patients should drain a minimum of 30 mL of urine per hour.
   b. In adults, the average amount of urine per void is 500 mL.
   c. Urinary output does not vary all that much between adults and children.
   d. In adults, the amount of urine voided typically does not depend on fluid intake and losses.

3. Which of the following is not true of urine color?
   a. Medications can alter urine's color.
   b. Someone's state of hydration affects the color.
   c. The color of urine ranges from light yellow to amber.
   d. The appearance of urine streaked with blood is always abnormal.

4. Which of the following is the test that would provide you with an accurate measurement of the kidney's excretion of creatinine?
   a. 24-hour specimen
   b. Clean-catch specimen
   c. Random specimen
   d. Intermittent specimen

5. Darwin is a 75-year-old man who was admitted to the hospital for altered mental status. He had been in his usual state of good health until this morning when a nurse at the long-term care facility that he lives at noticed that he was confused. Shortly after being admitted to the hospital, he became combative and had to be restrained. His bed linens have to be changed frequently because of urinary incontinence. Which nursing diagnosis best describes this patient's condition?
   a. Stress incontinence
   b. Urge urinary incontinence
   c. Functional incontinence
   d. Total urinary incontinence

6. Mr. Smith, a 57-year-old man, is suffering from polyuria. Which of the following can cause polyuria?

   a. Diabetes insipidus

   b. Renal disease

   c. Urinary tract infection

   d. Renal calculi

7. You are working primarily with adult and older adult patients. Which of the following lifespan considerations should you, as the nurse, keep in the mind when working with these populations?

   a. Older men may experience urinary hesitancy and difficulty starting the urinary stream.

   b. Older adults may try to manage incontinence by restricting intake of fluids.

   c. Because of decreased arterial perfusion, kidney function progressively decreases later in life.

   d. Urinary incontinence is a normal part of aging.

   e. Men have a higher risk of developing urinary incontinence than women.

   f. Symptoms of a urinary tract infection in an older adult include painful urination and a high fever.

8. Diet may affect urinary elimination. Which of the following contain diuretics that can increase urine output when they are ingested in large amounts? Select all that apply.

   a. Potato chips

   b. Pretzels

   c. Alcohol

   d. Coffee

   e. Tea

   f. Chocolate

9. A urinalysis has been ordered for your patient. When is the best time for the patient to provide a urine sample?

   a. Before bedtime

   b. Afternoon

   c. Evening

   d. First thing in the morning

Bowel Elimination

SECTION I: LEARNING OBJECTIVES

Upon completion of this chapter, the student will be able to do the following:

1. Identify factors that affect bowel elimination.

2. Describe the manifestations of altered bowel elimination.

3. Describe appropriate subjective and objective data to collect to assess bowel function.

4. Identify nursing diagnoses relating to altered bowel elimination.

5. Describe independent and collaborative nursing interventions to promote normal bowel function.

SECTION II: ASSESSING YOUR UNDERSTANDING

Activity A FILL IN THE BLANKS

1. The three parts of the small intestine are the duodenum, _____, and ileum.

2. Segmentation in the intestine allows for better food absorption, whereas _____ allows food contents to be moved through the intestine.

3. The internal anal sphincter is under the control of the _____ nervous system.

4. Approximately _____% of stool is composed of water. Thus it is necessary to consume about _____ mL of water per day to maintain a comfortable stool pattern.

5. Individuals with spinal cord injuries or neurologic disease like multiple sclerosis are at risk for fecal _____.

6. Postoperatively, the absence of bowel sounds for greater than _____ hours may indicate a paralytic ileus.

7. One way to consistently measure abdominal girth is to mark an "X" at the site of measurement; another is to measure at the _____ and document.

8. The _____ reflex is stimulated after a meal, resulting in the urge to defecate.

9. To properly administer a large volume enema and prevent unwanted side effects, slowly instill _____ water or saline solution directly into the rectum.

10. To promote the placement of a nasointestinal tube, the patient should lie on their _____ side and allow the mercury bag to float into place.

11. Skin protection is a key component of stoma care because _____ _____ cause skin breakdown.

Activity B   MATCHING

1. Match the stage in life listed in Column A with the description of normal stool listed in Column B.

Column A	Column B
____ **1.** Newborn	**A.** Bright yellow, soft and unformed with unobjectionable odor
____ **2.** Breastfed infant	
____ **3.** Older infant or toddler	**B.** Constipation is common due to physiologic changes
____ **4.** Adult	**C.** Thick, dark green, and tenacious
____ **5.** Pregnant women	**D.** Formed, varies depending on diet
	E. Formed, strong duodenocolic reflex

2. Match the medical terminology in Column A with its associated definition in Column B.

Column A	Column B
____ **1.** Borborygmi	**A.** The outpouching of blood vessels in the anus
____ **2.** Paralytic ileus	
____ **3.** Peristalsis	**B.** Movement that propels gastric contents through the intestine
____ **4.** Hemorrhoids	
____ **5.** Stoma	**C.** A loud "growl" of the stomach auscultated without the aid of a stethoscope
	D. A piece of intestine brought out to the abdominal wall
	E. Temporary paralysis of a section of intestine

Activity C   SEQUENCING

1. Sequence the proper order of the abdominal exam.

  a. Auscultation

  b. Palpation

  c. Percussion

  d. Inspection

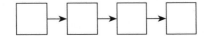

Activity D   SHORT ANSWER

1. What is *Clostridium difficile* (C-diff)?

_____

_____

_____

2. Describe some factors that lead to abdominal distention.

_____

_____

_____

3. Why is it important that palpation is the last part of the abdominal exam?

_____

_____

_____

4. Describe the purpose and process of a fecal occult blood test (FOBT).

_____

_____

_____

5. Discuss health promotion activities to prevent constipation.

_____

_____

_____

6. What is the numeric difference between low and high suction? When would you use continuous versus intermittent suction?

_____

_____

_____

SECTION III: APPLYING YOUR KNOWLEDGE

Activity E CASE STUDY

Mr. Ellis recently returned from a colonic diversion surgery. He has a transverse colostomy and a mucous fistula in the left upper quadrant of his abdomen. He also returned with a vented nasogastric tube in place. He is ordered to have the nasogastric tube to low intermittent suction.

1. Write two NANDA-I nursing diagnoses that apply to Mr. Ellis.

   _____

   _____

   _____

2. Describe the nursing activities you would perform prior to using Mr. El.'s nasogastric tube.

   _____

   _____

   _____

3. Describe the assessment of Mr. Ellis' transverse colonoscopy.

   _____

   _____

   _____

SECTION IV: PRACTICING FOR NCLEX

Activity F MULTIPLE CHOICE

Answer the following questions.

1. Sara is a 7-month-old infant who recently underwent a bowel resection for an isolated perforation. The surgeons removed most of Sara's ileum. The remaining small intestine was spared, and the large intestine remains intact. Based on your knowledge of digestion, you know that Sara will likely have problems with what type of nutrient absorption?

   a. Some vitamins and iron
   b. Electrolyte
   c. Fluid
   d. All nutrients

2. All of the following occur with the Valsalva maneuver except which?

   a. Taking a deep breath against a closed glottis
   b. Contracting abdominal muscles
   c. Contraction of the external sphincter
   d. Contracting pelvic floor muscles

3. You are caring for Mrs. Smith, a 65-year-old woman who has undergone a hernia operation. Mrs. Smith has a morphine PCA for post-surgical pain. She also receives sulfamethoxazole and trimethoprim (Bactrim) DS every 12 hours to treat a urinary tract infection, and an iron supplement for anemia. Mrs. Smith is on mobility restrictions because of the narcotics. She explains that while she usually stools once per day, she has stooled four times today. What is most likely contributing to her diarrhea?

   a. Morphine
   b. Iron supplement
   c. Immobility
   d. Bactrim DS

4. Mr. J. informs you that he has had difficulty defecating over the past 6 months. He describes his stools as firm and pebble-like and sometimes he is required to strain to relieve himself. In order to diagnose Mr. J. with constipation using the Rome III criteria, what percentage of stool must be affected?

   a. 50%
   b. 25%
   c. 75%
   d. 5%

5. Mr. Downs is a 68-year-old man who is in the hospital following an intestinal diversion. He has an ileostomy on his RUQ and a mucous fistula. Which of the following is the most important nursing activity for Mr. Downs?

   a. Assess the color of the stoma.
   b. Apply device for stool collection.
   c. Perform stoma irrigation.
   d. Teach the patient proper stoma care.

6. Mr. Jones is a paraplegic man who receives care in the rehabilitation facility where you work. He confides in you that he has trouble controlling his bowel movements. He tends to normally stool six to eight times per day. This has caused the skin around his rectum to become irritated. Which of the following is NOT an appropriate NANDA-I diagnosis for this patient?

   a. Fecal incontinence r/t decreased muscle tone and sphincter control

   b. The risk for impaired skin integrity r/t fecal incontinence

   c. The risk for disturbed body image r/t fecal incontinence

   d. Diarrhea r/t decreased muscle tone and sphincter control

7. James is a 5-year-old patient with a gastrointestinal infection. His mother plans to send him to school tomorrow. As the school nurse, you know which nursing outcome is most important to include in your care plan of James?

   a. The patient will demonstrate good health practices to prevent spread of infection.

   b. The patient will inform all contacts that he is ill.

   c. The patient will not return to school until he is completely symptom free for 7 days.

   d. The patient will demonstrate good health practices by isolating himself from others.

8. Mrs. M. is a 76-year-old woman who immigrated to the United States from the Middle East in her 40s. She speaks limited English. Her son has brought her to the clinic today because he is concerned that there is blood in her stool. Mrs. M. insists that he not worry as she is treating her condition with a mixture of herbs imported from her home. Which of the following applies to Mrs. M.? Select all that apply.

   a. Treatment for bowel changes with folk remedies is a common practice.

   b. Mrs. M. may be reluctant to discuss her bowel movements in front of her son.

   c. Mrs. M.'s son can be used to interpret because of the personal nature of the concern.

   d. Mrs. M. should continue to use her folk remedies and return in 6 months for follow up.

9. Which of the following are important goals of a bowel training program for patients with spinal cord injuries? Select all that apply.

   a. Maintain soft stool consistency.

   b. Develop a routine method for stool evacuation.

   c. Prevent fecal impaction.

   d. Regain previous level of bowel independence.

10. The risk for developing colorectal cancer during one's lifetime is 1 in 19. Nurses play an integral role in the promotion of colorectal cancer screening. Which of the following are risk factors for colorectal cancer? Select all that apply.

    a. Age 50 and older

    b. A positive family history

    c. A history of inflammatory bowel disease

    d. Smoking

11. Mr. Tompkins is an 86-year-old man with a history of constipation. He currently self-treats his constipation with over-the-counter laxatives. You know which to be true of these medications? Select all that apply.

    a. All older adults should use laxatives to promote normal defecation.

    b. Oral laxatives take longer to effect change than laxatives administered rectally.

    c. Older adults are at particular risk for laxative abuse.

    d. Rectal suppositories tend to work within 60 minutes of administration.

CHAPTER 33

Sleep and Rest

SECTION I: LEARNING OBJECTIVES

Upon completion of this chapter, the student will be able to do the following:

1. Describe NREM and REM sleep.

2. Describe normal patterns of sleep throughout the lifespan.

3. Identify factors that affect sleep and rest.

4. Conduct an assessment interview regarding normal sleep patterns, risk for disturbance, and actual sleep problems.

5. Develop a daily schedule with a patient, incorporating his or her unique needs and patterns for sleep and rest.

6. Discuss interventions to promote sleep.

7. Develop a nursing plan of care for a patient with sleep disturbance.

SECTION II: ASSESSING YOUR UNDERSTANDING

Activity A FILL IN THE BLANKS

1. Whereas sleep involves the whole body, _____ may involve total body relaxation or only a part of the body.

2. Sleep physiology involves electrophysiological recordings of changes in brain waves, eye movements, and muscle, known as _____.

3. An urge of varying intensity to go to sleep is called _____.

4. Biologic rhythms that follow a cycle of about 24 hours are termed _____ rhythms.

5. _____ is the need to void during the night.

6. _____ are medications that decrease sleep latency improve sleep maintenance.

7. _____ is a chronic disabling neurologic disorder of excessive daytime sleepiness characterized by short, almost irresistible daytime sleep attacks.

8. Activities that are normal during waking but abnormal during sleep such as sleeping walking, talking, night terrors, and bed-wetting are collectively called _____.

Activity B **MATCHING**

1. *Match the different sleep stages in Column A with the correct definition in Column B.*

Column A

____ **1.** N2

____ **2.** Rapid eye movement sleep

____ **3.** N3

____ **4.** N1

____ **5.** Non-rapid eye movement sleep

Column B

A. Comprises the largest percentage of a night's sleep time and is divided into three distinct stages

B. Constitutes approximately 40% to 50% of a night's sleep time during which a person can be more easily awakened

C. The transitional stage between drowsiness and sleep; muscles relax, respirations become even, and pulse rate decreases

D. Closely resembles wakefulness in the EEG and is characterized by very low or absent EMG muscle tone

E. Considered deep sleep, sometimes termed slow-wave or delta sleep after characteristic large amplitude EEG waves

2. *Match the different sleep disorders in Column A with the correct definition in Column B.*

Column A

____ **1.** Insomnia

____ **2.** Obstructive sleep apnea

____ **3.** Narcolepsy

____ **4.** Restless legs syndrome

____ **5.** Parasomnias

Column B

A. A disorder characterized by recurrent periods of absence of breathing for 10 seconds or longer which occurs at least five times per hour with sleep.

B. A neurological disorder that is characterized by an unpleasant sensation in the legs that leads to an irresistible urge to move them.

C. A cluster of symptoms as well as a complex of disorders of poor sleep quality, often associated with an inadequate amount of sleep.

D. A chronic disabling neurologic disorder of excessive daytime sleepiness characterized by short, almost irresistible daytime sleep attacks.

E. Activities that are normal during waking but abnormal during sleep such as sleepwalking, talking, night terrors, and bed-wetting.

Activity C **SEQUENCING**

1. Electrophysiologic recording of sleep shows a rhythmic pattern of 90 minute NREM/REM cycles during which people progress in sequence through the sleep stages. Sharon is a patient who is having a sleep study performed. Place the stages of sleep that Sharon goes through in the order in which they would occur. *Write the correct sequence in the boxes provided below.*

a. Sharon can be easily wakened.

b. Sharon transitions between drowsiness and sleep.

c. Sharon can again be easily wakened and her EEG shows readily recognized sleep spindles and K complexes.

d. Sharon's respirations are irregular and she is dreaming about flying over a city.

e. Sharon is in a "deep" sleep.

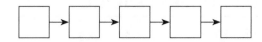

Activity D **SHORT ANSWER**

1. What do some cultural considerations have to do with sleep?

_____

_____

_____

2. Describe how shift work can affect sleep and rest.

_____

_____

_____

3. Why is sleep disordered breathing considered a major health and safety issue?

_____

_____

_____

4. What is meant by sleep hygiene?

_____

_____

_____

5. Why aren't medications used in all instances of a sleep disturbance?

_____

_____

_____

SECTION III: APPLYING YOUR KNOWLEDGE

Activity E CASE STUDY

Answer the following questions, which involve the nurse's role in caring for a patient with a sleep disorder.

You are a nurse working with Virginia, a 36-year-old mother of three children ages 6 months, 2 years, and 7 years. She has been diagnosed with onset insomnia and has experienced symptoms off and on since the birth of her first child. Her husband is with her and states that he feels it is getting worse recently.

1. How would you go about assessing this patient?

_____

_____

_____

2. Discuss interventions to promote sleep in this individual?

_____

_____

_____

3. If this was a patient in the hospital and you were her nurse what interventions could you implement to help her sleep?

_____

_____

_____

SECTION IV: PRACTICING FOR NCLEX

Activity F MULTIPLE CHOICE

Answer the following questions.

1. Which of the following patients could be diagnosed with insomnia?

   a. Danielle is a 45-year-old woman who has been complaining of fatigue for the last year. When asked about her sleep schedule she states that she usually goes to bed around 1 AM in the morning and gets up at 7 AM when her 5-year-old daughter gets up. She describes herself as a night owl.

   b. Mike is a 40-year-old obese man who is complaining of fatigue. He states that he goes to bed around 9 PM every night and wakes up between 5 and 6 in the morning. He feels like he gets a good night sleep but his wife says that she constantly has to poke him throughout the night because he "stops breathing."

   c. Susanna is a 50-year-old woman who is complaining of increased irritability for the past 2 months. She states that she goes to bed at 10 PM every night and tries to sleep in but, no matter what she does, she always wakes up at around 4 AM.

   d. John is a 20-year-old man who is complaining of excessive drowsiness at work to the point that he falls asleep while at his computer. He goes to bed at 11 PM and wakes up at 7 AM without difficulty. Twice in the last year he passed out after getting extremely angry.

2. Which of the following activities for rest break should not be incorporated into care planning for patients to aid in healing and recovery?

   a. Drinking an 8 oz cup of a caffeinated beverage

   b. Taking a short 15- to 30-minute nap

   c. Stretching exercises

   d. Focusing thoughts on a pleasant scene away from work

   e. Going for a short walk

3. Which of the following is a physiological change during NREM sleep?

   a. Muscle tone absent

   b. Body temperature is not regulated

   c. Sympathetic nerve activity increases from wakefulness

   d. Decreased brain activity from wakefulness

4. Which of the following is not a lifespan consideration for sleep cycles?

   a. By middle age, the frequency of nocturnal awakenings decreases, and satisfaction with sleep quality increases.

   b. Newborns can sleep up to 16 to 18 hours per day.

   c. Getting the toddler and preschooler to fall asleep is a common problem.

   d. In adolescents, there is a shift to late evening bedtime and late morning rise time.

5. Which of the following is a possible outcome criterion that addresses the goal that the patient will demonstrate physical signs of being rested?

   a. The patient reports a decrease in sleep latency to 10 to 15 minutes.

   b. The patient has decreases in circles under her eyes and excessive yawning by 1 week.

   c. The patient reports less anxiety regarding falling asleep.

   d. The patient verbalizes feeling less fatigued by 1 week.

   e. The patient reports the use of only one cup of coffee a day.

6. Which of the following are characteristics of rapid eye movement sleep? Select all that apply.

   a. Blood pressure and pulse rate show wide variations and may fluctuate rapidly.

   b. A person is unable to move during this stage.

   c. Theta waves often have a sawtooth or notched appearance.

   d. Muscles are relaxed but muscle tone is maintained.

   e. Sleepwalking and bed-wetting are most likely to occur during this stage.

7. Which of the following factors affect sleep and rest? Select all that apply.

   a. Relationships

   b. Nutrition and metabolism

   c. Vigilance

   d. Medications

   e. Shift work

8. Sadie is a nurse who is working with Torrence, a 60-year-old man who has been diagnosed with onset insomnia. He tells her that he wakes up at least once during the night. Which of the following are good examples of health promotion for this patient? Select all that apply.

   a. Sadie advises Torrance to exercise at least 6 hours before bedtime.

   b. Sadie encourages Torrance to remove the television from his bedroom.

   c. Sadie enocourages Torrance to minimize caffeine intake several hours prior to bedtime

   d. Sadie helps Torrance come up with a bedtime routine that he can implement each night.

   e. Sadie teaches Torrance that shorter unbroken sleep periods are not normal.

Pain Management

SECTION I: LEARNING OBJECTIVES

Upon completion of this chapter, the student will be able to do the following:

1. Explain the basic process of normal pain transmission.

2. Outline how pain transmission is facilitated or inhibited.

3. Describe the four dimensions of pain.

4. Examine nonpharmacologic methods of pain relief based on individual needs.

5. Describe the types, actions, and adverse effects of analgesics.

6. List nursing implications for various classes of drugs used for pain management.

7. Develop a nursing plan of care for a patient experiencing pain.

SECTION II: ASSESSING YOUR UNDERSTANDING

Activity A **FILL IN THE BLANKS**

1. Pain activates the _____ nervous system.

2. Serotonin and norepinephrine are examples of _____ opioid inhibitors.

3. Depression and anxiety often _____ pain perception.

4. A _____-aged child exposed to persistent pain may regress to thumb sucking or loss of bladder control.

5. The most common type of pain in older adults is _____ pain.

6. While pain is a response to tissue damage, _____ is an emotional response to noxious stimuli.

7. The Wong-Baker FACES scale is used to assess pain in _____.

8. The most common reason for undertreatment of pain is an incomplete or inadequate _____.

9. The use of two different medications to attack two different sources of pain is known as _____ drug therapy.

10. The _____ must always administer patient-controlled anesthesia.

Activity B MATCHING

1. Match the term listed in Column A with its definition in Column B.

Column A

___ 1. Somatic pain

___ 2. Visceral pain

___ 3. Neuropathic pain

___ 4. Nociceptive pain

___ 5. Hyperalgia

Column B

A. Arises from damage to peripheral nerves

B. Exaggerated response to a painful stimuli

C. Internal pain that results from stretching or distention of organs

D. Originates in tissues other than the nervous system

E. Pain in the bone, skin, or soft tissue that is well localized

2. Match the medication type in Column A with its nursing implication in Column B.

Column A

___ 1. NSAIDs (nonsteroidal anti-inflammatory)

___ 2. Opioid agonist (i.e., hydromorphone)

___ 3. Naloxone

___ 4. Acetaminophen

Column B

A. Constipation is the most common side effect

B. Has analgesic but not anti-inflammatory properties

C. Use with caution in patients with a history of GI bleeds or renal dysfunction

D. Used to treat respiratory depression that results from oversedation

Activity C SEQUENCING

Place the events in the process of nocioception in the order in which they occur.

a. Signals are carried through the dorsal root of the spinal horn.

b. The thalamus receives pain signals.

c. A painful stimulus is encountered.

d. Signals are transmitted via the spinothalamic tract toward the brain.

e. Pain is perceived in the cerebral cortex.

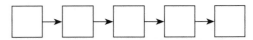

Activity D SHORT ANSWER

1. Discuss the risks of untreated pain in the older adult population.

   _____

   _____

   _____

2. Describe some common physiologic responses to pain.

   _____

   _____

   _____

3. What is the difference between tolerance and addiction?

   _____

   _____

   _____

4. Describe symptoms of physical withdrawal from an opioid.

   _____

   _____

   _____

5. Describe some nonpharmacologic pain relief strategies for patients with back pain.

   _____

   _____

   _____

SECTION III: APPLYING YOUR KNOWLEDGE

Activity E CASE STUDY

You are caring for Sahib, a 3 year old who has just come out of surgery following a serious motor vehicle accident. He is awake and oriented to person, place, and time. However, he is crying inconsolably indicating that his leg is bothering him. His mother and father are present at his bedside.

1. Describe how you might assess Sahib's pain.

_____

_____

_____

2. You plan to contact the licensed provider to place an order for pain medication. List some possible options for pain relief.

_____

_____

_____

3. Sahib's father stops you in the hall. He tells you that he is worried that his son will become addicted to pain medications. What is your best response?

_____

_____

_____

4. What do you need to monitor when administering an opioid intravenously to Sahib?

_____

_____

_____

SECTION IV: PRACTICING FOR NCLEX

Activity F MULTIPLE CHOICE

Answer the following questions.

1. Jorge is a 54-year-old man recovering from an outbreak of Herpes zoster on his left chest. He tells you that even his shirt touching him causes a horrible pain on the left side of the chest. What term would best describe Jorge's pain?
   a. Chronic pain
   b. Nociceptive pain
   c. Hyperalgia
   d. Somatic pain

2. Charles is an 86-year-old man with chronic lower back pain. He asks you what some appropriate treatments might be for his back pain. Which would you not expect to be ordered as first-line therapy?
   a. Physical therapy referral
   b. A walking aid
   c. Acupuncture
   d. A chronic opioid therapy plan

3. You are a nurse in an outpatient cancer center. You know that which ethnic group is most likely to request narcotics for chronic cancer pain relief?
   a. Caucasian
   b. African American
   c. Hispanic American
   d. Asian American

4. Alex is a 35-year-old with chronic back pain. What condition would exacerbate Alex's pain?
   a. Depression
   b. Constipation
   c. Smoking
   d. Exercise

5. Evelyn is a 90-year-old woman who just returned from the operating room to your medical unit. She is otherwise healthy and has a history of some mild arthritis. As you examine Evelyn, you know that all of the following are signs of pain EXCEPT which?
   a. Elevated blood pressure
   b. Elevated serum glucose
   c. Elevated lactic acid production
   d. Elevated kidney function

6. You are a new nurse in an ambulatory care setting. You know that the Joint Commission requires that pain be addressed at each visit. When is the most appropriate time to do so?

   a. When obtaining patient vital signs

   b. Before the patient is discharged

   c. The first question you ask the patient

   d. At several points throughout your history-taking

7. Which of the following medications would you most likely see on the medication administration record (MAR) of a patient with diabetic neuropathy?

   a. Morphine

   b. Gabapentin (Neurontin)

   c. Hydromorphone (Dilaudid)

   d. Lorazepam (Ativan)

8. Andre is a 38-year-old man in your outpatient clinic who complains of chronic back pain. As you review his chart, you notice that he has required escalating doses of hydromorphone (Dilaudid) to treat his pain. He tells you that the old dose "just doesn't work anymore". What term best describes Andre's situation?

   a. Addiction

   b. Tolerance

   c. Withdrawal

   d. Whining

9. You are working with James, a 12-year-old boy after being involved in an MVA. He has several broken bones and contusions. He rates his pain as a 7/10. You plan to administer intravenous hydromorphone to relieve the pain. What side effect are you most worried about?

   a. Itching

   b. Cardiac arrest

   c. Respiratory depression

   d. Addiction

10. Samuel is an 18-year-old man who sprained his ankle yesterday. He rates the pain as a 3/10. Which nonpharmacologic pain measures would be appropriate for Samuel to implore?

    a. Rest

    b. Heat

    c. Ice

    d. Range of motion

11. You are conducting a pain assessment on a post-operative surgical unit. Your patient, Larry, has just arrived following a cholecystectomy. When should you assess his pain? Select all that apply.

    a. With your first set of vital signs

    b. Within 2 hours of administering a PRN morphine dose

    c. Once per day

    d. Every hour for the first 8 hours

12. Lee has just returned from surgery. He asks you for an extra dose of pain medication. What would be some signs that Lee is in pain? Select all that apply.

    a. Elevated heart rate

    b. Elevated respiratory rate

    c. Decreased blood pressure

    d. Decreased temperature

13. Cecilia is a 92-year-old woman on your inpatient unit following hip replacement surgery. You ask her if she is in pain, and she tells you that she is fine. You know which of the following to be true regarding pain in the older adult? Select all that apply.

    a. Older adults are less likely to feel pain than younger adults.

    b. Older adults have decreased opioid receptors.

    c. Older adults often believe that pain is a consequence of growing older.

    d. Older adults are more likely to be disabled by pain than younger adults.

CHAPTER 35

Sensory Perception

SECTION I: LEARNING OBJECTIVES

Upon completion of this chapter, the student will be able to do the following:

1. Associate stress and sensoristasis with the sensory/perceptual process.

2. Describe the five senses and their role across the lifespan in sensory perception.

3. Summarize factors affecting sensory perception.

4. Specify how sensory overload, deprivation, and deficit can occur, with interventions for each.

5. Relate manifestations of altered sensory function to their causes.

6. Identify patients who are at risk for altered sensory function in healthcare settings and in the home.

7. Discuss the relationship of safety to sensory dysfunction.

SECTION II: ASSESSING YOUR UNDERSTANDING

Activity A FILL IN THE BLANKS

1. The _____ activating system is responsible for bringing together information from the cerebellum and other parts of the brain with that obtained from the sense organs.

2. _____ are nerve endings in the skin and body tissue.

3. The _____ sense receives stimuli that affect awareness related to the body's large interior organs.

4. Vision, hearing, smell, and taste are termed _____ senses.

5. Touch, kinesthetic sensation, and visceral sensation are termed _____ senses.

6. _____ is a state of optimum arousal.

7. Sensory _____ occurs when a person is unable to process and manage the intensity or quantity of incoming sensory stimuli.

8. Sensory impressions that are based on internal stimulations and have not basis in reality are called _____.

9. The _____ sense influences awareness of the placement and action of body parts.

10. _____ is the time needed to think about, evaluate, and come to terms with an activity after it happens.

11. Sensory _____ is a lessening or lack of meaningful sensory stimuli, monotonous sensory input, or an interference with the process of information.

Activity B MATCHING

1. *Match the life stage in Column A with the correct sensory perception characteristics in Column B.*

Column A

____ **1.** Newborn

____ **2.** Toddler

____ **3.** Adolescent

____ **4.** Adult

____ **5.** Older adult

Column B

A. Sensory perception function is at its peak

B. Need to explore their environment by using all five senses

C. Need to feel objects in the environment in order to process them

D. Eyesight is diminished, sounds are muffled, and other sensory systems are decreased

E. Make independent responses based on what is perceived through the senses

Activity C SEQUENCING

1. You are a community health nurse who was assigned to visit the home of a new patient whose name is Mia. Mia is 20 years old and was in a car accident 2 months ago that left her deaf. She was discharged from the hospital 2 days ago and is now living with her parents. As her nurse, you diligently apply the nursing process to come up with the best plan for Mia. Place these actions in the correct order so that they logically follow the nursing process for someone with a sensory deficit. *Write the correct sequence in the boxes provided below.*

a. You ask Mia how she is feeling psychologically to determine if she is experiencing any depression or anxiety related to her change in functioning.

b. You give Mia the nursing diagnosis of disturbed sensory perception related to loss of auditory function.

c. You perform a quick whisper test to determine, grossly, to what extent her hearing has been impaired.

d. Together with Mia, you decide that one goal will be to achieve normal maintenance of self-care within 1 month and you provide information on a support group within her community.

e. You interview Mia to gather subjective information on how she is able to function on a day-to-day basis.

f. When you see her in a week, you observe again how her self-care is being performed.

☐ → ☐ → ☐ → ☐ → ☐ → ☐

Activity D SHORT ANSWER

1. Describe the process of adaptation that occurs beyond sensoristasis.

_____

_____

_____

2. When performing patient education, why is it important to consider internal factors, the amount of information you are giving, and the environment you are giving it in?

_____

_____

_____

3. How can depression lead to sensory deficits?

_____

_____

_____

4. Why is it important to gather subjective information when assessing someone's sensory perception?

_____

_____

_____

5. What topics should be addressed during patient teaching that relate to sensory perception?

_____

_____

_____

Activity E CROSSWORD

Use the clues to complete the crossword puzzle.

Down

1. The point beyond sensoristasis when sensory receptors respond to repeated stimulation.
2. The sense that detects the body's position.
5. This can be prevented by preparing patients before procedures.

Across

3. Beliefs not based in reality, they reflect an unconscious need or fear.
4. It results from not being able to interact with the environment due to sensory deficit
6. Part of the nursing diagnosis for altered sensory perception accepted by the North American Nursing Diagnosis Association.

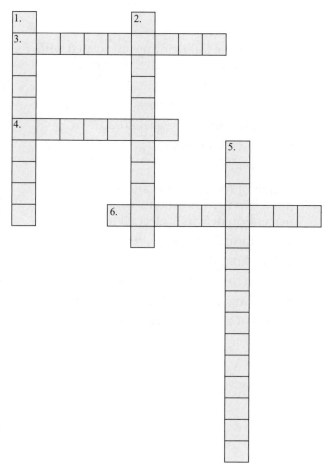

SECTION III: APPLYING YOUR KNOWLEDGE

Activity F CASE STUDY

Answer the following questions, which involve the nurse's role in caring for a patient with a sensory deficit.

Georgia is a 38-year-old paraplegic. She is currently in the hospital with a diagnosis of pneumonia. She lives in a skilled nursing facility but is normally able to do much of her own activities of daily living. Although she has been in the hospital many times she is always a bit anxious because of all the noise and from not having any privacy.

1. From this scenario what do you know about this person's normal pattern of sensory perception?

   _____

   _____

   _____

2. What other information do you need for risk identification in this patient?

   _____

   _____

   _____

3. What interventions could you implement to address her with the sensory overload she appears to be feeling?

   _____

   _____

   _____

SECTION IV: PRACTICING FOR NCLEX

Activity G MULTIPLE CHOICE

Answer the following questions.

1. Which of the following is not a lifespan consideration for sensory perception?

    a. Toddlers explore their environment by seeing, hearing, touching, tasting, and smelling.

    b. Preschoolers seek out information using organized play.

    c. School-aged children learn to make independent responses based on what is perceived through the senses.

    d. A newborn's sensory perception is very refined.

    e. As people reach middle age, they begin to notice certain changes in their sensory system.

2. Altered sensory reception is category of occurrences that can lead to sensory deprivation. Which of the following is an example of altered sensory reception?

    a. Tracy is a 35-year-old man who was diagnosed and is being treated for tuberculosis. He has been in an isolation room for 1 week and is starting to get anxious.

    b. Marcus has multiple sclerosis, a degenerative neuromuscular disease. Up until 1 year ago Marcus was a very social person. Now, he is bedridden and cannot get out to see his friends. This dramatic change in his environment, from stimulating to asocial, is causing Marcus to feel depressed.

    c. Lydia is a 2 month old who spends much of her day in a crib. Her mother suffers from post-partum depression and is not able to interact with Lydia except to change her diaper and feed her. Lydia cries most of the day.

    d. Laney is an 87-year-old woman who is losing her eyesight. She is not able to leave her assisted living apartment without help. She is becoming more and more confused.

3. The characteristics of somatic senses include discrimination of which of these? Select all that apply.

    a. Touch

    b. Pressure

    c. Vibration

    d. Positioning

    e. Auditory acuity

    f. Odors

4. Which of the following are associated with normal vision? Select all that apply.

    a. Vision intensity

    b. Extraocular movement

    c. Visual acuity at or near 20/20

    d. Full field of vision

    e. Tricolor vision

5. Which of the following are sensory aids a nurse can use for patients with sensory perception deficits? Select all that apply.

    a. Literature with large print

    b. Speaking slowly

    c. Fresh food served for meals

    d. Turning and repositioning

    e. Sips of water between foods

Cognitive Processes

SECTION I: LEARNING OBJECTIVES

Upon completion of this chapter, the student will be able to do the following:

1. Identify key components of cognition and communication.

2. Describe characteristics of normal cognition.

3. Describe influences on cognitive function related to the lifespan.

4. Explain factors that can affect cognitive processes.

5. Identify manifestations of altered cognitive processes.

6. Apply the nursing process to the care of persons experiencing altered cognitive processes.

7. Discuss socialization needs of people with altered cognition and their families.

8. List resources available to families of people with altered cognitive processes.

9. Communication is the exchange of information between at least two people and involves the use of language to store, process, and transmit _____ content.

10. _____ is the tendency of synapses and neural circuits to change as a result of activity.

SECTION II: ASSESSING YOUR UNDERSTANDING

Activity A FILL IN THE BLANKS

1. _____ is the systematic way in which a person thinks, reasons, and uses language.

2. Perception depends on functioning sensory receptors, _____, and central processing.

3. Change in nerve transmission from one neuron to the next due to previous neural activity results in _____.

4. The process of creating vocal sounds is called _____ and occurs when air from the lungs moves through the oral and nasal cavity during exhalation.

5. The enunciation of words and sentences is called _____.

6. _____ is the process of receiving and interpreting sensory stimuli that function as the basis for understanding, knowing, or learning.

7. Concrete _____ involves objects that can be perceived by the senses.

8. _____ is acute confusion in comparison to dementia which is a chronic, irreversible confusion.

9. _____ is the complete or partial loss of language abilities including understanding speech, reading, speaking, writing, arithmetic, and expression through pantomime.

Activity B MATCHING

1. *Match the anatomical structures involved in cognition in Column A with the correct function in Column B.*

Column A	Column B
___ **1.** The optic nerve	**A.** Carries impulses to the brain's visual receiving area
___ **2.** The reticular formation	**B.** Dominant for language function in most right-handed people
___ **3.** The brain's left hemisphere	
___ **4.** Wernicke's area	**C.** Maintains wakefulness and controls portions of vital cardiovascular and respiratory reflexes
___ **5.** Cerebral cortex	
	D. Is associated with specific sensory and motor function
	E. Is associated with the interpretation of language and understanding

Activity C ORDERING

1. Place the following characteristics of cognitive developmental phases in the order in which they should occur chronologically. *Write the correct sequence in the boxes provided below.*

a. Understand conservation, the idea that the properties of an object stay the same even if the object is altered in certain ways.

b. Become less rigid.

c. Learn that objects have constancy.

d. Develop compensatory mechanisms for adapting to changes in senses.

e. Learning occurs through interaction with the environment using the five senses.

f. Struggle for independence from family and belonging within a peer group.

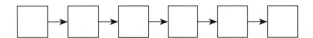

Activity D SHORT ANSWER

1. Describe the importance of the hippocampi in the formation of memories.

_____

_____

_____

2. In what way does blood flow affect cognitive function?

_____

_____

_____

3. Describe what Sundown syndrome is?

_____

_____

_____

4. Why can it be hard to identify mild-to-moderate cognitive impairment in a patient assessment?

_____

_____

_____

5. Why should a review of someone's medications be included in a patient assessment of someone with a cognitive impairment?

_____

_____

_____

SECTION III: APPLYING YOUR KNOWLEDGE

Activity E CASE STUDY

Answer the following questions, which involve the nurse's role in caring for a patient with a sensory deficit.

Li Chin is a 70-year-old man who is originally from China but has been living in the United States for 10 years. He lives with his son and daughter-in-law but is currently in the hospital to be evaluated after a fall. You are the nurse taking care of him and are talking with him and his son. His son states that Li Chin's health in general is pretty good. He doesn't take any medication and takes a daily multivitamin. His son has noticed that he has been getting quite forgetful recently. Once, 2 months ago, he found the patient wandering down the street from where they live and was apparently lost. He has also left the house and forgotten to close the door behind him. Otherwise, Li Chin has been performing his activities of daily living without any problems.

1. What sort of nursing interventions would be appropriate for this patient and his family?

_____

_____

_____

2. Why would an intelligence test not be appropriate to use in an assessment of this patient?

_____

_____

_____

SECTION IV: PRACTICING FOR NCLEX

Activity F   MULTIPLE CHOICE

Answer the following questions.

1. Which of the following anatomic structures coordinates consciousness, thought, memory, learning, and communication?
   a. The cerebral cortex
   b. The cochlea
   c. The reticular activating system
   d. Broca's area

2. Which of the following is used to describe a person's level of arousal?
   a. Delirium
   b. Sundown syndrome
   c. Aphasic
   d. Obtunded

3. Which of the following is not true regarding proprioceptors?
   a. They are located in the inner ear.
   b. They are located in tendons.
   c. They sense the relative position of different body parts.
   d. They sense pressure in the skin.

4. Which of the following is true regarding dementia?
   a. It is a progressive impairment of intellectual function and memory.
   b. It is the rapid decline in all cognitive processes.
   c. It is a normal process of aging.
   d. It is associated with disturbance in level of consciousness.

5. Which of the following is not a characteristic of normal cognition?
   a. Intelligence
   b. Reality perception
   c. Communicating
   d. Recall
   e. Judgment

6. Which of the following is true regarding how fluid and electrolyte balance can affect cognitive functioning?
   a. Diet has little effect on electrolyte balance and therefore cognition.
   b. The brain's cellular processes depend on the active and passive movement of water and electrolyte movement across cell membranes.
   c. Too little ammonia, a byproduct of protein metabolism, can cause delirium.
   d. Increased serum potassium levels (hyperkalemia) can lead to hepatic encephalopathy.
   e. The blood-brain barrier blocks all electrolytes from entering cerebrospinal fluid but allows normal fluid, which does not cause damage to sensitive nerve cells.

7. Jane is an 87-year-old woman who has just moved into a nursing home after being in an independent retirement facility. Since the move, she has been experiencing a progressive decline in her cognitive functioning. Her room is located across from a nursing station so that she can be observed at all times. Her daughter continues to visit every day for breakfast and has noticed that Jane is showing signs of depression. Since moving, she has become increasingly confused. Which of the following is not contributing to this increase in confusion?

   a. Jane's daughter continues to visit at the same time each day.

   b. Jane is in an unfamiliar environment.

   c. Jane's room is close to the nursing station.

   d. Jane is most likely depressed.

8. Which of the following illustrates someone with anomic aphasia?

   a. Dan is a 55-year-old man who recently suffered a cerebrovascular accident or stroke. He is growing increasingly angry because it has been 2 weeks and although he knows exactly what he wants to say he can't seem to come up with the words to say it. When asking his partner where their daughter was he said, "Who … gone … she … house."

   b. Susan is a 60-year-old woman who has recently been having problems coming up with certain words. Just yesterday, she was trying to tell her husband that she already had her keys but ended up saying "I have, you know, those things that go in the car. The thing that you turn and the car works." This seems to happen once or twice a day.

   c. Garrett is a 21-year-old man who was in a motor vehicle accident 2 months ago. Because of the accident he has lost the ability to both speak to those around him and to understand what they are saying to him.

   d. Jenny is a 35-year-old woman who is recovering after a procedure to resect a tumor in her brain. Since her surgery she hasn't been able to read or write and she does not understand why people are saying things that don't make sense.

9. Which of the following are forms of socialization therapies for people with cognitive impairment? Select all that apply.

   a. Pets

   b. Music

   c. Recreation

   d. Reminiscence

10. Which of the following structures are involved in speech production? Select all that apply.

    a. Larynx

    b. Nasal cavity

    c. Tongue

    d. Semicircular canals

    e. Organ of Corti

CHAPTER 37

Self-Concept

SECTION I: LEARNING OBJECTIVES

Upon completion of this chapter, the student will be able to do the following:

1. Describe the functions of self and self-concept.

2. Define self-concept, self-perception, self-knowledge, self-expectation, social self, and self-evaluation.

3. Identify the four patterns of self-concept.

4. Discuss how self-concept develops throughout the lifespan.

5. Discuss factors that can affect self-concept.

6. Identify possible manifestations of altered self-concept.

7. Apply theory to assess for self-concept functioning.

8. Plan care for a person with an altered self-concept.

SECTION II: ASSESSING YOUR UNDERSTANDING

Activity A FILL IN THE BLANKS

1. _____ may be defined as a person's unique dimensions, potentials, and purposes.

2. _____ is the mental image a person has of oneself.

3. _____ is how a person explains behavior based on self-observation.

4. How people feel about themselves is termed _____.

5. _____ is an organizing principle of the self, the awareness that one is a distinct individual separate from others.

6. A person's expected characteristic behavior in a social situation is called their _____.

7. Role _____ occurs when the person lacks knowledge of role expectations, which fosters anxiety and confusion.

Activity B MATCHING

1. *How one perceives oneself has several dimensions. Match the dimensions of self-perception in Column A with the correct description in Column B.*

Column A

___ 1. Self-knowledge

___ 2. Self-expectation

___ 3. Social self

___ 4. Self-evaluation

Column B

A. Involves the self a person wants to be

B. Involves the conscious assessment of self, leading to self-respect or self-worth

C. Involves how a person sees themselves in relation to social situations, including behavior and interaction with others

D. Involves a basic understanding on oneself, involving facts such as age, weight, and sex

2. *Match the developmental period in Column A with the correct nursing intervention for development of self-concept in Column B.*

Column A

____ **1.** Newborn

____ **2.** Preschooler

____ **3.** Infant

____ **4.** Toddler

Column B

A. Teach parents about the need to allow for movement, stimulation, and safety

B. Provide an environment that allows practice of newly developing skills, especially movement-related skills

C. Assist family members to adapt to their new roles and self-concept related to these roles

D. Provide education and support concerning health maintenance behaviors such as personal hygiene and healthcare visits

Activity C   SEQUENCING

1. It is important to keep in mind someone's developmental level when tailoring your nursing intervention. *Write the correct sequence of interventions, progressing from the school-aged child to the older adult, in the boxes provided below.*

   a. Treat with respect and allow independence and individuality. Help them integrate recent losses.

   b. Educate about sexual health, drug, and alcohol use. Offer choices in care to maintain autonomy.

   c. Use therapeutic relationship to support them as well as support decisions they make in relationships and activities.

   d. Allow for privacy, socialization, and belonging. Allow liberal visitations and age-appropriate activities if hospitalized.

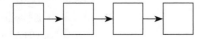

Activity D   SHORT ANSWER

1. Briefly describe what body image is and why it is so important to consider when addressing a person's self-concept.

_____

_____

_____

2. What are some lifespan considerations for the infant regarding self-concept?

_____

_____

_____

3. In what way does self-concept change after retirement?

_____

_____

_____

4. How does coping and stress tolerance influence self-concept?

_____

_____

_____

5. What should you consider when assessing a person's risk for self-concept dysfunction when they are ill?

_____

_____

_____

SECTION III: APPLYING YOUR KNOWLEDGE

Activity E   CASE STUDY

Answer the following questions, which involve the nurse's role in facilitating a healthy self-concept in their patient.

Richard is a 15-year-old man who is admitted to the hospital for a bone marrow transplant. You are a nurse caring for Richard on a pediatric floor before his procedure. He has been non-communicative and seems angry at everyone who comes into the room.

1. What developmental level should Richard be in and why is this important to know?

_____

_____

_____

2. What are the ways in which you can help Richard's self-concept?

_____

_____

_____

SECTION IV: PRACTICING FOR NCLEX

Activity F **MULTIPLE CHOICE**

Answer the following questions.

1. Jose is a 24-year-old man who is suffering from depression. He has come to the clinic today for a follow-up visit with his provider and you have been asked to provide some patient education on the antidepressants he has been prescribed. When you ask him how he is feeling today, he responds that he is feeling down because he feels as if he is a failure. This scenario best describes which dimension of self-perception?
   a. Self-knowledge
   b. Self-expectation
   c. Social self
   d. Self-evaluation

2. Biologic makeup comprises many characteristics that affect self-concept. Which of the following is not part of one's biology?
   a. Environment
   b. Sex
   c. Height
   d. Appearance

3. Jeremy is an 18 year old who tells you that it was just bad luck that he got in a motor vehicle accident and broke his arm. Which of the following is Jeremy demonstrating by this?
   a. Internal locus of control
   b. Control reasoning
   c. External locus of control
   d. Expectancy

4. Which of the following is a situational transition?
   a. The transition working to being retired.
   b. The transition from prepubescence through puberty.
   c. The transition from being in high school to being a college student.
   d. The transition from being married to being divorced.

5. Liz just started a nursing program. She is trying to balance going to school full-time, a part-time job, and spending time with her family. Recently she has been feeling a lot of stress and doesn't feel as if she is able to do any of the three very good. Which role problem is Liz experiencing from this role transition?
   a. Role strain
   b. Role ambiguity
   c. Role conflict
   d. Role agreement

6. Which of the following is objective data related to self-concept?
   a. The person states, "I am worthless."
   b. The person refuses to make eye contact.
   c. The person's mom tells you that they are never happy.
   d. The person admits that she always wears baggy clothes in order to hide her body.

7. Austin is a 2-year-old boy who has had a bowel repair for gastroparesis. He is doing well but has a colostomy to aide in healing of the surgical bowel. Which of the following would be an appropriate nursing intervention for Austin to enhance self-concept?
   a. Provide Austin with room to move around in and lots of toys to interact with while securing his colostomy so it does not get in his way.
   b. Assist Austin's parents to accept their role as caregivers to a child with a colostomy.
   c. Teach Austin's parents about how to provide a safe environment for him.
   d. Support and educate Austin about health maintenance behaviors such as person hygiene.

8. Micah is a nurse working on a pediatric psychiatry floor. One of his patients is a 17-year-old girl who was admitted to the hospital for anorexia nervosa. Micah decides, based on his assessment of this patient, that he is going to help her accept responsibility for herself, help her define realistic goals, help her utilize resources to enact change, and he is going to reward positive outcomes. Which nursing intervention is Micah using with this patient?

   a. Therapeutic relationship
   b. Self-evaluation
   c. Behavioral change
   d. Developmental

9. Which of the following illustrates interrole conflict?

   a. A nurse is asked to provide birth control teaching even though they do not believe in using birth control.
   b. A husband decides he wants to quit his job in order to try something new and his wife values financial security.

   c. A father is expected to play the role of father, wage earner, and cook for the family and is unsure of how to fulfill all of them.
   d. A doctor is asked to decide whether an ex-alcoholic patient is a liver transplant candidate.

10. Which of the following describes an ascribed role?

   a. Son
   b. Nurse
   c. Husband
   d. Mother

11. Which of the following developmental stages does Erikson term autonomy vs. shame?

   a. Toddler
   b. Adolescent
   c. Preschooler
   d. School-age child

Families and Their Relationships

SECTION I: LEARNING OBJECTIVES

Upon completion of this chapter, the student will be able to do the following:

1. Describe variations in family structure and function.

2. Identify demographic, sociocultural, and economic factors that affect family relationships.

3. Describe manifestations of altered family function.

4. Evaluate the possible impact of altered family function on activities of daily living.

5. Differentiate subjective and objective data needed to assess family function.

6. Identify nursing diagnoses and related factors associated with altered family function.

7. Discuss evidence-based nursing interventions to promote family health and function.

8. Discuss evidence-based nursing interventions for altered family function.

9. List family-centered healthcare services in the community.

SECTION II: ASSESSING YOUR UNDERSTANDING

Activity A FILL IN THE BLANKS

1. Autonomy is developed by allowing _____ within established limits.

2. Stable family relationships during the developmental stage of "initiative" foster _____.

3. The number of children living in a home maintained by a grandparent _____ over the past 35 years.

4. Socioeconomic status and marital disagreements are predictive of _____ problems in children.

5. Adults who have difficulty achieving generatively because they are caring for older parents and their children are said to be part of the _____ generation.

6. Problems with _____ health can be found in all generations when individuals do not receive support, nurturing, and encouragement.

7. Abuse of the _____ continues to be a growing problem in the United States.

8. In order to deliver _____ care, the wishes of the caregivers and extended family must be considered.

9. A nurse can teach skills and offer emotional support for someone who is new to the _____ role.

10. When developing an intervention for altered family function, a _____ approach is often helpful.

Activity B   MATCHING

1. *Match the key terminology in Column A with its definition in Column B.*

Column A

___ 1. Nuclear family

___ 2. Blended family

___ 3. Cohabitated family

___ 4. Communal family

___ 5. Non-traditional family

Column B

A. One birth parent and one non-birth parent raising a child

B. A group who shares a bond such as a religious affiliation

C. Same sex partners raising a child, for example

D. One man, one woman, and their children

E. Two people residing in a residence outside of a legal marriage

2. *Match Erickson's stage of development listed in Column A with its appropriate age in Column B.*

Column A

___ 1. Trust

___ 2. Autonomy

___ 3. Initiative

___ 4. Industry

___ 5. Generativity

Column B

A. Preschool

B. Adult

C. Toddlers

D. Newborn and infant

E. School age

Activity C   SHORT ANSWER

1. How does Western lifestyle affect families?

_____

_____

_____

2. Define role strain and explain how it can affect families.

_____

_____

_____

3. Describe how chronic illness affects family function.

_____

_____

_____

4. List some common signs of child and elder abuse.

_____

_____

_____

5. How is problem solving used as a nursing intervention for family dysfunction?

_____

_____

_____

SECTION III: APPLYING YOUR KNOWLEDGE

Activity D   CASE STUDY

Jim is a 55-year-old steel worker who was recently laid-off due to budget cuts. He was separated from his wife 6 months ago because "my wife couldn't live with me anymore". Jim admits that he has been drinking more than usual. He also confides that he is struggling to make his housing payments. Jim tells you that he would like to get his life back on track, starting with marital reconciliation.

1. List two NANDA-I nursing diagnoses that apply to Jim and his family.

_____

_____

_____

2. When planning an intervention with Jim, what is a potential outcome?

_____

_____

_____

3. Discuss why you would consider an interdisciplinary approach for Jim and his family.

_____

_____

_____

SECTION IV: PRACTICING FOR NCLEX

Activity E MULTIPLE CHOICE

Answer the following questions.

1. You are meeting with Mrs. G., a 35-year-old woman who is in your office today for treatment of headache. She mentions that she recently returned to the workforce after a 10-year absence because her husband is recently unemployed. She is having difficulty coping with her new work schedule. Which factor is affecting this family function?

   a. Lifestyle
   b. Cultural beliefs
   c. Previous life experience
   d. Role strain

2. You are working with Jenna, age 16, her boyfriend of 2 years, and baby Alex, age 1 month. Part of your assessment is to ascertain the parents' feelings about the birth and their emotional attachment to Alex. You know that these are critical contributing factors to which of Erickson's stages of development for Alex?

   a. Autonomy
   b. Trust
   c. Industry
   d. Generativity

3. You are working with the family of Samantha, age 4. The family recently experienced the loss of Samantha's grandmother who was a caregiver for Samantha. What is the most important intervention that the family can do for Samantha at this developmental stage?

   a. Assure Samantha that the death was not her fault.
   b. Avoid talking about this loss.
   c. Ask Samantha every day if she remembers her grandmother.
   d. Hire a nanny to immediately assume the role of the grandmother.

4. You are caring for Amy in the hospital following a femur fracture. She tells you all about her best friend Katie, who is planning to come over and work on a puzzle with her. Amy also tells you how she loves school, especially math, and always completes all of her math problems so that she will receive a sticker. Based on this description, Amy is likely how old?

   a. 3 years
   b. 8 years
   c. 12 years
   d. 6 months

5. Mrs. A. is a new mother to 2-month-old Amelia. When discussing her return to work, she states "I have to stay home. My mother stayed home, my aunts stayed home. That is what we do". What factor is most influencing Mrs. A.'s decision to stay home?

   a. Religion
   b. Previous life experience
   c. Lifestyle
   d. Stress tolerance

6. Which of the following situations is most concerning for abuse?

   a. An infant who is in the fifth percentile for weight.
   b. A 2 year old with bruising on his knees.
   c. An adolescent with a broken tibia.
   d. A pregnant woman with bruising on her ribcage.

7. Mrs. F. is a 56-year-old mother of two. She describes her husband as a frequent drinker, but states that it is not a big deal. Only on the weekends will he start to drink in the morning. He has also had a hard time keeping a job, so Mrs. F. cleans houses after her 9 to 5 job in order to make ends meet. What term would best describe Mrs. F.?

   a. Helpful
   b. Caretaker
   c. Enabler
   d. Responsible

8. Dana is a 20-year-old mother to baby Hanna, age 6 months. Dana was in a relationship with the Hanna's father until she was 8 months pregnant. She has not seen him in 7 months and has not received any child support. She states that she is having difficulty caring for Hanna and worries that she will lose her job. Which NANDA-I nursing diagnosis could be applied to this situation? Select all that apply.

   a. Impaired parenting r/t lack of support from significant other AEB lack of paternal involvement.

   b. Compromised family coping r/t exhaustion of persons capabilities AEB concerns for job security.

   c. The risk of impaired parenting r/t dead beat dad.

   d. Exhaustion r/t lack of support from significant other.

9. Which of the following are signs of child abuse? Select all that apply.

   a. Failure to thrive

   b. Lack of attachment

   c. Rigid role expectations

   d. Bruising on a child's knees

10. Mrs. P. is a 45-year-old woman in your outpatient clinic today for her well woman exam. As you go to take her blood pressure, you notice bruising in the shape of a hand on her forearm. You suspect that she is being abused. Which of the following place Mrs. P. at risk for abuse? Select all that apply.

   a. Unemployment

   b. Substance abuse

   c. Chronic illness

   d. College education

CHAPTER 39

Loss and Grieving

SECTION I: LEARNING OBJECTIVES

Upon completion of this chapter, the student will be able to do the following:

1. Discuss the importance of self-care and hygiene in health and illness.

2. Describe the effects of health and illness on the ability to perform self-care.

3. Discuss important subjective and objective areas of assessment when identifying self-care deficits and individualizing a plan for self-care.

4. Demonstrate basic hygiene skills such as bathing, shampooing hair, perineal care, foot care, back massage, toileting, and bed making.

5. Demonstrate proper care of eyes, ears, and teeth, including aids such as dentures, eyeglasses, contact lenses, and hearing aids.

6. List beneficial patient teaching for each of the four areas of self-care.

SECTION II: ASSESSING YOUR UNDERSTANDING

Activity A FILL IN THE BLANKS

1. _____ is the characteristic pattern of psychological and physiologic responses a person experiences after the loss of a significant person, object, belief, or relationship.

2. _____ is a state of desolation that occurs as the result of a loss, particularly the death of a significant other.

3. _____encompasses the socially prescribed behaviors after the death of a significant other.

4. _____ grief is the characteristic pattern of psychological and physiologic responses a person makes to the impending loss of a significant person, object, belief, or relationship.

5. Grief that falls outside the normal response range and may be manifested as exaggerated grief, prolonged grief, or absence of grief is called _____.

6. _____ care is a viable alternative for dying patient and their families and focuses on relieving symptoms and supporting patients with life expectancy of 6 months or less.

7. _____ is defined in three ways: as irreversible cessation of heart–lung function, or of whole-brain function, or of higher-brain function.

8. When a patient is _____, the lungs become less efficient for has diffusion and oxygenation.

9. _____ is defined as the experience of parting with an object, person, belief, or relationship that one values; the loss requires a reorganization of one or more aspects of the person's life.

Activity B **MATCHING**

1. *Match the models of grief listed in Column A with the correct self-care activities in Column B.*

Column A

____ **1.** Engel's model

____ **2.** Parkes' model

____ **3.** Demi's grief cycle model

____ **4.** Kubler-Ross' stages of dying

Column B

A. Shock, protest, disorganization, and reorganization

B. Denial, anger, bargaining, depression, and acceptance

C. Numbness, yearning, disorganization, and reorganization

D. Shock and disbelief, developing awareness, restitution, resolving the loss, idealization, and outcome

2. *Match the stages/phases of grief listed in Column A with the correct functional manifestations in Column B.*

Column A

____ **1.** Shock

____ **2.** Protest

____ **3.** Disorganization

____ **4.** Reorganization

Column B

A. Slowed thinking, emotional outbursts, unaware of others

B. Aimlessness, loss of interest, depression, restlessness

C. Nightmares, sadness, seeks help from others, searching for deceased

D. Realistic memory of deceased, feels life has meaning, renewed social relationships

Activity C **ORDERING**

1. You are a nurse providing care for an 81-year-old woman who recently lost her husband of 60 years. According to Engel's model, this patient is expected to experience six phases of grief. Place the following experiences and emotions in the order that they would occur.

  a. She is angry and can't stop crying over her loss.

  b. She has brought out a box of pictures with him and her together and looks at them for hours on end.

  c. She refuses to accept that he is gone.

  d. She tells you that she may be ready to seek companionship again.

  e. She tells you that he was the most kind-hearted, good natured, man who could do no wrong.

  f. She states that she needs to make preparations for his funeral.

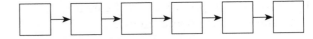

Activity D **SHORT ANSWER**

1. What are the two main categories of losses and give some examples of each?

_____

_____

_____

2. Describe the disorganization stage in Parkes' model of grief.

_____

_____

_____

3. What are some lifespan considerations for loss and grieving for toddlers?

_____

_____

_____

4. What are some lifespan considerations for loss and grieving for a school-aged child?

_____

_____

_____

5. Why is it important to reflect on your own cultural beliefs and traditions surrounding loss and grieving when caring for patients?

_____

_____

_____

SECTION III: APPLYING YOUR KNOWLEDGE

Activity E CASE STUDY

Answer the following questions, which involve the nurse's role in assessing a patient.

You are a nurse taking care of a patient who is dying of metastatic pancreas cancer with approximately 5 months to live. She states that she is okay with dying and has reached the acceptance phase. She is having a significant amount of pain. Her family is in the room and it is obviously distressing for them to see her in so much pain.

1. Is hospice care appropriate for this patient and why?

_____

_____

_____

2. What skills do you need as a nurse to help this patient and their family experience a "good death?"

_____

_____

_____

SECTION IV: PRACTICING FOR NCLEX

Activity F MULTIPLE CHOICE

Answer the following questions.

1. The grieving process has several important functions. Which of the following is not one of these functions?

   a. To make the outer reality of the loss into an internally accepted reality.

   b. To allow one to move on from their sadness.

   c. To alter the emotional attachment to the lost person or object.

   d. To make it possible for the bereaved person to become attached to other people or objects.

2. Lila is a 22-year-old woman who was recently in a motor vehicle accident which resulted in an amputation of her right leg. Since that time, she has been withdrawn and has been crying a lot. She does not wish to get out of bed and refuses to perform self-care activities. Which of the following is Lila exhibiting?

   a. Anticipatory grief

   b. Bereavement

   c. Mourning

   d. Grief

3. You are a nurse taking care of Esther, a 24-year-old woman who was recently in a motor vehicle accident during which she lost her beloved golden retriever. She tells you that when she thinks of him, her heart aches. She does not want to eat and can't sleep even though she is exhausted. Which of the following stages of the grief cycle model is Esther experiencing?

   a. Reorganization

   b. Depression

   c. Disorganization

   d. Protest

4. Which stage of the Parkes' model of grief lasts the longest?

   a. Numbness

   b. Yearning

   c. Disorganization

   d. Reorganization

5. Chandler has recently lost his father. He spent about 6 months deeply mourning his loss and is just now able to function at his pre-loss level. He was helped in this process by his strong social support. Which of the following category is Chandler most likely a member?

   a. Adult

   b. Infant

   c. Toddler

   d. School-aged child

6. You are a nurse taking care of a patient who was hospitalized for an ulcerative colitis flare. Her father recently died of colon cancer. Which of the following questions would be essential to ask this person at the start of your assessment of her loss reaction?

   a. What did your father do for a living?

   b. How close were you to your father?

   c. Did your father also have ulcerative colitis?

   d. How old was your father?

7. You are taking care a patient who is obviously going through the shock phase of grieving. Which of the following nursing interventions is best for this patient?

   a. Help them create new patterns of behavior.

   b. Helping them to express their thoughts and feelings.

   c. Helping them to mobilize support systems.

   d. Help them to accept the reality of the loss and to begin to reorganize their life.

8. Which of the following is Kubler-Ross' third stage of grief?

   a. Depression

   b. Bargaining

   c. Denial

   d. Anger

9. Which of the following describes lower-brain death?

   a. Results in the inability to maintain circulation and respiration and is ventilator dependent.

   b. Results in a vegetative state in which the patient has no consciousness, speech, or feelings but is able to breathe independently.

   c. Results in an irreversible cessation of heart–lung function.

   d. Results in a coma state.

10. Which of the following is an example of dysfunctional grieving?

    a. Weeping

    b. Outbursts of anger

    c. Emotional blunting

    d. All of the above

    e. None of the above

11. Which of the following factors affect the grieving process? Select all that apply.

    a. Meaning of loss

    b. Determination of loss

    c. Circumstances of loss

    d. Personal stressors

    e. Sociocultural resources

12. Which of the following are proper actions to take when preparing a child for death?

    a. Know your own feelings and beliefs

    b. Praise stoicism

    c. Encourage remembrance of deceased

    d. Compare the child to the deceased

    e. Expect the child to alternate between grieving and normal functioning

CHAPTER 40

Stress, Coping, and Adaptation

SECTION I: LEARNING OBJECTIVES

Upon completion of this chapter, the student will be able to do the following:

1. Identify physiologic signs and symptoms of stress.

2. Identify psychological responses to stress.

3. List examples of biophysical and psychosocial stressors.

4. Give examples of variables that affect a person's ability to cope with stress.

5. Describe various types of coping patterns people typically use to handle stress.

6. Identify stress management techniques that nurses can use to help patients adapt to stress.

SECTION II: ASSESSING YOUR UNDERSTANDING

Activity A FILL IN THE BLANKS

1. The body's maintenance of a physiologic set point is known as _____.

2. The outcome of coping is _____, or the adjustment made in response to a stressful event.

3. The Everyday Hassles Scale was created to quantify and evaluate both positive and negative _____ in one's life.

4. Ultimately the _____ is responsible for emotional processing of information and activation of the hypothalamic–pituitary–adrenal (HPA) axis.

5. The release of cortisol during stress impairs _____ activity and subsequently contributes to development of infections and cancers.

6. In adults, stress is known to inhibit _____ and lead to difficulty coping and development of depression.

7. _____ is a coping strategy that reduces feelings of anxiety as well as improves muscle tone and bone density.

8. Increased heart rate and altered sleep patterns are examples of _____ reactions to stress.

9. Reducing caffeine intake or initiating an exercise program is an example of _____ modification.

10. The body has the ability to elicit the _____ response to directly oppose the physiologic arousal response.

11. Depression, cardiovascular disease, and HIV/AIDS progression are all associated with _____ stress.

Activity B MATCHING

1. *Match the defense mechanism listed in Column A with its definition in Column B.*

Column A

____ **1.** Regression

____ **2.** Projection

____ **3.** Introjection

____ **4.** Rationalization

____ **5.** Denial

____ **6.** Repression

Column B

A. Attributing one's own thoughts or actions onto another

B. Refusing to accept something as it is but instead wishing it to be another way

C. Covering the meaning of an action with a more socially acceptable rationale

D. Behavior more appropriate for an earlier stage of development

E. Placing something in the subconscious level of thought

F. Adopting the personality characteristics of someone else

Activity C SHORT ANSWER

1. Describe the role of the HPA axis.

_____

_____

_____

2. How does cortisol affect emotional health under acute and chronic stress?

_____

_____

_____

3. Describe how the autonomic nervous system (ANS) reacts during stress.

_____

_____

_____

4. Discuss some of the physical manifestations of stress.

_____

_____

_____

5. What are the three steps to changing internal messages?

_____

_____

_____

6. Describe some nursing activities that can help a patient in time of altered function.

_____

_____

_____

SECTION III: APPLYING YOUR KNOWLEDGE

Activity D CASE STUDY

David is a 40-year-old car salesman who is happily married with two children. David's life recently changed when his mother-in-law moved in with the family. David's wife had to leave her job in order to care for her mother. David now feels that he must do everything perfectly in order to maintain his job to support his family.

1. What would be some clues in your patient history that David is experiencing physiologic stress? What might you see on physical exam?

_____

_____

_____

2. Write two appropriate NANDA-I diagnosis for David.

_____

_____

_____

3. What are some health promotion activities you could suggest for David?

_____

_____

_____

SECTION IV: PRACTICING FOR NCLEX

Activity E MULTIPLE CHOICE

Answer the following questions.

1. John is a 78-year-old widower who recently relocated to your assisted living facility. His aunt used to live in this facility and always talked fondly about her fellow residents and the staff. However, you've noticed that John has spent most of his time in his room alone. What type of stress are you most concerned about with John?

   a. Sociocultural stress
   b. Physiologic stress
   c. Psychological stress
   d. Environmental stress

2. Jemma is a 15-year-old student on the high school soccer team. She tells you how she has really started to take a leadership role on the team. When you talk with Jemma's mother, she tells you that Jemma's best friend, Claire, is a natural leader and may be voted team captain next year. Jemma's behavior is an example of what defense mechanism?

   a. Introjection
   b. Projection
   c. Denial
   d. Lying

3. Aleah is a 22-year-old college student who recently engaged in sexual intercourse with a new partner. When you tell her that she is pregnant, she tells you "that's not possible, I got my period last week". This is an example of what defense mechanism?

   a. Regression
   b. Denial
   c. Rationalization
   d. Suppression

4. You are working with Ms. N. on a stress management program. Ms. N. states that she is open to trying a guided meditation class. When helping her gets started, you tell her that all of the following are important except which?

   a. A quiet environment
   b. An open attitude
   c. Soft music
   d. A focus of attention

5. Josephina is admitted to the oncology unit with a diagnosis of leukemia. Her sister, Carla, comes to visit. She tells you that Josephina is sick because "I got mad at her and wished she would go away". Based on this information, you would estimate Carla's age to be what?

   a. 7 years
   b. 15 years
   c. 3 years
   d. 21 years

6. You are working with Mrs. K., a 67-year-old Asian-American woman about diet changes to help with weight loss. She is explaining her role in the family as the one who prepares the meats for the family, while her daughter is responsible for preparing vegetables. Based on your knowledge of traditional Asian cultures, you know what to be true?

   a. Families operate in a collectivistic manner.
   b. Families operate in an individualistic manner.
   c. Family the only thing that is important.
   d. Older adults never change their eating patterns.

7. James is a 56-year-old construction worker in your office for his annual physical. As you take his vital signs, he tells you that his blood pressure may be a little off this morning. He tells you that he is recently unemployed, is quite stressed, and is having a hard time coping. He feels like he needs to numb the pain. What are you most concerned about regarding James?

   a. Cocaine use
   b. Projection
   c. Exercise
   d. Alcohol abuse

8. Alex is a single mother of two small children. In order to make ends meet, Alex is working two part-time jobs. She comes into your community health center looking disheveled and fatigued. She asks you to make this appointment quick because she must go home and make dinner. Which of the following health promotion activities would Alex benefit from? Select all that apply.

   a. Reducing stressors

   b. Perfection reduction

   c. Using aggressiveness

   d. Cognitive behavioral therapy

9. Ella is a 55-year-old widow who recently assumed care of her 85-year-old mother, Jane. Ella had to cut back on her hours at work in order to be present in the home because she is concerned about her mother's safety. She is struggling to make mortgage payments as a result. Which of the following are applicable NANDA-I nursing diagnosis for this situation? Select all that apply.

   a. Caregiver role–strain r/t change in family dynamics

   b. Anxiety r/t change in family dynamics

   c. Compromised family coping r/t change in family dynamics

   d. Readiness for enhanced family process r/t change in family dynamics

10. Olivia is a 2 day old, 28-week gestation pre-term infant being cared for in the Neonatal Intensive Care Unit. Her mother is recovering from a cesarean section and comes in to visit her for the first time today. You know that stress can affect infant development. Which of the following are likely to be true in this situation? Select all that apply.

    a. Mother's increased cortisol levels leads to increased anxiety and decreased attachment.

    b. The inability to hold and touch can lead to delay in bonding between mother and infant.

    c. Excessive noise and lights can increase cortisol levels in the neonate.

    d. The mother's cesarean section will impair her ability to hold and bond.

11. Jamal is a 33-year-old secondary education teacher. Lately, Jamal tells you there was several incidence of violence in the school where he teaches. What symptoms on history and physical exam would indicate that Jamal is experiencing physical manifestations of stress? Select all that apply.

    a. A blood pressure of 110/68.

    b. Difficulty viewing objects more than 100 feet away.

    c. An extra heart sound every fourth to sixth beat.

    d. Report of frequent evening headaches relieved by sleep.

CHAPTER 41

Human Sexuality

SECTION I: LEARNING OBJECTIVES

Upon completion of this chapter, the student will be able to do the following:

1. Describe the structures of the male and female reproductive systems.

2. Discuss sexual expression, menstruation, and reproduction as functions of human sexuality.

3. Compare the male and female sexual response cycles.

4. Relate sexuality to all stages of the life cycle.

5. Identify factors that affect sexual functioning.

6. Describe common risks and alterations in sexuality.

7. Understand the nursing process as it relates to sexual functioning.

8. Teach patients to perform breast self-examination or testicular self-examination.

SECTION II: ASSESSING YOUR UNDERSTANDING

Activity A FILL IN THE BLANKS

1. _____ includes function of the sexual organs and the person's perceptions of his or her own functioning, sexual expression, and preferences.

2. The loose skin that covers the glans of the penis is called the _____.

3. _____ is a cyclic, periodic discharge of bloody fluid from the uterus through the vagina during a woman's reproductive years.

4. A _____ person is someone who appears as, may have had surgery for, or desires to be a member of the opposite sex.

5. A key point in the development of adolescent girls is the onset of menstruation which is termed _____.

6. The _____ refers to the period during which significant sexual changes occur in the transition from middle age to old age.

7. _____ is the inability to attain or maintain an erection long enough for satisfactory sexual intercourse.

8. _____ is painful intercourse as a direct result of physical or structural problems or the result of psychological traumas or problems.

9. The involuntary contraction of the muscles surrounding the vaginal orifice so that penetration may be impossible and very painful is called _____.

10. _____ occurs exactly 1 year after a woman's last menstrual period.

Activity B MATCHING

1. _Match the method of contraception listed in Column A with the correct description in Column B._

Column A

___ 1. Fertility awareness methods

___ 2. Hormonal methods

___ 3. Intrauterine devices

___ 4. Barrier methods

Column B

A. The use of estrogen and progesterone or progesterone only to avoid pregnancy

B. Understanding when a women is most likely to get pregnant an refraining from having sexual intercourse at those times

C. Include diaphragms, cervical caps, and condoms

D. A small "T"-shaped device that is inserted through the cervix into the uterine cavity

2. _In order to evaluate effectiveness of nursing interventions and how a patient is progressing, it is important to set goals with specific outcome criteria. Match the goal in Column A with the appropriate outcome criteria in Column B._

Column A

___ 1. The patient/ couple will recognize symptoms of sexual dysfunction.

___ 2. The patient will have decreased symptoms of altered sexual functioning.

___ 3. The patient/ couple will express satisfaction with level of sexual functioning.

Column B

A. Patient describes male and female reproductive anatomy after next teaching session with the nurse.

B. Within 6 months, patient states success in using alternate method of sexual functioning.

C. Within 6 months, patient verbalizes to nurse that symptoms are decreasing.

Activity C ORDERING

1. Menstruation depends on interplay between various hormones. This happens in a specific order and acts as a feedback loop. _Write the correct sequence in the boxes provided below._

   a. The hypothalamus secretes gonadotropin-releasing hormone.

   b. The pituitary gland is stimulated to secrete follicle-stimulating hormone and luteinizing hormone.

   c. The ovaries are stimulated to produce estrogen and progesterone.

   d. Target organs (vagina, breast, uterus) are stimulated to prepare for pregnancy. If pregnancy does not occur, menses ensue.

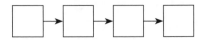

Activity D SHORT ANSWER

1. Why are breasts considered a sexual organ?

   _____

   _____

   _____

2. In what way does sexual expression differ from person to person?

   _____

   _____

   _____

3. Why is it important to consider the intrauterine period related to sexuality?

   _____

   _____

   _____

4. Why is it important to keep an open, nonjudgmental attitude with respect for the beliefs and values of others?

   _____

   _____

   _____

5. How does self-concept affect someone's sexual response?

_____

_____

_____

SECTION III: APPLYING YOUR KNOWLEDGE

Activity E CASE STUDY

Answer the following questions based on the scenario below.

You work as a school nurse in a middle school. Sasha is a 13-year-old girl who has come to your office to talk about different birth control methods. She states that she has had sex two times in the last month and used a condom only with the first partner.

1. What are some important things to keep in mind when talking with Sasha about birth control?

_____

_____

_____

2. Why would assessing Sasha for her level of self-confidence be important?

_____

_____

_____

SECTION IV: PRACTICING FOR NCLEX

Activity F MULTIPLE CHOICE

Answer the following questions.

1. Which of the following does not help to stimulate milk production in a nursing mom?
   a. Estrogen
   b. Prolactin
   c. Glucocorticoids
   d. Insulin
   e. Parathyroid hormone

2. Difficulty achieving orgasm has been reported by what percentage of women?
   a. 10% to 20%
   b. 5% to 10%
   c. 30% to 40%
   d. 20% to 30%

3. Which of the following diagnostic test is used to diagnose a chlamydial infection?
   a. Cervical culture
   b. Pap smear
   c. Blood work
   d. Wet preparation with KOH

4. Traditionally, the male sexual response is thought to be broken up into three phases. Which of the following is part of the plateau phase?
   a. A rapid erection of the penis occurs.
   b. The circumference of the penis thickens at the coronal ridge and a few drops of fluid appear at the urethral meatus.
   c. A decrease in vasocongestion occurs.
   d. The spermatic cords shorten, causing a partial elevation of both testes.

5. Which of the following is true regarding the female sexual response?
   a. All females follow the same pattern of sexual response.
   b. During the excitement phase, the clitoris becomes smaller and the vagina becomes lubricated in response to vasocongestion.
   c. The plateau phase involves full elevation of the uterus and the cervix.
   d. During the refractory period, women are unable to be restimulated.
   e. During the plateau phase, the clitoris retracts under the clitoral hood, the labia minora increase, and the uterus becomes fully elevated along with the cervix.

6. The female reproductive system is made up of both external and internal organs. Which of the following are external organs in this system? Select all that apply.
   a. Mons pubis
   b. Labia majora
   c. Clitoris
   d. Skene's glands
   e. Ovaries

CHAPTER 42

Spiritual Health

SECTION I: LEARNING OBJECTIVES

Upon completion of this chapter, the student will be able to do the following:

1. Explore philosophic questions about life.

2. Discuss his or her personal spiritual journey.

3. Identify spiritual needs in self and others.

4. Identify major religious faiths and their traditions.

5. Incorporate age-appropriate spiritual assessment questions into nursing assessment.

6. Use appropriate nursing diagnoses in writing plans of care for patients with spiritual problems.

7. Plan how to use self in spiritual support.

SECTION II: ASSESSING YOUR UNDERSTANDING

Activity A FILL IN THE BLANKS

1. One of the major characteristics of _____ is harmony with oneself, others, and a higher being.

2. Nurses often strive to deliver _____ nursing care, or care that treats the mind, body, and soul.

3. The way that an individual acts out their beliefs in life is a demonstration of _____.

4. Religious practices are often times tied to _____ of origin.

5. A sudden acute illness or the loss of a loved one can precipitate a spiritual _____.

6. An _____ committee may become involved when a religious organization says "no" to a therapy but the healthcare system says "yes".

7. The acceptance of a wide spectrum of beliefs and practices is known as religious _____.

8. The role of the parish nurse is to promote the _____ of the parish by working with the ministry.

9. All persons suffering from ill health are at risk for spiritual _____.

10. A nurse should not attempt to change a patient's faith but instead _____ on that faith.

11. Nurses may provide inadequate nursing care if they have not addressed their own _____.

Activity B MATCHING

1. *Match the religion in Column A with the commonly held religious belief in Column B. Each choice in Column A may be affiliated with multiple choices in Column B. Select all that apply.*

Column A

____ **1.** Orthodox Jew

____ **2.** Roman Catholic

____ **3.** Islam (Muslim)

____ **4.** Protestant

____ **5.** Jehovah's witness

____ **6.** LDS (Mormon)

Column B

A. Opposed to abortion

B. Abstinence from alcohol

C. Organ transplant unquestionably permitted

D. Kosher dietary practices

E. Birth control is a personal choice

F. Receipt of blood products is prohibited

2. *Match the age in Column A with the appropriate religious-affiliated developmental task in Column B.*

Column A

____ **1.** Toddlers

____ **2.** School age

____ **3.** Young adult

____ **4.** Adult and older adult

Column B

A. Establish one's own commitment to faith

B. Renewed questioning based on world view

C. Introduction of lore, legends, and story

D. Introduction of faith rituals

Activity C SHORT ANSWER

1. What is the difference between religion and spirituality?

_____

_____

_____

2. Differentiate between a spiritual crisis and separation from spiritual ties.

_____

_____

_____

3. What questions might you ask to identify a person's normal religious practices?

_____

_____

_____

4. Provide some examples of appropriate nursing outcomes for a person in spiritual distress.

_____

_____

_____

5. Discuss how you can appropriately provide spiritual support for a toddler and their family.

_____

_____

_____

SECTION III: APPLYING YOUR KNOWLEDGE

Activity D CASE STUDY

Paul is a 23-year-old man recently diagnosed with non-Hodgkin's lymphoma. Paul is active in his Episcopal church. However, since admission to the hospital 6 weeks ago, Paul has refused visits from the hospital chaplain. He tells you that "no God he prays to would allow this to happen".

1. What do you think is contributing to Paul's lack of interest in religious practice?

_____

_____

_____

2. Formulate an appropriate NANDA-I diagnosis for Paul.

_____

_____

_____

3. What are some nursing activities that would be appropriate in your care plan for Paul?

_____

_____

_____

SECTION IV: PRACTICING FOR NCLEX

Activity E MULTIPLE CHOICE

Answer the following questions.

1. Caleb is an inpatient on your hospital unit. He was recently diagnosed with metastatic pancreatic cancer and was told that any treatment would be palliative. He tells you that there is no God that he knows of who would subject someone to this. Caleb's statement is most reflective of what?

   a. Spiritual crisis

   b. Change in beliefs

   c. Separation from spiritual ties

   d. Depression

2. Allen is an 82-year-old retiree who recently relocated to senior apartments. The apartments are not affiliated with any religious beliefs. Allen was raised in the Roman Catholic Church and has attended mass every Sunday since childhood. He has not attended mass for 3 weeks. What best describes Allen's situation?

   a. Change in beliefs

   b. Spiritual crisis

   c. Separation from spiritual ties

   d. Depression

3. Nurse Hudson is a practicing Baptist. She works with Nurse Hassan who is active in the Muslim community. Nurse Sanchez was raised Roman Catholic. The three of them often assist each other in understanding different practices when caring for a patient of a different faith. This is best described as what?

   a. Open-mindedness

   b. Spiritual crisis

   c. Cooperation

   d. Pluralism

4. Mr. V. is recovering from pneumonia. You know that a well-balanced diet will help him to recover. However, Mr. V. informs you that it is Ramadan and he must fast from sunrise to sunset. What is your most appropriate nursing action?

   a. Work with the nutrition staff to provide nutritious meals at off hours.

   b. Encourage Mr. V. to speak with a religious leader to grant a medical exception.

   c. Provide liquid nutrition only as this does not interfere with religious practice.

   d. Tell Mr. V. he must eat to maintain his health.

5. You are the nurse caring for Mr. U., a 55-year-old man found unconscious at a construction site. He has not regained consciousness in 6 days and is on full life support. His wife and children are present at his bedside. The family is practicing Orthodox Jews. Based on this information, how would you expect the family to respond to a discussion regarding Mr. U.'s care?

   a. The family will plan to withdraw support in the next few days.

   b. The family will do whatever is necessary to continue life support.

   c. Continued life support is appropriate as long as the measures are not heroic.

   d. The Orthodox Jewish faith does not speak to the use of life support.

6. Mr. J. is a 78-year-old man, who is actively dying of unknown causes. Mr. J. is a practicing Muslim. His wife, children, and grandchildren are present. The physician in charge of Mr. J.'s care plans to discuss Mr. J.'s impending death with the family. Based on your knowledge of the Muslim faith, which of the following is NOT true?

   a. The body is washed and cared for by the family.

   b. The family will likely want an autopsy.

   c. The family will want to read from the Koran at the time of death.

   d. Organ donation is generally not permitted.

7. You are caring for Mr. Z., a 55-year-old man admitted to the hospital for liver failure. He is an active member in the LDS (Mormon) church. Mr. Z. tells you that he strictly adheres to the religious practices that are condoned by the church. However, you overhear two of his physicians discussing that Mr. Z.'s liver failure is likely due to chronic alcohol use. You suspect that they are wrong. Which of the following is an appropriate nursing activity?

   a. Know that the physicians are wrong; the Mormon faith does not permit alcohol use.

   b. Engage Mr. Z. in a discussion about past and present religious practices.

   c. Accuse Mr. Z. of lying and find out why he lied to you.

   d. Order several laboratory tests looking for genetic defects that affect the liver.

8. Ezekiel is the 3-year-old son of a practicing Protestant family. They are interested in teaching Ezekiel some of their religious traditions. Based on his age, which of the following activities would be appropriate? Select all that apply.

   a. Bedtime prayer

   b. Prayer before meals

   c. Holy day celebrations

   d. Stories about religious symbols

9. You are conducting a spiritual assessment on Jake, a patient recently admitted to your hospital unit. Which of the following questions would be appropriate to ask Jake about his religious and spiritual practices? Select all that apply.

   a. Is religion a significant part of your life?

   b. Are there any spiritual practices that you would like to continue while hospitalized?

   c. You would like the priest to come and visit you, right?

   d. Does the present situation interfere with any spiritual or religious practice?

10. Eleanor is a 3-year-old girl who is hospitalized following repair of a fractured femur. Her parents have asked that the hospital chaplain visit her room this Sunday. Based on Eleanor's age, what activities would be appropriate during the chaplain's visit? Select all that apply.

    a. Recitation of a simple prayer

    b. Singing church hymns

    c. Drawing pictures of religious figures

    d. Stories of biblical legends

CHAPTER 1

SECTION II: ASSESSING YOUR UNDERSTANDING

Activity A FILL IN THE BLANKS

1. American Nursing Association (ANA)
2. Baccalaureate
3. Certification
4. Licensure
5. Scholarship
6. Nurse-prescribed
7. Advocates
8. Maslow's
9. Change
10. Patterns

Activity B MATCHING

1 – D,   2 – B,   3 – C,   4 – A,   5 – E

Activity C ORDERING

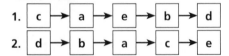

1. c → a → e → b → d
2. d → b → a → c → e

Activity D SHORT ANSWER

1. Each new graduate must take and pass the national NCLEX exam to qualify for nursing licensure. The state board of nursing then sets any additional requirements for licensure. These requirements are enumerated in the states Nurse Practice Act. Once a nurse is licensed, he/she may gain licensure in another state through reciprocity. The nurse is not required to retake the NCLEX exam, but may be asked to complete educational requirements deemed appropriate by the state. Twenty-four states currently participate in the Nurse Licensure Compact. This allows nurses to practice in another participating state without obtaining a separate nursing license.
2. Membership in the ANA consists of registered professional nurses. The ANA sets the standards of practice for nurses and decides the activities, functions, and goals of the nursing profession. The ANA also acts as the national voice for nurses by advo-

cating for the issues and wishes expressed by its members.
3. Florence Nightingale's *Notes on Nursing: What It Is, What It Is Not* addresses the fundamental needs of the sick and basic principles of good healthcare. This theory identifies the person as an individual with their own reparative processes to deal with disease. The environment refers to that persons' external condition that affect their reparative process, such as warmth, light, and odor. Health is the focus on the reparative process of getting well. Nursing then is the goal of placing the individual in the best possible condition to obtain good healthcare.
4. According to Maslow, there is esteem that is derived from others and there is self-esteem. Esteem derived from others is a person's sense that others think well of them. Self-esteem is the sense of a person's own adequacy and worth.
5. Many changes in the healthcare industry have led to the broadening scope of nursing practice. These changes include a shift in healthcare settings, technological advances, and a growing concern for healthcare costs and access. Nurses have moved from simply observing and giving prescribed medications to coordinating clinical information for the entire healthcare team.

SECTION III: APPLYING YOUR KNOWLEDGE

Activity E CASE STUDY

1. According to Maslow's hierarchy of human needs, physiological needs are fundamental motivating forces and provide the base for Maslow's pyramid because they are essential for existence. If one of these needs is not met, illness or death may occur. Thus, John's lack of food consumption should take priority when developing a plan of care for John.
2. The need for love and belonging is the third tier on Maslow's hierarchy of needs. Once John's physiological and safety concerns are met, this need must be addressed to avoid isolation. A nurse may consider an interdisciplinary team to brainstorm ideas on how to best approach John's feelings of loneliness.

SECTION IV: PRACTICING FOR NCLEX

Activity F MULTIPLE CHOICE

1. **Answer: a**
   RATIONALE: An associate degree in nursing is a two-year degree that can be attained at a junior or community college. A diploma in nursing program that is usually 3 years of study where the emphasis is on clinical experience and college credit is not awarded for nursing courses. The baccalaureate degree is a full college or university education. Licensed practical nurse is someone who has attended a 1-year program, which prepared them to perform technical skills under the supervision on a registered nurse.

2. **Answer: d**
   RATIONALE: Nightingale established nursing as a profession with two missions. "Sick nursing" was helping patients use their own reparative processes to get well and "health nursing" was to prevent illness.

3. **Answer: b**
   RATIONALE: (A) describes the role of the nurse researcher, (C) describes a nurse anesthetist, and (D) is a nurse administrator.

4. **Answer: d**
   RATIONALE: The Nurse Practice Act of each state defines the practice of nursing within that area. The National League for Nursing is an organization that supports nursing education. The American Nurses Credentialing Center certifies nurses in various specialties. The ANA is nursing's professional organization in the US and sets standards of practice for nurses.

5. **Answer: c**
   RATIONALE: Spirituality is not one of the four central concepts in nursing. The four central concepts in nursing practice include person, environment, health, and nursing.

6. **Answer: a**
   RATIONALE: Oxygen, food, water, and rest are all examples of physiologic need according to Maslow's hierarchy of need. Physiologic need is the most fundamental and essential need for existence.

7. **Answer: b**
   RATIONALE: Mark is in the unfreezing state where he has recognized the need to change a long-standing pattern but has not yet taken action.

8. **Answer: a**
   RATIONALE: Health perception–health management pattern focuses on health values and beliefs, as well as the resources in the community that are available to meet health needs. Elimination pattern is closely related to nutrition and metabolism.

9. **Answer: c**
   RATIONALE: According to Maslow's hierarchy of needs, physiological needs come first, followed by safety, then love and belonging, then esteem, and then self-actualization.

10. **Answer: a**
    RATIONALE: The competent nurse consciously and deliberately plans nursing care in terms of long-range goals.

11. **Answer: d**
    RATIONALE: Hidlegard Peplau developed the theory of Interpersonal Relations in Nursing whose purpose was to develop an interpersonal interaction between the patient and the nurse.

CHAPTER 2

SECTION II: ASSESSING YOUR UNDERSTANDING

Activity A FILL IN THE BLANKS

1. Social
2. Actions
3. Spirit
4. Primary
5. Values
6. Peer
7. Lifestyle
8. Reflection
9. Plants
10. Energy

Activity B MATCHING

1 – B,   2 – E,   3 – A,   4 – C,   5 – D

Activity C ORDERING

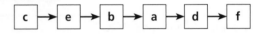

$$c \rightarrow e \rightarrow b \rightarrow a \rightarrow d \rightarrow f$$

Activity D SHORT ANSWER

1. According to the Health Belief Model, factors that can affect a person's response to illness include personal expectations in relation to health and illness, earlier experiences with health and illness, sociocultural context, and age and developmental state. Expectations that the person has can either positively or negatively affect someone's health. Previous experiences will influence how someone reacts to future challenges related to illness. A person might rely on information about a given illness they get from peers in order to process what they are or will be experiencing. And, age and developmental stage influence how a person might understand an illness as well as cope with that illness.

2. Holism takes into consideration a person's mind, body, and spirit and how these interact with the environment. Holism sees people as ever-changing systems of energy that must be examined in the context of their environment and not just in parts. From as early as Florence Nightingale, nursing has developed this model of healthcare by manipulating the environment in which care is provided and by incorporating many ideas and practices from

various traditions and cultures to support patients self-healing.

3. Allopathic medicine is described as Western medicine and includes such advances as antibiotics and surgery. Complimentary and alternative medicines are therapies that are generally thought of as unconventional and include such practices as meditation, acupuncture, and therapeutic touch. Integrative medicine focuses on the whole person and emphasizes the therapeutic relationship. Integrative medicine utilizes both conventional and alternative therapies.

4. In the Theory of Integral Nursing, integral nursing is the incorporation the multidimensional aspects of human experience to provide a philosophy of care that incorporates all aspects of healing. It challenges the healthcare provider to reflect on his or her own personal self-care in order to grow on a personal and professional level.

5. Safety issues surrounding botanicals include the lack of studies on herb–drug interactions. Standardization is attempted by herbal manufacturers but is limited in value because not all compounds that can be used as a comparison or the required levels needed for that comparisons are known. Since 1994 herbal products have had to follow guidelines set forth by the U.S. Dietary Supplement Health and Education Act (DSHEA). In order to ensure quality, consumers are encouraged to buy products that have certain seals of approval.

SECTION III: APPLYING YOUR KNOWLEDGE

Activity E CASE STUDY

1. By approaching this patient with an open and nonjudgmental attitude, the nurse is able to accurately collect information about this patient. If the patient feels comfortable with the practitioner and observes that the practitioner is at least aware of CAM therapies, they are more likely to report their use.

2. I want to ask her about her use of CAM and specifically is she taking any vitamins or supplements which could potentially interact with any medications she is prescribed. I would also want to ask her about her dietary practices. I would also want to know if she has been using any CAM therapies to treat either her hypertension or any other conditions.

3. There are several CAM therapies that this person might want to try. Meditation is one therapy that I might suggest. Meditation can be used to decrease anxiety and stress that often lead to tension-type headaches. Cynthia can choose from concentrative, receptive, reflective, and expressive meditations to find what would best suit her.

SECTION IV: PRACTICING FOR NCLEX

Activity F MULTIPLE CHOICE

1. **Answer: a**
RATIONALE: According to the Clinical Model, health is the absence of signs and symptoms of disease. In the Health Belief Model, a person's level of health is influenced by many factors. These factors include personal expectations, prior experiences, a person's sociocultural context, and their age/developmental state. The High-Level Wellness Model asserts that a person's lifestyle and the choices they make determine a person's level of health. The Holistic Health Model acknowledges that there is an interaction between a person's mind, body, and spirit within the environment. This person may no longer have any symptoms of bronchitis but the fact that he still smokes means that he is not healthy on the whole.

2. **Answer: a**
RATIONALE: Tertiary prevention occurs when diagnosis of a long-term disease or disability has already been made. The goal is to minimize complications and maximize function in any way possible for these patients.

3. **Answer: a**
RATIONALE: Integrative medicine is healing-oriented medicine that takes account of the whole person (body, mind, spirit, and community), including all aspects of lifestyle. It does not reject allopathic medicine and CAM practices. It includes establishing a partnership between patient and practitioner, facilitating the body's innate healing abilities, and focusing on promoting health and preventing illness, as well as treating disease.

4. **Answer: a**
RATIONALE: Concentrative meditation is most familiar to people. The person focuses on an object such as prayer, a chant, or visualization.

5. **Answer: c**
RATIONALE: Integrative systems

6. **Answer: b**
RATIONALE: Diagnosis in Traditional Chinese Medicine is based in the balance, or lack thereof, of Yin and Yang. Yin and Yang are both aspects of qi which is considered a vital life force.

7. **Answer: d**
RATIONALE: Martha has moved beyond the Preparation and Action stages and is now in the Maintenance stage where she is trying to prevent lapses and maintain her weight loss. Terminations will come when she no longer worries about overeating.

8. **Answers: a, b, c, d, e**
RATIONALE: The Health Belief Model asserts that certain factors influence a person's health and the way they respond to illness. These factors include personal expectations in relation to health and illness, earlier experiences with health and illness, sociocultural context, and age and developmental state.

9. **Answers: d, e**
   RATIONALE: Emptying a colostomy bag and changing a wound dressing are both "doing" therapies as they both have measurable, linear outcomes. "Being" therapies such as prayer, concentrative medicine, and imagery recognize the less measurable effects of consciousness both within the person and as a bridge betweenindividuals.

CHAPTER 3

SECTION II: ASSESSING YOUR UNDERSTANDING

Activity A FILL IN THE BLANKS

1. Secondary
2. Communities
3. Populations
4. Workplace
5. Chronic
6. Standardized
7. Social
8. Information
9. Self-care
10. Disruption
11. Assets

Activity B MATCHING

1 – C,   2 – D,   3 – A,   4 – B,   5 – E

Activity C ORDERING

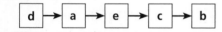

d → a → e → c → b

Activity D SHORT ANSWER

1. Primary healthcare is focused on health promotion, education, protection, and screening. Secondary healthcare is directed a problem that already exists and includes services such as emergency care, acute and critical care, diagnosis and treatment. Tertiary care involves rehabilitation, long-term care, and hospice care.
2. In general, the focus of nursing is on the health of the whole person. In community-based nursing, this could mean of an individual or a population. The community-based nurse uses information gained from a thorough assessment of the patient or patients in order to provide prioritized and holistic care.
3. Discharge planning occurs either when a patient is moving from one setting to another or when they no longer require services. The discharge planner, usually a health or social services professional, coordinates the transition and serves as a link between the discharging facility and the community. Discharge planning can reduce readmissions, minimize residual effects of the health condition, and improve patient and family satisfaction with the healthcare team.

4. A nurse that is familiar with community resources is able to provide their patient with a more realistic and individualized nursing plan of care. Services that should be assessed include emergency care, equipment rental stores, chore and homemaker services, home-delivered meals, and visiting nurse services. Availability of these services also gives the nurse important insight into the community's economic stability, the patient's neighborhood, and the community's cultural norms.
5. The major areas requiring assessment by a home care nurse are the individual, the family, risk level, the home, and community resources. By assessing the individual, the nurse can determine the patient's ability to manage at home, from self-care tasks to what equipment they might need. An assessment of the family provides information about the person's support system or lack thereof. The risk for impaired ability to manage at home is determined by the relationship between functional impairments and available internal and external supports. A home assessment should include safety, sanitation, mobility, temperature, and personal space. All of these can be used to determine whether the home is a safe environment for the patient to live and function in. An assessment of community resources gives the nurse information about the community's economic stability, the patient's neighborhood, the social and health resources available, and the cultural norms of the community.

SECTION III: APPLYING YOUR KNOWLEDGE

Activity E CASE STUDY

1. I would assess Daren from a systems point of view. This would include assessing him as an individual, assessing his family, his risk, his home, and his community resources. By looking at the individual, I am able to assess how this person is able to manage in the home. Assessing the family would give me important information on how involved his wife is able to be in his care and how they function together. There are several risk factors that Daren has that would necessitate home care for Daren. He might have multiple illnesses with multiple medications and decreased mental and physical functioning following his stroke. Assessment of his home would elicit information on the safety of his living environment as well as tell me whether or not he has all the equipment he might need for his care.
2. Following Stanhope and Lancaster, I would go through the five phases of the home visit with Daren. After having clarified the purpose of the referral and calling Daren and his wife to schedule a home visit, I would then take the opportunity of being face to face with them to start to develop a therapeutic relationship.
3. Based on my holistic assessment of Daren I would use the four steps of the educational process to assure that

Daren and his wife are getting the education they need and want. Patient education would be based on shared goals with measurable outcomes. Uptake of the educational material would be evaluated to ensure that my teaching plan was appropriate.

SECTION IV: PRACTICING FOR NCLEX

Activity F MULTIPLE CHOICE

1. Answer: e
RATIONALE: Multiple area rugs are considered a tripping hazard and should be removed from the house.

2. Answer: c
RATIONALE: Asthma should not hinder the patient's ability to live independently as chronic severe pain, dementia, substance abuse, or blindness would.

3. Answer: d
RATIONALE: The simple referral is the second type of discharge planning that involves referring a patient to community services and is a request for services outside of the scope of the nursing professional.

4. Answer: a
RATIONALE: A systems view acknowledges that a person's healthcare occurs within the context of family, friends, and the community around them. These factors affect the wellbeing of the individual and vice versa. John's illness affects those that live in his neighborhood and how they react to him can affect how John copes with his symptoms.

5. Answer: a
RATIONALE: According to Koerner, the capacities that are hallmarks of a nursing leader within the community include the capacity to negotiate and be authentic with a patient, the capacity to see relationships and create new systems from chaos, the capacity for having an upstanding character, and the capacity for creativity.

6. Answer: a
RATIONALE: The three discharge planning elements for the patient are goal setting, transition, and continuity of care. Goal setting focuses on measurable and realistic outcomes that the patient thinks that they can achieve. Transition addresses both the physical change from one place to another and the emotional change. A change occurs in how people see themselves and interact with others in a new role. Continuity of care is assuring that a person will still receive the services they need in their new setting. Discharge planning elements for the nurse are collaboration, facilitation, and negation.

7. Answers: a, b, c
RATIONALE: Screening, health promotion, and protection are components of primary healthcare; emergency care is a component of secondary healthcare, and rehabilitation and treatment are components of tertiary healthcare.

8. Answers: a, b, c, f
RATIONALE: Coordinating, making referrals, monitoring medical progress, and filing and completing paperwork are just a few of the tasks that the case manager performs on a regular basis.

9. Answers: a, b, c
RATIONALE: Martha is a part of an aging population that is much bigger than anything our country has dealt with before. She is also a single-person household without a lay caregiver who might have otherwise been able to assist her. By choosing to stay in her own home, she is taking a greater responsibility for making healthcare choices.

CHAPTER 4

SECTION II: ASSESSING YOUR UNDERSTANDING

Activity A FILL IN THE BLANKS

1. Family
2. Different
3. Key informants
4. Habituation
5. Rituals
6. Health disparities
7. Biologic, social
8. Individualized
9. Words
10. Clarification

Activity B MATCHING

1. 1 – D,   2 – A,   3 – E,   4 – C,   5 – B
2. 1 – B,   2 – E,   3 – D,   4 – A,   5 – C

Activity C SHORT ANSWER

1. Cultural diversity increases the plurality of ideas with a society. Cultural diversity also increases the number of behaviors that members of society are exposed to. These factors increase the society's potential for varied human resources.

2. Cultural diversity within groups refers to the differing cultural characteristics of individuals who all categorize themselves under one group. An example of this is that varying educational backgrounds and countries of origin have led to varying health beliefs of registered nurses in the United States.

3. In Tuskegee, Alabama poor, rural, or imprisoned African American men who were known to be infected with syphilis were observed, rather than treated, by physicians under the guise that they were receiving free health care. The goal was to study the natural course of the disease. However, this already stigmatized group has caused decades of unnecessary death and suffering. As a result, many African Americans who were directly or indirectly impacted by the Tuskegee project continue to be mistrustful of the Western healthcare system.

4. Stereotypes are preconceived, untested, and often exaggerated beliefs about a culture or subculture. Stereotypes are potentially harmful to the nurse–patient interaction because they cause the holder of

such beliefs to negate the individuality of the patient. Stereotypes can also lead to an incorrect assessment and thus incorrect and potentially harmful intervention on the part of the nurse.

5. The American Nurses Association highlights the importance of culturally competent nursing in its draft of the second edition of the *Nursing: Scope and Standards of Practice* (2010). In this document, they describe that the nurse should partner with the patient and/or family to develop an individualized plan of care that encompasses the patient's "beliefs, spiritual and health practices, preferences, choices, developmental level, coping style, culture and environment and available technology". Teaching methods should also be individualized and address a patient's "values, beliefs, health practices, developmental level, learning needs, readiness and ability to learn, language preference, spirituality, culture, and socioeconomic status".

SECTION III: APPLYING YOUR KNOWLEDGE

Activity D CASE STUDY

1. The Joint Commission (2010) states that hospitals are obliged to provide trained language interpreters for patients "who do not speak or understand the predominant language of the community". While Mohammed is well-intentioned, the use of a family member as an interpreter can lead to intentional or unintentional additions or omissions in the information that is communicated to the patient and subsequently can result in harm or improper care. Interpretation often goes beyond the literal meaning of the words, and trained language interpreters are well-versed in translating cultural idioms as well as verbatim conversation.

2. When possible, arrange for an interpreter who is of the same gender as the patient. Meet with the interpreter outside of the room prior to meeting with Fatima and Mohammed. Discuss with the interpreter what the context of your discussion will entail. You may also discuss any concerns that you have about this interaction. If the interpreter is familiar with the particular culture of the patient (not just the language) they may offer insights as a key informant of the culture on how to engage in a culturally appropriate interaction. Speak directly to Fatima and Mohammed rather than the interpreter. Watch how both the patient and her husband respond to your comments, how they interact with you and with one another. Speak slowly and use brief phrases to allow the interpreter time to relay the message. The interpreter may not directly interpret English idioms or embarrassing questions; allow the interpreter to ask questions in a culturally appropriate manner. If you ask a question of Fatima or Mohammed and the answer does not match the question, try rephrasing.

SECTION IV: PRACTICING FOR NCLEX

Activity E MULTIPLE CHOICE

1. **Answer: c**
RATIONALE: "Despite continued advances in health care and technology, racial and ethnic minorities continue to have higher rates of disease, disability and premature death than non-minorities." ("What Are Health disparities?" 2010).

2. **Answer: a**
RATIONALE: Cultural relativity suggests an underlying explanation for behavior, particularly for behavior that is repeated by different people of the same culture or ethnic group.

3. **Answer: b**
RATIONALE: Stereotypes are exaggerated descriptors of character or behavior that are commonly reiterated in mass media, idiomatic expressions, and folklore.

4. **Answer: a**
RATIONALE: Patients and families often express rituals during times of stress, such as during an acute hospitalization. Keeping the body covered and warm is a home remedy used by many cultures to help heal the body. As in this example, cultural rituals may conflict with Western medical beliefs.

5. **Answer: a**
RATIONALE: Culture shock occurs when a person is immersed in an environment different from the one they are accustomed to, resulting in rapid disorientation and distress.

6. **Answers: b, c, d**
RATIONALE: It is important to speak directly to the patient as this enables the patient to read your nonverbal language.

7. **Answer: c**
RATIONALE: According to The American Nurses Association's draft of the second edition of the *Nursing: Scope and Standards of Practice* (2010), "The registered nurse develops in partnership with the person, family and others an individualized plan considering the person's characteristics or situation, including but not limited to, values, beliefs, spiritual and health practices, preferences, choices, developmental level, coping style, culture and environment and available technology." (p. 31).

8. **Answer: b**
RATIONALE: A culturally sensitive nurse is one who respects a patient's requests while ensuring that their requests reflect safe medical practice. Mrs. A.'s request does not interfere with patient safety. Thus, her request should be respected and communicated through documentation to other healthcare personnel.

CHAPTER 5

SECTION II: ASSESSING YOUR UNDERSTANDING

Activity A FILL IN THE BLANKS

1. Patient
2. Incongruent
3. Feedback
4. Language
5. Informal
6. Empathy
7. Confidentiality
8. Restatement
9. Transcript
10. Children

Activity B MATCHING

1. 1 – B,   2 – D,   3 – A,   4 – C
2. 1 – C,   2 – A,   3 – B

Activity C SHORT ANSWER

1. The relationship between types of communication describes whether verbal, nonverbal, written, and metacommunication fit together (are congruent) or do not fit together (noncongruent). An example of a congruent relationship between types of communication is a patient who has just received the news that she is pregnant. She is beaming and states "we have tried to get pregnant for years. I cannot believe this finally happened". In this example, the patient's words match her expressions. An example of a noncongruent relationship between communication is the patient who states "I am perfectly content with my life. I wouldn't change a thing" with a completely flat affect and tears in his eyes. He appears unkept and exhausted. As a nurse, you astutely recognize that his verbal communication does not match his nonverbal communication.

2. The patient is always the focus in the nurse–patient relationship. The goal of the relationship is to meet the patient's needs. These needs may be immediate such as needing to use the bathroom, or they may require problem solving to help the patient cope and adapt with the healthcare environment. The nurse–patient relationship is limited to the needs incurred by the healthcare situation and should be terminated when the healthcare goals are met and service is no longer needed.

3. Open-ended questions provide an excellent starting point for a therapeutic nurse–patient conversation. Something as simple as "how did you come to be here in the hospital?" can encourage a patient to begin speaking openly. Opening remarks can also initiate a conversation. Verbalizing a simple observation "you seem uncomfortable, why don't we discuss what is bothering you" can help a patient feel as if they will be listened to and respected.

4. Silence offers both the nurse and the patient a moment to reflect on what has been stated in the conversation. Silence can also provide the patient with the opportunity to alter the conversation as they see fit. Often silence feels very uncomfortable, especially for a newly practicing nurse.

5. Age-related changes such as hearing or vision impairment may require the nurse to use special skills when conversing with the older adult. In the inpatient setting, patients may be without their glasses or hearing aids. This is especially true if the patient has just undergone a surgical procedure.

SECTION III: APPLYING YOUR KNOWLEDGE

Activity D CASE STUDY

1. Begin the communication with an informal contract. This would include a brief introduction and description of your role. The patient is grieving the loss of this pregnancy. A thoughtful, open-ended question might initiate a conversation, but an opening remark may be preferable. Such statements are assessment based; in this case, you've assessed that the patient is quite sad and perhaps contemplative. Try stating: "I know this is a very difficult time for you. I am here to listen if you would like to talk". Such statements do not place pressure on the patient to engage in conversation if she is not ready, but invite a discussion if desired.

2. Answers will vary.

SECTION IV: PRACTICING FOR NCLEX

Activity E MULTIPLE CHOICE

1. **Answer: c**
   RATIONALE: The patient's actions, expressions and words all are fitting following the receipt of a difficult diagnosis.

   Incongruent communication – The patient's actions, expressions and words all "fit" together. Her communication would be incongruent in this same scenario but she was described as beaming from ear to ear.

   Verbal communication – This is not the best choice because it does not take into account the whole picture. Although verbal communication is used as a part of the patient's response, the nurse must also consider her posture and her facial expressions.

   This is not the best choice because it does not take into account the whole picture. Although nonverbal communication is used as a part of the patient's response, the nurse must also consider the patient's words.

2. **Answer: a**
   RATIONALE: The focus of the nurse–patient interaction is on the patient. The nurse should only disclose personal information if it is necessary or benefits the patient. Answers b, c, and d are all part of daily social interaction.

3. **Answer: d**
RATIONALE: The nurse advocates for the patient by offering the patient choices based on the current situation. Answers a and c are examples of guilt inducement and answer b is an example of an authoritarian interaction as there are no choices presented to the patient.

4. **Answer: a**
RATIONALE: Language barrier, fatigue and having too many family members are not conducive to good communication and can lead to what is perceived as difficult behaviors in a patient. Taking time to reflect on one's own triggers as well as environmental triggers, leads to reduction of difficulties.

5. **Answer: c**
RATIONALE: Empathy, positive regard, and a comfortable sense of self were among the key ingredients.

6. **Answer: a**
RATIONALE: Rephrasing, reflection, and active listening are essential for accurate assessment and interventions.

7. **Answer: d**
RATIONALE: Encouraging elaboration helps the patient to describe more fully the concerns or problems under discussion.

8. **Answer: b**
RATIONALE: False reassurance minimized the patient's situation and is providing assurance not based on fact.

9. **Answers: a, b**
RATIONALE: Nurses who talk too much with patients about themselves and their own goals and problems are being nonprofessional. The purpose of a professional relationship is to meet the patient's needs, not the nurse's.

10. **Answer: a**
RATIONALE: When utilizing an interpreter, speak clearly in a conversational tone and directly address the patient. While a patient may be more comfortable having a family member present, this is not required. Interpreters should not be asked to translate written information; instead the nurse should verbally explain the brochure or a copy should be obtained in Mrs. Singh's native language.

CHAPTER 6

SECTION II: ASSESSING YOUR UNDERSTANDING

Activity A FILL IN THE BLANKS
1. Values
2. Older adulthood
3. Self
4. Ethics
5. Beneficence
6. Entitled
7. Confidential

8. Outcomes
9. Libel
10. Duty
11. Hospital
12. Liability
13. Evil
14. Authorized

Activity B MATCHING
1. 1 – G, 2 – C, 3 – H, 4 – B, 5 – A, 6 – E, 7 – F, 8 – D
2. 1 – C, 2 – A, 3 – F, 4 – E, 5 – B, 6 – D

Activity C SHORT ANSWER
1. Personal values are ideas or beliefs that an individual deems important. These ideas or beliefs may be shared with coworkers or patients but should not be placed or transferred onto others. Personal values are learned and adapted over a lifetime through social interactions. In contrast, professional ethics are held by a group and are deemed to be generalizable and are used to uphold standards of conduct by that group of people. Professional ethics can be transferred onto a group of people, say a patient population.
2. Beneficence is the act of doing good, or of promoting the patient's best interests. The nurse acts on the behalf of the patient when engaging in beneficence. For example, when a nurse dims the lights to promote a therapeutic healing environment, that nurse is practicing beneficence. Nonmaleficence is the act of doing no harm or to prevent harm. The act of premedication prior to a painful procedure, such as a wound dressing change, is an example of a nurse practicing nonmaleficence.
3. Patients in the United States have a right to receive emergency medical care regardless of their ability to pay. No one can be discriminated against based on gender, race or social status. Patients have varying backgrounds with healthcare and medical terminology but have a right to informed consent, meaning they need to understand and approve the medical care that they receive. Patients for whom English is not their primary language have a right to interpreter services.
4. Licensure is the legal ability of a nurse to practice in a state. In order to receive compensation for practice, a nurse must be licensed. Licensure commits the nurse to abide by the nurse practice act of that state. The nurse practice act describes the scope and expectations of nursing practice, and details how nursing will be governed, and outlines the criteria for nursing education.
5. Code status refers to the extent to which an individual decides they would like to be resuscitated in the event of respiratory or cardiopulmonary status. Do Not Resuscitate is a common term used to describe a patient who does not wish to have extraordinary measures taken to extend their life. A "full code" describes a person who wishes to have all measures taken to extend their life no matter the circumstance. A "modified code" can be created in which the patient directs healthcare providers to which measures (i.e., yes to CPR but no to intubation)

they would like to have taken. It is important to understand the code status of a patient not only to comply with their wishes but because legal action can be taken against a nurse who fails to follow the patient's expressed wish.

SECTION III: APPLYING YOUR KNOWLEDGE

Activity D CASE STUDY

1. In order to be found liable for a patients injuries, the four elements of negligence must be proven. Those four elements are: Duty to the patient, a breach of duty or failure to meet the standards of care, causation, and damages. Based on the information provided in the case study, the four conditions were not met. Ms. Montrose was a full code status and your job as a Registered Nurse is to carry out her wishes. In this case, you followed her wishes by working with the team to perform CPR and stabilizing her medical condition. You did not deviate from the standards of care. However, just because it does not appear that you are liable for injuries, you still need to seek legal protection. In this example, you are employed by a hospital; you should make an appointment to speak to the hospital legal department.
2. A nurse can follow several steps to protect herself/himself legally. First, the nurse should maintain current practice by attending seminars and continuing education events. The nurse should also maintain meticulous documentation. In this example, one nurse should be designated to document during the code. After the code is completed, you should document how the chain of command was used during this emergency situation. You can always go back and amend documentation after an emergency situation. This ensures that documentation is complete and accurate. Codes can also be practiced so that it is ensured that all nursing staff are up to date on standards of care for a code situation. More nurses are finding that malpractice insurance is a reasonable option. Your own insurance ensures your representation and financial protection. Contact your state board of nursing to inquire about individual insurance.

SECTION IV: PRACTICING FOR NCLEX

Activity E MULTIPLE CHOICE

1. **Answer: b**
   RATIONALE: The preconventional stage is characterized by learning right from wrong and understanding the choice between obedience and punishment. The conventional stage is characterized by conformity and learning behaviors from others. Values and Will are not stages in Kohlberg's theory.
2. **Answer: a**
   RATIONALE: The United States healthcare system allows the patient to make medical decisions. In the

case of a minor, the patient is Anna and her primary caregivers, her parents. United States law also gives patients the autonomy to make decisions about medical care that are culturally appropriate. This affords patients the right to share or to not share any information about treatment. It is the responsibility of the healthcare team to uphold the request of patients.
3. **Answer: c**
   RATIONALE: This example illustrates the principle of fidelity. The patient has asked that you assist him by not administering any narcotics. Thus, he has already made his wishes known and you do not need to ask him again. While it is important to pass this information on to the next nurse, this is not the best choice because verbally passing on patient information can cause that information to accidentally be changed or left out during report. Thus, it is important to be proactive and have the order discontinued. You should also document the patient's wishes in his plan of care.
4. **Answer: a**
   RATIONALE: A family conflict can arise when values differ between family members. This often occurs when various family members are in different stages of development. A healthcare conflict occurs when the values of the individual patient or family differ from the healthcare system as a whole.
5. **Answer: d**
   RATIONALE: This example illustrates the four components of nursing malpractice. The nurse had a duty to this patient as he was assigned to her care. The nurse did not act in a manner that a reasonably prudent nursing professional would do by failing to check the patient's allergies prior to administering a medication. The act of the nurse resulted in harm to the patient as he was intubated. It is clear that causation exists because the patient had a documented allergy and exhibited signs of an allergic reaction.
6. **Answer: a**
   RATIONALE: The Good Samaritan Law offers legal immunity for healthcare professionals who assist in an emergency and render reasonable care under such circumstances. A nurse who helps is obligated to remain until additional assistance is obtained. The nurse should then relinquish care to official rescue personnel unless asked to remain.

CHAPTER 7

SECTION II: ASSESSING YOUR UNDERSTANDING

Activity A FILL IN THE BLANKS

1. Transitional
2. Research
3. Outcome
4. Fundamental
5. Qualitative
6. Foreground
7. Variables
8. Confidentiality

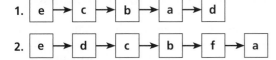

Activity B MATCHING

1 – A,   2 – B,   3 – B,   4 – B,   5 – A

Activity C ORDERING

1. e → c → b → a → d

2. e → d → c → b → f → a

Activity D SHORT ANSWER

1. A literature review allows the researcher the opportunity to see what research has already been done on the subject they want to explore. This prevents duplication of research efforts and can reveal areas where little is known on the subject. Literature can be based on evidence by varying degrees so it is important that the research know what study qualities to look for.

2. Institutional review boards (IRBs) protect the rights of study participants. IRBs were developed in response to inhumane studies that were performed on human subjects in concentration camps during World War II. Other similar historical studies have placed subjects at risk and have profoundly illustrated the need for governing bodies to protect study participants.

3. Within a problem statement, a relationship is expressed between two or more variables which can be described as independent for dependent. Independent variables are presumed to have an effect of the dependent variable and can be manipulated by the researcher. Dependent variables are supposed to change in relationship to the independent variable.

4. Dissemination can occur by several means. Results can be communicated by oral or poster presentation or by publication in a widely distributed journal.

5. The goal of evidence-based practice (EBP) is to provide patients with the best care possible. In EBP, the practitioner uses research evidence to guide their care and to ensure favorable outcomes.

SECTION III: APPLYING YOUR KNOWLEDGE

Activity E CASE STUDY

1. Some examples of a foreground question for this patient and others like him include:
   A. In patients predisposed to type II diabetes, what is the effect of dieting and exercise in comparison to diet alone, on lowering hemoglobin A1c levels?
   B. For patients predisposed to type II diabetes, does hemoglobin A1c yield more accurate diagnostic information than random blood glucose level testing for type II diabetes?
   C. For patients predisposed to type II diabetes, does having a diagnosis of hypertension and hyperlipidemia compared to having no medical conditions, increase the risk of developing type II diabetes.

2. The first step to finding the most up-to-date information to give patient's like Bill is to know where to look to find up-to-date research. There are many sources of information out there and much information can be found through the internet. But, not all sources are reliable. Indexes such as Cumulative Index to Nursing and Allied Health Literature are good places to find primary studies. Books can offer overviews of areas as well as provide sources for original articles. Also, once pertinent studies are found, it is important to be able to critically appraise each one as not all studies are created equal.

SECTION IV: PRACTICING FOR NCLEX

Activity F MULTIPLE CHOICE

1. **Answer: b**
   RATIONALE: Qualitative research is the systematic collection of subjective data. Information such as thoughts or feelings that this population might have regarding the care that they receive cannot be quantified and very little control is imposed on the research participants by the researcher. Although Kathleen has not placed a lot of control over her research subjects, nurses, she is collecting numeric data that can be analyzed statistically. This would be considered a quantitative research project. Because Jason is measuring a change in knowledge by analyzing quiz scores, this would be considered a quantitative experiment. Marta is relying on serum levels to look for a statistical correlation between Crohn's disease and iron deficiency anemia, which would be considered quantitative.

2. **Answer: a**
   RATIONALE: Dorothea identified a problem that she saw in her practice. She then performed a literature review on respected medical sites. Next she took the information she gained and applied it to patients in her practice. Although there may be a vast amount of research done on the use of central line dressing kits, Jared has not taken the time to critically look for the evidence. Maggie is choosing to ignore research finding because, anecdotally, ciprofloxacin works. Unfortunately, if a resistant strain infected one of her patients she would be undertreating them and serious sequelae could occur. We are not given enough information to determine if the information regarding aspirin use in this population is based on research. Dora's argument might be strengthened if she cited some valid studies.

3. **Answer: a**
   RATIONALE: Cytochrome P450 are required for metabolism of medications. Nursing research is defined as a systematic inquiry into the problems encountered in nursing practice and into the modalities of patient care such as health appraisal, prevention of trauma, promotion of recovery, and coordination of healthcare (Gortner, 1975).

4. **Answer: e**
   RATIONALE: Authority, Currency, Objectivity, and coverage are just a few of the criteria used to determine is website content is valid, accurate, and reliable.

5. Answer: a

RATIONALE: The nurse with an associate degree will assist in collection of data within an established, structured format. The nurse with a bachelor's degree will read, interprets, and evaluate research for applicability to nursing practice. They will identify nursing problems that need to be investigated and participates in implementation of scientific studies. The nurse with a master's degree in nursing will analyzes and reformulates nursing practice problems so that scientific knowledge and scientific method can be used to find solutions.

6. Answer: c

RATIONALE: A problem statement identifies the direction that a research project will take. It should be introduced at the beginning of a research project and include a population to be studied as well as express a relationship between two or more variables. A problem statement that contains a judgment or that is asking about ethics, morals, or values, is not amenable to the research process.

7. Answers: a, b, c, d

RATIONALE: The first step is the nurse assesses the problem; the second step is to determine the appropriate nursing diagnosis, the third step involves the nurse planning an intervention. In this case, Marion starts a group therapy session for the residents so they can discuss their experiences with depression. Finally, the nurse evaluates the outcome.

CHAPTER 8

SECTION II: ASSESSING YOUR UNDERSTANDING

Activity A FILL IN THE BLANKS

1. Shared
2. Psychomotor
3. Wellness, prevent
4. Baseline
5. Priority
6. Adherence
7. Literacy
8. Role play
9. Model
10. Outcomes

Activity B MATCHING

1. 1 – C,   2 – A,   3 – D,   4 – B
2. 1 – B,   2 – D,   3 – C,   4 – E,   5 – A

Activity C SEQUENCING

1.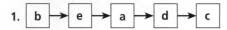

Activity D SHORT ANSWER

1. Patient focus means that teaching is geared toward the patient's needs or knowledge gaps. This means that teaching needs can vary from patient to patient, even if the diagnosis is the same. A

patient's background and their own experience with the diagnosis will affect the focus of teaching. Also, a patient's personal belief about wellness or a disease process, their value of the healthcare system and personal values will affect teaching needs.

2. Health promotion and disease prevention both share the common goal of improving one's health. Health promotion is a means to help patient's take control of their health. The focus is on global improvement of health and well-being. Disease prevention typically focuses on avoidance of one particular disease process.

3. Primary prevention is an activity that promotes health and wellness. An example is engaging in exercise five times per week. Secondary prevention targets the prevention of a specific disease or illness. An example is vaccination against influenza. Tertiary prevention aims to restore optimum function after a disease has already occurred. An example is adherence to a low sodium diet following a myocardial infarction.

4. Language is a major barrier in healthcare. Language discrepancy can interfere with informed consent, teaching, and patient's expression of their wishes. Spiritual and cultural beliefs affect how patient's views a disease process and the treatment for that process. This affects adherence to medication or therapeutic regimens and understanding of teaching instructions.

5. Always read any written material prior to distribution and make sure that your verbal communication matches what is distributed. If the patient has a low literacy level, use written material that has short sentences and small words. Typically, written material should be below a sixth-grade reading level. Assess the size of print for visual impairment. Provide a patient with one or two carefully selected documents rather than barraging them with massive amounts of literature. If possible, highlight key phrases for the patient.

6. The patient should be awake, alert, and comfortable. Identify if the patient would like to have any friends or family members present. Teaching should be scheduled so that it is not interrupted; it should not be scheduled during mealtime or if the patient plans to have visitors or a procedure. Teaching should not be done immediately prior to a major event, such as a surgery. The patient is unlikely to focus on teaching if they are concerned about such an event. Teaching should also be time limited to about 20 to 30 minutes. Have any written information ready to distribute.

SECTION III: APPLYING YOUR KNOWLEDGE

Activity E CASE STUDY

1. Mr. Morgan is in the preparation stage of the Transtheoretical Model of Change. He is planning for

change by asking for a prescription for a new medication to help him.

2. Health-seeking behavior RT increased awareness from media information AEB patient seeking a new medication that he learned about on television.

3. Middle-aged learners appreciate praise, and Mr. Morgan should be praised for his decision. Adult learners like to feel respected and that the baseline knowledge they bring to the conversation is appreciated. However, misconceptions may need to be corrected. Adult learners respond well to straightforward approaches where they can apply the knowledge immediately.

4. First, Mr. Morgan's learning needs must be assessed. Engage Mr. Morgan in a discussion to determine his baseline knowledge about the medications' side effects. You may also ask Mr. Morgan what tools he would like to help inform him of these side effects. This will help you determine how Mr. Morgan prefers to learn. Come prepared with written information that is at a sixth-grade reading level. Highlight key passages, particularly noting side effects that may decrease adherence to the medication regimen.

SECTION IV: PRACTICING FOR NCLEX

Activity F MULTIPLE CHOICE

1. **Answer: c**
   RATIONALE: The precontemplation stage is the first stage change in which the patient does not indicate that he will make any changes within the next 6 months. Mr. Milner gives no indication that he will be ready to change his diet within the next 6 months.

2. **Answer: a**
   RATIONALE: The education that you provide has influenced the value some of her patient place on their food choices. This is the definition of affective learning.

3. **Answer: c**
   RATIONALE: Secondary prevention seeks to identify specific illnesses or conditions at an early stage with prompt intervention to prevent or limit disability.

4. **Answer: a**
   RATIONALE: Mrs. Shields is in the preparation stage as she is actively making changes to lose weight. She has moved beyond the contemplation stage by obtaining a gym membership and enrolling in classes.

5. **Answer: a**
   RATIONALE: Preschool age children (2 to 5 years) have short attention spans. Five- to ten-minute blocks of time are age appropriate. A 30-minute block is more appropriate for an older patient.

6. **Answer: a**
   RATIONALE: Using the zero to ten scale is a key aspect of assessing importance with motivational interviewing. It helps you to understand the patient's feelings toward the recommended activ-

ity and can help start a conversation about why they chose that number and what they could do to increase the number.

7. **Answer: a**
   RATIONALE: Peers are often more influential than parents, nurses or teachers at this age. It is often appropriate to include a close friend in on the teaching session.

8. **Answers: a, b, c**
   RATIONALE: Allowing Zach to practice his own insulin injections is developmentally appropriate. However, Zach is not developmentally ready to be solely responsible for his own medication administration. Since his mother is Zach's primary caregiver, you would need to work with Zach's mother to help her become comfortable with administration of this new medication.

9. **Answers: a, b, c**
   RATIONALE: The internet can be a wonderful resource for patients to learn about a new diagnosis. However, there are reports of websites not maintaining up-to-date information. A reputable website should provide the date in which it was last updated and reviewed.

10. **Answers: a, d**
    RATIONALE: There is no evidence of cognitive limitations or lack of motivation in this example.

CHAPTER 9

SECTION II: ASSESSING YOUR UNDERSTANDING

Activity A FILL IN THE BLANKS

1. 12.8
2. Southern
3. Delirium
4. Depression
5. Urge
6. Integrity
7. Nutritional
8. Double
9. Emotion
10. Palliative

Activity B MATCHING

1. 1 C,   2 – E,   3 – B,   4 – A,   5 – D

Activity C SHORT ANSWER

1. Antipsychotic medications carry the risk of side effects that place the older adult at risk for adverse events. These events include falls, increased confusion, and cardiovascular events.

2. Self-care activities are also referred to as "activities of daily living". Self-care refers to a wide range of activities from shopping and managing finances to bathing and brushing ones teeth. Typically, dementia tends to affect higher level functioning first. These activities include managing

finances, shopping and driving. As dementia progresses, basic self-care activities are affected such as the ability to bathe, use the toilet, and feed oneself.

3. Falls are the number one cause of injury-related disability and death in the older adult. Changes in gait and balance, delays in reaction time, and changes in vision all contribute to falls. Additionally, many older adults have increased need to urinate, especially in the middle of the night. Medications can contribute by causing confusion, orthostatic hypotension, and cognitive changes.

4. Older adults may experience losses related to health, significant others (spouses, family, friends, pets), finances, geography (e.g., moves to assisted living or long-term care facilities), and leisure activities. Initial grief reactions include shock, disbelief, anger, or denial of the loss. The severity and length of the grieving (or bereavement) varies with the individual and the type of loss. Social support, therapy, and religious faith are sources of adaptive coping. Nursing interventions that focus on developing or enhancing coping strategies are appropriate in this scenario.

5. Persistent depressed mood (most days for 2 weeks) or loss of interest in previously pleasurable activities must be present. Other symptoms include significant change in weight or appetite; sleep disturbance (increased or decreased); psychomotor retardation or agitation; fatigue; feelings of worthlessness or inappropriate guilt; poor cognitive performance or diminished ability to think or concentrate, or indecisiveness; and recurrent thoughts of death or suicidal ideation.

SECTION III: APPLYING YOUR KNOWLEDGE

Activity D CASE STUDY

1. A history of the original incident including events that lead up to the fall. History of musculoskeletal conditions including arthritis, gait disturbance or previous surgeries. List of medications including those that affect cognition, balance, dieresis or blood pressure. Perceived environmental hazards including stairs, loose cords, loose carpeting or piles of personal items. Presence and use of assistive devices. History of cognitive or mood impairments.

2. Older women are twice as likely to suffer from incontinence than men. Urge incontinence results from an overactive detrusor muscle causing increased bladder contractions. Stress incontinence results from a weakened pelvic floor and is particularly common in women who have had multiple pregnancies. Incontinence often causes patients to rush to the bathroom, setting them up for a risk of falls.

3. Persistent depressed mood or loss of interest in previously pleasurable activities must be present. Other symptoms include significant change in weight or

appetite; sleep disturbance (increased or decreased); psychomotor retardation or agitation; fatigue; feelings of worthlessness or inappropriate guilt; poor cognitive performance or diminished ability to think or concentrate, or indecisiveness; and recurrent thoughts of death or suicidal ideation.

4. Deficits in self-care are signs of cognitive impairment. Early signs of cognitive impairment include avoidance of shopping, cooking, and management of finances. Late signs include the inability to bathe, feed oneself, or ambulate. These late signs often require that the patient be placed in an institution.

SECTION IV: PRACTICING FOR NCLEX

Activity E MULTIPLE CHOICE

1. **Answer: a**
   RATIONALE: Hydromorphone is a narcotic agent which is often constipating in older adults. Psyllium helps promote regular bowel elimination. Acetaminophen is not linked to constipation. Furosemide is used as a diuretic. It does not cause constipation.

2. **Answer: c**
   RATIONALE: Hemiparesis is weakness on one side of the body.

3. **Answer: b**
   RATIONALE: As mobility impairment increases in persons over the age of 65, the risk of falls increases. Hip fractures are a particular risk factor for disability and death.

4. **Answer: a**
   RATIONALE: Medications are typically the last choice for treating sleep disturbance because they can interact with other medications or have paradoxical effects on the older adult.

5. **Answer: d**
   RATIONALE: The Braden scale is an evidence-based tool used to assess for pressure ulcers. Pressure ulcers can result from urinary incontinence, particularly if the skin is moist and skin integrity is impaired. Ruth would likely require assistance every time she uses the toilet. A Foley catheter is an extreme solution to this problem.

6. **Answer: a**
   RATIONALE: One sign of depression is a lack of interest in previously enjoyable activities. Further investigation is necessary to make a formal diagnosis.

7. **Answer: c**
   RATIONALE: Decongestants can worsen insomnia in the older adult.

8. **Answers: a, b**
   RATIONALE: As people age, their immune system becomes less efficient. Their humoral immunity declines due to diminished T cell function and older adults have lower antibody response following respiratory infections to fight off pneumonia. Nutrition does not contribute to immune system function in older adults and alcoholism may contribute to depression by not diminished immune function.

9. **Answers, a, b, c**
   RATIONALE: Depression is often under diagnosed in the older adult. Patients suffering from multiple health issues are more likely to report depression than their healthier counterparts. If the patient has recently changed housing that, will also put a patient at risk for depression. Older Caucasin males have the highest rate of suicide in the United States.

CHAPTER 10

SECTION II: ASSESSING YOUR UNDERSTANDING

Activity A FILL IN THE BLANKS

1. Individualized
2. Patient
3. Reasoning
4. Diagnosis
5. Evaluation
6. Nonverbal
7. Reasoning
8. Reflection
9. Expert
10. Competence
11. Patient centered
12. Process
13. Proficient

Activity B MATCHING

1. 1 – D,   2 – E,   3 – C,   4 – A,   5 – B

Activity C SHORT ANSWER

1. Primary sources of information come from the patient herself. This is gathered from observation, interview, or examination. Primary sources also include diagnostic tests and laboratory data. A secondary source is any source of information about the patient that is obtained via another source. Examples of secondary sources include information from family members, significant others, other healthcare professionals, and healthcare records.
2. The nursing process serves as a systematic template to develop a nursing care plan for any patient in any situation. The nursing process helps the nurse tailor the plan of care to the unique needs of the patient. Thus, the patient and nurse are a team when setting priorities and goals and developing appropriate interventions.
3. The nurse can anticipate questions that a patient, physician, or fellow nurse would ask and mentally prepare an answer. The nurse can also anticipate what the patient might do next and think through the scenario. For instance, what would the nurse do if the patient suddenly decompensate? What if they suddenly improve? A nurse who engages in critical thinking actively looks for answers to questions rather than accepting the fact that they do not know. When a critical thinker makes a mistake, that nurse turns the mistake into a learning opportunity

and thinks through ways to prevent the error from happening again.
4. Reflection-in-action occurs in the moment of clinical practice. This skill allows the nurse to analyze the appropriateness of nursing actions and interventions as they happen. Reflection-on-action occurs after an event is completed. A nurse can take time to consider what went well and what could be improved upon in any given situation. Both skills are critical when developing critical thinking skills.
5. A *novice* has little to no experience to base their clinical judgment and thus must rely on rules and guidelines to guide clinical practice. An *advanced beginner* also relies on guidelines and rules. However, the advanced beginner can now use clinical experience to question rules when they do not seem to apply to their patient. A nurse develops *competence* through experience, learns to question rules, and feels responsible for outcomes. As a nurse becomes *proficient,* she realizes that events, context, and situation are as important as the nurses' knowledge and resources and thinking that is fluid, flexible, and intuitive. The *expert* nurse can effortlessly link theory, practice, and intuition to provide care.

SECTION III: APPLYING YOUR KNOWLEDGE

Activity D CASE STUDY

1. Mr. Simmons may find that he wants to use his time with family and friends to focus on their experiences rather than the end of his life. Perhaps the role of Mr. Simmons within the family is that of the listener, and he is using his last days to provide support to his family as he has for many years. In the evenings, he again may wish to reflect on the joyful times in his life. He may also be quite social, but worries that he will cause grief for his family if he reflects on their time together.
2. Information from a primary source is information from the patient himself. An example of primary information would be his quiet demeanor during family visits. An example of information from a secondary source is his wife telling you that this is the most at peace she has seen Mr. Simmons in a long time.

SECTION IV: PRACTICING FOR NCLEX

Activity E MULTIPLE CHOICE

1. **Answer: c**
   RATIONALE: The novice must rely on rules and guidelines to guide clinical judgment. The novice does not yet have the clinical expertise to use previous experiences to think outside of the box.
2. **Answer: a**
   RATIONALE: Active listening is a skill that requires you as the nurse to pay attention to both nonverbal cues and spoken responses.

3. Answer: c
   RATIONALE: Nurse Chen assessing relevant information to formulate a nursing diagnosis and plan for her patient. Information obtained from the literature is an example of a secondary source of information.
4. Answer: b
   RATIONALE: The patient is always considered the primary source of information. Primary information is obtained through interview, examination, laboratory, and diagnostic findings. Secondary information is obtained via sources external to the patient such as family members or outside health records.
5. Answer: b
   RATIONALE: This example illustrates several phases of the nursing process. You evaluated that your plan of ambulating twice that day was unsuccessful. Your next step is to revise the plan based on this evaluation.
6. Answer: d
   RATIONALE: Assessment is the first phase of the nursing process and refers to the evaluation or appraisal of the patient's health state.
7. Answer: c
   RATIONALE: Clinical reasoning occurs when you apply textbook knowledge to an actual patient scenario. In this case, you recognize a drop in blood pressure and the inability to orient to person, place, and time as signs of clinical deterioration.
8. Answers: a, b
   RATIONALE: Interpretation of evidence is a task of analysis. The revision of a plan is a skill in explanation.

CHAPTER 11

SECTION II: ASSESSING YOUR UNDERSTANDING

Activity A FILL IN THE BLANKS

1. Assessment
2. Observation
3. Interviewing
4. Inspection
5. Auscultation
6. Objective
7. Secondary
8. Frameworks
9. Admission
10. Palpation

Activity B MATCHING

1. 1 – B,   2 – D,   3 – A,   4 – C
2. 1 – C,   2 – A,   3 – B,   4 – D,   5 – E

Activity C ORDERING

1.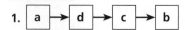

Activity D SHORT ANSWER

1. Setting and environment are important because how much a patient shares depends greatly on how comfortable they feel. They can give you their full attention if there are not distractions and the area needs to be quiet and provide for the patient's privacy. Taking all of this into consideration allows the freedom to talk opening and honestly and to focus on the questions you are asking.
2. Smell is a part of the observation process. Certain odors are indicative of someone's physical condition. For example, someone who smells of urine could have issues with cleanliness or with urinary incontinence.
3. The nursing history elicits subjective data from the patient or family. It helps the nurse clarify the patient's perception of their health status, compare the patient's health status currently to what is was like in the past, identify nursing diagnoses, develop a plan of care for this patient, and implement interventions specific to this patient.
4. Data gathered from secondary sources can help to clarify information obtained from the patient. Family members can give other perspectives and may have details that the patient might have forgotten about. Health records, which include written reports from other health team members, provide information on the person's past and current medical conditions and give the current nurse a point of comparison for their assessment. Laboratory tests and diagnostic procedures offer supplemental information about the person's physical status and can be used to monitor interventions. A literature review can provide current information on medical diagnoses, treatments, and follow-up.
5. Data that are collected can often be interpreted in many ways. In order to properly analyze the data, and to then come up with an appropriate nursing diagnosis, the information must be confirmed.

SECTION III: APPLYING YOUR KNOWLEDGE

Activity E CASE STUDY

1. Because this is an admission assessment, I know that I am going to have to be thorough. This assessment will provide a comparison for all subsequent assessments. I want to first set up an environment where the patient feels comfortable enough to share in-depth information about herself. Next, I will look through her chart to gather any information that I can before meeting with her. When I introduce myself, I will explain my role and begin to establish rapport. During the maintenance phase of the interview I will focus on gathering information by encouraging the patient to be an active participant and by keeping focused on the task at hand. Next we will review the information together. After completing the interview, I will move to the physical exam portion where I will utilize the four techniques of inspection, palpation, percussion, and auscultation to gather objective data. After validating the information that I gather, I will then organize and analyze the data in order to come up with a nursing diagnosis.

2. There are various frameworks that one could use to gather all pertinent information about this patient. For this patient I would choose to use a combination of the three models mentioned in this chapter. During the interview process, the functional health patterns model would help me identify Natalia's normal function as well as her risk for altered function. For example, I would want to talk to her about how she is coping with this new diagnosis. This would allow me to identify if she is coping well or if one of my nursing diagnosis would need to focus on improving her coping skills. I could utilize the body systems model to go through each body system and identify any other symptoms she might have. Besides possibly having an enlarged thyroid, she may have scattered symptoms such as lethargy, weight gain or loss, a cough, and difficulty swallowing. I would also want to utilize the head-to-toe model to guide me through a systematic physical examination of this patient.

SECTION IV: PRACTICING FOR NCLEX

Activity F MULTIPLE CHOICE

1. Answer: a

RATIONALE: In the functional health patterns model, the patient's strengths, talents, and functional health patterns are an integral part of the assessment data. This framework identifies strengths as well as deficits. The body systems' model starts with an assessment of the patient's general state of health and then moves to a systematic assessment of each body system. By systematically assessing each organ system using the body systems' model, the nurse may reveal information that the patient did not consider important.

2. Answer: b, d

RATIONALE: Assessing your own feelings or reactions regarding previous patients that might interfere with this relationship is addressed in the preparatory phase of the interview. The nurse will review the goal or task attainment in the concluding phase of the interview.

3. Answer: c

RATIONALE: Symptoms such as muscle pain or myalgia are considered subjective cues in a patient's health history. Signs of illness, such as temperature, leukoplakia, ptosis not oriented to time or situation, are considered objective cues in a health history.

4. Answer: a

RATIONALE: Auscultation is the technique of listening to body sounds with a stethoscope placed on the body surface. A visual examination is conduction in the inspection phase of assessment. Palpation is the specialized use of touch for data collection. Percussion is the technique in which one or both hands are used to strike the body surface in a precise manner. The physical examination is the systematic data collection method that uses the four senses to detect health problems.

5. Answer: d

RATIONALE: A time-lapse reassessment is performed in ordered to reevaluate any changes in the patient's health from a previous assessment. It is used to monitor the status of an already identified problem.

6. Answers: a, b, c

RATIONALE: Using broad opening statements, sharing observations and using silence are just a few of the techniques nurses use to establish rapport, elicit patients' thoughts and feelings, and encourage conversation and understanding.

CHAPTER 12

SECTION II: ASSESSING YOUR UNDERSTANDING

Activity A FILL IN THE BLANKS

1. Interpretation
2. Disease, Response
3. Collaborative
4. Cues
5. Interpretation
6. Mentor
7. "as evidenced by"
8. Specificity

Activity B MATCHING MATCHING

1. 1 – C,   2 – A,   3 – D,   4 – E,   5 – B
2. 1 – D,   2 – A,   3 – B,   4 – C,   5 – E

Activity C ORDERING

1.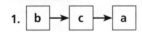

Activity D SHORT ANSWER

1. Nursing diagnoses carry legal ramifications. A nurse can only make a diagnosis that can be identified within the scope of nursing practice. The nurse must be able to act on these problems independently. A nurse cannot make a medical diagnosis or prescribe treatment unless the nurse has an advanced practice license.

2. Individually, each clue provides insight into a patient's condition. When these clues are clustered together a nurse is given a picture of the patient's condition. Clustering therefore helps the nurse derive meaning from the cues.

3. The nurse is collecting cues throughout the course of care for a patient via verbal and nonverbal communication and environmental observation. The nurse must intellectually synthesize these cues in order to formulate appropriate nursing diagnoses and care plans. It is only by clustering cues that the nurse is able to see the entire picture.

4. An actual diagnosis describes a patient's response to a health problem that is currently manifesting itself. A risk for diagnosis describes a patient who's condition makes them particularly vulnerable to a health problem. A wellness diagnosis describes the human response to levels of wellness or readiness for enhancement. A possible nursing diagnosis describes a health problem that the nurse is not sure the patient has but would like to collect more evidence to determine if it is a true problem.

5. The focus of assessment of a nursing diagnosis is to monitor the human response to actual and potential health problems. In collaborative diagnoses, the focus of the assessment is on the pathophysiology. A nursing diagnosis is both identified and treated independently of a physician or advanced practice provider, where a collaborative diagnosis is addressed with the advanced practice team.

SECTION III: APPLYING YOUR KNOWLEDGE

Activity E CASE STUDY

1. Grieving related to loss of normal feeding behavior as evidenced by maternal expressed sorrow. Ineffective breastfeeding related to lip and palate anomaly as evidenced by patient's inability to latch. Impaired tissue integrity related to congenital anomaly as evidenced by visualization of cleft lip and palate.
2. Risk for ineffective role performance related to change in the physical ability to breastfeed. Risk for situational low self-esteem related to unanticipated congenital defect. Risk for disturbed body image related to lip anomaly and postoperative scarring.

SECTION IV: PRACTICING FOR NCLEX

Activity F MULTIPLE CHOICE

1. **Answer: c**
   Both gastroesophageal reflux and cellulitis are medical diagnosis. Ineffective airway clearance is an appropriate diagnostic label. However, a patient not speaking does not match the diagnosis.
2. **Answer: a**
   Any of these choices could be a clue to caregiver role strain when clustered with other evidence. However, the inability to care for oneself strongly indicates that this woman is not coping well.
3. **Answer: d**
   This is the definition of a possible nursing diagnosis. The statement is phrased the same way as an actual problem except that the "related to" phrase is "unknown etiology".
4. **Answer: a**
   When considering the responses, first check for sentence structure. Only one of the choices contains the three elements of the nursing diagnosis: the diagnostic label, the related factors and the defining characteristics. The question asks for an actual diagnosis; this eliminates any risk, wellness, or potential diagnoses.

5. **Answer: b**
   RATIONALE: Premature closure is when the nurse selects a nursing diagnosis before analyzing all of the pertinent information in the patient's case. The nurse did not investigate any other information in this case before making her diagnosis. Inconsistent cues occur when the meaning attached to one cue may be altered based on another cue. The patient did not provide any additional cues for this to be the correct answer. Clustering of cues is a clustering of data.
6. **Answer: a**
   RATIONALE: This is an actual diagnosis as it contains the diagnostic label (acute pain), related factors (instillation of peritoneal dialysate), and defining characteristics (wincing, grimacing during procedure, stabbing). Risk Diagnosis is a two-part statement includes diagnostic label and risk factors. Wellness diagnosis is one-part statement that includes diagnostic label. Potential diagnosis is a two-part statement that includes diagnostic label and unknown related factors.
7. **Answer: d**
   RATIONALE: Risk for falls related to altered mobility is an accurately phrased risk diagnosis. It is a two part statement that contains the diagnostic statement (altered mobility) and risk factors (risk for falls).
8. **Answer: b, c, e, f**
   RATIONALE: Defining characteristics are the observable "cues or inferences that cluster as manifestations of an actual illness or wellness health state." (NANDA, 2009). Related factors describe the condition, circumstances, or etiologies that contribute to the problem. Descriptors are words used to give additional meaning to a nursing diagnosis. Each approved NANDA-I nursing diagnosis have a definition that describes the characteristics of the human response under consideration. Rick factors describes the clinical cues in risk nursing diagnoses and are not used in actual nursing diagnosis.

CHAPTER 13

SECTION II: ASSESSING YOUR UNDERSTANDING

Activity A FILL IN THE BLANKS

1. Outcomes
2. Life-threatening
3. Week
4. Treatment
5. Decision-making
6. Priority
7. Patient
8. Cost-efficient
9. Multidisciplinary
10. Variance

Activity B MATCHING

1. 1 – D,   2 – A,   3 – B,   4 – E,   5 – B

Activity C SHORT ANSWER

1. Outcome identification serves four purposes. It allows nurses to provide individualized care, promote patient participation, plan care that is realistic and measurable and allow for the involvement of family or support people.
2. The five components of outcome criteria are: 1. *Subject:* Who is the person expected to achieve the goal? 2. *Verb:* What actions must the person do to achieve the goal? 3. *Condition:* Under what circumstances is the person to perform the action? 4. *Criteria:* How well is the person to perform the action? 5. *Specific time:* When is the person expected to perform the action? All five of these must be included in an outcome criteria statement.
3. The plan of care is a critical aspect of focusing patient care. The plan of care helps to set up the evaluation criteria and reflects the standards of practice of the institution. A documented plan of care is required by the Joint Commission, Medicare, and Medicaid.
4. The individual healthcare agency is responsible for developing a critical path. Critical paths may be shared between institutions, however, and agencies like Medicaid have influence on the critical path. The purpose of the critical path is to determine an expected course for a patient's hospitalization based on the patient's diagnosis. The critical path helps the nurse develop a plan of care because it provides critical information such as when a patient is expected to be ambulatory after surgery and when discharge is expected.
5. Variance occurs when the patient's condition or an unforeseen complication causes the patient to deviate from the critical path. Variance should be well documented because it helps with retrospective analysis and may modify and agencies critical path. Documentation of variance may also help with third-party reimbursement for extended hospital stay.

SECTION III: APPLYING YOUR KNOWLEDGE

Activity D CASE STUDY

1. A critical path assists the multidisciplinary team understand what to expect from most of the patients who undergo a particular procedure or have a particular diagnosis. In this case, the critical path may dictate when a patient is expected to be ambulatory, resume enteral feeding, and helps the team develop a plan for discharge.
2. (Answers will vary). *Use of SCD's:* Prolonged immobility leads to venous stasis. *Use of incentive spirometer:* Prolonged immobility leads to increased susceptibility to respiratory infections. *Offer moist toothette sponges:* Oral hygiene helps to prevent respiratory complications.

3. The patient will take 100 cc clear liquids by mouth without evidence of gastrointestinal distress at 12 PM.

SECTION IV: PRACTICING FOR NCLEX

Activity E MULTIPLE CHOICE

1. **Answer: a**
   RATIONALE: A sickle cell crisis is an extremely painful event. Most patients with sickle cell have an individualized narcotic plan that will help them to receive narcotics in an expedited manner when they present in crisis. The slight elevation in Jamal's BP and HR are likely secondary to pain. There is no evidence of respiratory illness based on the information given. Tylenol is not strong enough to treat pain. Further, Jamal does not have a fever.
2. **Answer: c**
   RATIONALE: Airway impairment is considered a life-threatening emergency. This must be assessed and resolved before proceeding with other tasks.
3. **Answers: a, b**
   RATIONALE: The action is one of the essential pieces of a nursing outcome criteria statement.
4. **Answer: d**
   RATIONALE: Outcome criteria are specific, measurable, realistic statements that can be evaluated to judge goal attainment.
5. **Answer: a**
   RATIONALE: The nursing rationale is the "why". Students will often reference textbooks and journal articles to justify their actions in a care plan, and the rationale is termed "scientific rationale".
6. **Answer: c**
   RATIONALE: The critical path is based on large bodies of research and provides information on the expected course of a patient's treatment or illness. Deviations from the critical path are documented in the individualized plan of care.
7. **Answer: b**
   RATIONALE: Documentation should be specific. The evaluation is a form of communication with the multidisciplinary healthcare team.
8. **Answer: a**
   RATIONALE: Nursing outcomes should include five components: Subject, Verb, Condition, Criteria, Specific time.
9. **Answers: a, b**
   RATIONALE: Patient's on bed rest must have a medical order to begin ambulation. Acetaminophen must be prescribed by a licensed practitioner in the inpatient setting.
10. **Answers: b, c, d**
    RATIONALE: Feedings should begin slowly with clear liquids as the first food. Immediately resuming a standard diet after a period of NPO is likely to result in GI distress.

11. Answers: c, d
RATIONALE: Ambulation is not a developmentally appropriate task, nor is it appropriate s/p femoral fracture. Complete resolution of a pressure ulcer is not likely to be realistic; more information is needed.

12. Answers: a, b, c
RATIONALE: The goal of outcome identification is to provide individualized care, not standardized care.

CHAPTER 14

SECTION II: ASSESSING YOUR UNDERSTANDING

Activity A FILL IN THE BLANKS

1. Implementation
2. Intellectual
3. Priorities
4. Delegate
5. Collaborative
6. Coordinating
7. Maintenance
8. Effectiveness
9. Response
10. Structure
11. Ambiguous
12. Removed

Activity B MATCHING

1. 1 – E,   2 – A,   3 – B,   4 – D,   5 – C
2. 1 –D,   2 – A,   3 – C,   4 – E,   5 – B

Activity C SHORT ANSWER

1. Assessment is an ongoing part of the nursing process. Reassessment is actively searching for changes in the patient condition. Recognition of subtle cues allows the nurse to recognize emerging problems early on.
2. Nurses use theoretical teaching and learning models to educate patients and families about their healthcare needs. These teaching methods are often used during a hospital stay and planning for discharge. In the community setting, nurses may use teaching to educate patients about their home or the environment in which they live. Nurses base their teaching on their assessment of a patient's knowledge, willingness to carry out a plan, and physical and psychological ability to carry out a plan.
3. The nurse is responsible for overseeing the patient's overall care. However, nurses cannot act alone on a healthcare team. A nurse may need to delegate tasks to support staff in order to accomplish all tasks for the day. However, the nurse remains responsible for the completion of the tasks; she must ensure that the task is completed and that it is completed correctly. Nurses also supervise patients and families as they transition from a dependent patient role toward independence. A nurse must work with the patient by demonstrating tasks with patients performing return demonstrations.

4. Coordinating interventions are those in which a nurse may act as a patient advocate, collaborate with other members of the healthcare team, or ensure that a patient's schedule is therapeutic to allow plenty of time for rest and healing. Supportive interventions emphasize the nurses' role of supporting the patient with good communication skills and caring behavior. Psychosocial interventions focus on solving the patient's emotional, psychological, or social problems.

5. Evaluation is the nurses' judgment of the effectiveness of an intervention. Such information is vital when planning future interventions and allows the nurse to alter the plan of care if necessary. Evaluation is also a part of the learning process and will help the nurse learn how to plan interventions for patient populations.

6. Knowledge of the standards of care serves as a necessary framework to evaluate nursing practice. Formal education can provide a tremendous amount of knowledge about normal physiologic response. Awareness of current research helps nurses sharpen their assessment and diagnostic skills.

7. The ANA published an updated version of *Nursing: Standards of Practice* in 2004. The ANA included six standards of providing care to all patients. The ANA also included nine "standards of professional performance". These standards are used as measures of evaluation and nursing performance. Nurses who work in specialty groups have also developed their own process and outcome evaluations for specific nursing diagnoses. These were developed in conjunction with the ANA and are also considered standards for practice. The Joint Commission focuses on institutional policies and ensures that the institution functions within specific guidelines. Since the guidelines are general, institutions set up their own quality improvement programs to ensure that they meet the Joint Commission's general requirements.

SECTION III: APPLYING YOUR KNOWLEDGE

Activity D CASE STUDY

1. The risk for deficient fluid volume secondary to absence of IV or enteric fluid intake. The risk for infection secondary to presence of synthetic, externalized drain.
2. (Answers will vary). Based on the information provided, "risk for deficient fluid volume" as your nursing priority. One intellectual activity you could do is to analyze Mr. P's fluid status. You may come to the conclusion that Mr. P may need interim IV fluid until the bag of TPN arrives. This may lead you to collaborate with your physician colleagues to suggest ordering an interim fluid. One technical skill

you could apply in this situation is to assess the patency of the IV in Mr. P's hand. If the IV is not patent, you may start a new IV in anticipation of needing IV fluids.

SECTION IV: PRACTICING FOR NCLEX

Activity E MULTIPLE CHOICE

1. Answer: a
RATIONALE: Each of these factors contributes to the prioritization of nursing diagnoses except the patient's finances. The nursing code of ethics states that patients receive the same treatment regardless of their ability to pay.

2. Answer: c
RATIONALE: ABCs (Airway, Breathing and Circulation) are always top priority in patient care. In this example, ensuring that the patient maintains a patent airway will always be top priority. Each of these nursing tasks is important and will need to be accomplished at some point during patient care.

3. Answer: c
RATIONALE: An outcome evaluation determines the extent to which a patient's behavioral response to a nursing intervention reflects the outcome criteria.

4. Answer: b
RATIONALE: This question asks specifically about evaluation. Modeling self-care behaviors is an intervention, not an evaluation or assessment technique. When considering the responses, first check for sentence structure. Only one of the choices contains the three elements of the nursing diagnosis: the diagnostic label, the related factors, and the defining characteristics. The question asks for an actual diagnosis; this eliminates any risk, wellness, or potential diagnoses.

5. Answer: a
RATIONALE: Supportive interventions emphasize use of communication skills, relief of spiritual distress, and caring behaviors. Psychosocial interventions focus on resolving emotional, psychological, or social problems. Coordinating interventions involve many different activities such acting as a patient advocate, and making referrals for follow-up care. Supervisory interventions refer to overseeing the patient's overall healthcare.

6. Answer: a
RATIONALE: The nurse is supervising the patient's skill performance with regard to assuming responsibility for the self-management of his diet.

7. Answer: d
RATIONALE: Surveillance interventions include detecting changes from baseline data and recognizing abnormal response. Nurses rely on the senses to detect changes: observing the appearance and characteristics of patients; hearing by auscultation, pitch, and tone. Nurses use these surveillance

activities to determine the current status of patients and changes from previous states.

8. Answers: a, b, c
RATIONALE: Nurse Sanchez is exhibiting educational intervention as she is demonstrating to her patients how to prepare appropriate foods; psychosocial interventions in that she is focusing on resolving her patients cultural and social views on preparing foods that may not be healthy; supervisory intervention in that she is overseeing and encouraging patient changes regarding diet.

9. Answers: a, b, c
RATIONALE: Additionally, the NIC helps to expand the knowledge of similarities and differences across nursing diagnoses and explore nursing care information systems.

CHAPTER 15

SECTION II: ASSESSING YOUR UNDERSTANDING

Activity A FILL IN THE BLANKS

1. Documentation
2. Reporting
3. Confidentiality
4. Batch
5. Flowsheets
6. Variance
7. Handoff
8. Consults
9. Incident
10. Audit

Activity B MATCHING

1 – B,   2 – D,   3 – A,   4 – E,   5 – C

Activity C ORDERING

1.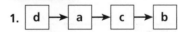

Activity D SHORT ANSWER

1. Timely documentation promotes efficiency and accuracy. Documentation that is done as care occurs, called point of care documentation, helps avoid errors that might occur from waiting and relying on memory. It also allows all other healthcare team members to have the most up-to-date information when considering future actions.
2. A nursing discharge summary is a plan that is started at the initiation of care, which indicates potential discharge needs and patient teaching that will take place. It also notes the patient's condition at discharge and provides information about care after discharge. A copy of this summary is given either to the patient or the patient's caregiver upon discharge.
3. Home care of patients on Medicare and Medicaid is documented by using the Outcome and Assessment Information Set. This tool measures the patient's status at various specified points during an episode

of care. These points put together provide the basis for measuring patient outcomes.

4. The Resident Assessment Instrument is a tool used to document in long-term care settings. It tracks goal achievement among residents of long-term care facilities. It can be used to collect minimum data sets which are mandated by Medicare, triggers, resident assessment protocols, and utilization guidelines. It helps to coordinate the efforts of all members of the healthcare team in order to optimize the resident's quality of life.

5. A care plan conference is a time when care team members gather together to discuss patient care. This is usually an interdisciplinary meeting that facilitates the coordination of services in an efficient manner. Patients who have complex issues involving multiple disciplines benefit the most from these conferences.

SECTION III: APPLYING YOUR KNOWLEDGE

Activity E CASE STUDY

1. Jan is a 38-year-old woman, c/o 1/10 pain in lower back. Denies any current burning with urination or blood in urine. Vital signs BP 122/63, HR 58, Temp. 102.8, O_2 saturations 99%. Currently febrile secondary to infectious process. Will notify primary provider of elevated temperature, draw blood cultures if warranted, and provide acetaminophen.

2. Jan has a temperature of 102.8, otherwise asymptomatic with normal BP and HR. She is a 38-year-old woman with a diagnosis of pyelonephritis, on 2 days of IV antibiotics. Elevated temperature secondary to recurrent versus resistant infection. Would recommend ordering for blood cultures and a urine culture. I will give acetaminophen and recheck temperature.

SECTION IV: PRACTICING FOR NCLEX

Activity F MULTIPLE CHOICE

1. **Answer: c**
   RATIONALE: Medical records are legal documents, communication tools, and assessment tools. They are used for care planning purposes, quality assurance purposes, for reimbursement, research, and education.

2. **Answer: a**
   RATIONALE: Quality assurance is when records are randomly selected to determine whether certain standards of care were met and documented. Care planning is when the nurse considers all data on the patient record when developing, goals, outcome criteria, interventions, and evaluation criteria for and with patients. Research is performed when data are gathered from groups of records to determine significant similarities in disease pre-

sentation, to identify contributing factors, or to determine the effectiveness of therapies. The medical record can be used for educational purposes such as when it is used, by a student, to learn how a disease might present itself in certain patients.

3. **Answer: b**
   RATIONALE: Information commonly found in a the patient care summary or kardex include, demographic data, code status, safety precautions, basis care needs such as activity status or diet, treatment such as vital sign schedule, IV therapy, and diagnostic or laboratory tests.

4. **Answer: b**
   RATIONALE: Charting by exception charts only that which falls outside the standard of care and norms.

5. **Answer: a**
   RATIONALE: A SOAP note consists of subjective information, objective information, an assessment, and a plan.

6. **Answer: c**
   RATIONALE: SBAR stands for Situation, Background, Assessment, and Recommendations.

7. **Answer: d**
   RATIONALE: FOCUS charting permits documentation on any significant topic. It is organized around data, action, and response.

8. **Answer: a**
   RATIONALE: PO signifies by mouth.

9. **Answer: b**
   RATIONALE: For legal reasons you should not attach a copy of the incident report to the chart. You should, however, fill out an incident report, stop the infusion and document the time, and report the error to the primary provider.

10. **Answer: a**
    RATIONALE: If a patient refuses a dose, it is important to circle that dose and write a note as to why you did not administer it.

11. **Answer: b**
    RATIONALE: A variance occurs when the patient does not proceed along a clinical pathway as planned.

12. **Answers: a, b, c, e**
    RATIONALE: Although batch charting is not ideal, it is not considered a high-risk error made in documentation. High-risk errors that are made include falsifying patient records, failure to record changes in patient's condition, failure to document that physician was notified when patient's condition changed, inadequate admission assessment, failure to document completely, failure to follow agency's standards or policies on documentation, and charting in advance.

13. **Answers: b, c, d, e**
    RATIONALE: The principles of proper documentation include confidentiality, accuracy, completeness, concise, objective, organized, timely, and legibility.

CHAPTER 16

SECTION II: ASSESSING YOUR UNDERSTANDING

Activity A FILL IN THE BLANKS

1. Subjective
2. Secondary
3. Metabolic
4. Coping
5. Expression
6. Resonance
7. Receptive
8. Nystagmus
9. Aortic
10. Objective
11. Physical

Activity B MATCHING

1. 1 – A,   2 – E,   3 – C,   4 – B,   5 – D
2. 1 – B,   2 – A,   3 – C

Activity C ORDERING

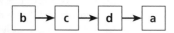

Activity D SHORT ANSWER

1. A complete assessment provides the nurse with a complete picture of the patient. Having this information aide in coming up with a nursing diagnosis and plan that fits the needs of the patient.
2. The environment in which the patient assessment is performed should be comfortable for both the patient and the nurse. It also should ensure privacy for the patient and allow for confidentiality. Both these measures help to ensure the collection of all relevant data and put the patient at ease.
3. As a nurse you encounter many different people from many different cultures. It is important to acknowledge one's own culture because it effects how you respond to others, both consciously and subconsciously. It is important not to let biases get in the way of providing care to patients.
4. Sexuality is an integral aspect of human nature. Sexual dysfunction can be seen in chronic illness and need to be addressed. Bringing the topic up with a patient lets them know that it is an important area to discuss and that their concerns are legitimate. It also gives them permission to ask sexually related questions.
5. When performing an assessment of the school-aged child, it is important to keep in mind that they can be asked direct questions but should be asked at a language level that is easy to understand. Adolescents are often examined alone and are often very sensitive about their body. It is important to discuss the changes that are rapidly occurring during this maturation process.

Activity E CROSSWORD

Across
2. Scoliosis
4. Frequency
5. Inspection
6. Edema

Down
1. Percussion
3. Overstimulation

SECTION III: APPLYING YOUR KNOWLEDGE

Activity F CASE STUDY

1. We know from the scenario that Jordana plays, at the least, the roles of daughter and long-time patient. At this moment, she is also filling the role of a support person to her mother. This last role could be either rewarding for Jordana or overwhelming and stressful, and therefore be exacerbating the problem. It is important to know this before getting involved in the situation.
2. I would want to perform an exam that focuses on assessing Jordana's respiratory status. Throughout the exam I would pay close attention to draping her so that her modesty is maintained. My assessment of her skin will be performed throughout the exam as each body part is uncovered. I would first perform a general survey to give me a good idea of Jordan's overall health and to look for any signs of distress that need to be dealt with. I would then gather her vital signs. If she is alert and oriented I would move on to assessing her skin for any signs of cyanosis and her nails for any clubbing, a sign of chronic hypoxia. I would inspect the configuration of her thorax, her breathing pattern, and the use of any accessory muscles. I would then palpate her chest wall for any pain, asymmetry, or abnormal areas such as masses or bulging. I could also apply tactile fremitus and check for respiratory excursion. Next, I would perform percussion to look for any areas that sounds abnormal in her lung fields. Then, I would auscultate for any adventitious breath sounds.

SECTION IV: PRACTICING FOR NCLEX

Activity G MULTIPLE CHOICE

1. **Answer: c**
   RATIONALE: Communicating the patient's pain level is only something the patient can state and validate. Subjective data are those symptoms, feelings, perception, preferences, values, and information that only the patient can describe. The rest of the options can be directly observed or measured and are known as objective data.
2. **Answer: a**
   RATIONALE: The skin over the dorsum of the hand is sensitive to temperature because it is thin and its nerve density is great. The palm of the hand is sensitive to vibration and is useful in locating a vibration associated with a heart murmur. The fingertips

are concentrated with nerve endings and can sense fine difference in texture and consistency. The knuckles are not used in palpation.

3. **Answer: b**
   RATIONALE: Regular physical activity contributes to a person's physical and psychological well-being.
4. **Answer: c**
   RATIONALE: Oriented × 3 indicates that the person is oriented to person (one's own name, the names of significant others, or knowing the nurse), place (location, city, or state), and time (time of day, day of week, or date).
5. **Answer: d**
   RATIONALE: When using a translator it is important to remember that the patient still comes first. This means that all information is directed at them and not the translator. Also, there are certain circumstances where it is not appropriate to use a family member such as when you are talking about an emotional topic. Talking loudly not only does not help with better understanding, but it can also come across hostile and rude. It is true that even professional translators don't understand all medical terms and may need some clarification at times.
6. **Answer: a**
   RATIONALE: Cranial nerve I is important for a person's sense of smell. Cranial nerve II, III, and IV are important for vision.
7. **Answer: a**
   RATIONALE: Although acute pancreatitis can be fatal if Dana is asking for pain medications, she is at the very least alert. Patients who are being treated for a stroke, brain tumor, or who are recovering from brain surgery need to be monitored closely for level of consciousness.
8. **Answers: a, b, c, d, e**
   RATIONALE: All of the above are helpful to the health team in soliciting subjective information concerning the patient's pain experience and how it affects daily life and other health patterns.
9. **Answers: a, c, d, f**
   RATIONALE: You are evaluating the pupils bilaterally for size, shape, accommodation, and reaction to light. Normally, pupils are black, round and they constrict briskly when exposed to a bright light source. You will observe both pupils and estimate initial size and reaction size.

CHAPTER 17

SECTION II: ASSESSING YOUR UNDERSTANDING

Activity A   FILL IN THE BLANKS

1. Afebrile
2. Tachycardia
3. Bradypnea
4. Apnea
5. Stroke
6. Auscultory
7. Hypertension
8. Hypotension
9. Bradycardia
10. Eupnea

Activity B   MATCHING

1. 1 – F,   2 – A,   3 – D,   4 – E,   5 – C,   6 – B
2. 1 – C,   2 – D,   3 – A,   4 – E,   5 – B

Activity C   ORDERING

1.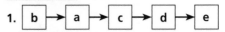

Activity D   SHORT ANSWER

1. People at different ages of the lifespan have varying degrees to which they are able to regulate their body temperature. Newborns have immature thermoregulatory mechanism and thus have unstable body temperatures. Older adults may have baseline temperatures below what is considered the normal range. They also may not mount a fever response in the setting of an infection.
2. Some medications decrease respiratory rate and depth such as opioids. Others dilate the bronchioles which increase a person's ability to move air into and out of the lungs. These are called sympathomimetics. Inhaled corticosteroids decrease airway inflammation which can improve airway clearance.
3. It is important to observe someone's respirations first without them knowing you are doing so because they may alter their breathing pattern or rate if they are aware of what you are doing.
4. Blood flow resistance is caused by friction among the cells and other blood components and between the blood and the vessel walls. It is also caused by contraction and relaxation of the smooth muscle in the vessel walls which control the diameter of the blood vessels. Greater overall resistance leads to increased blood pressure.
5. Orthostatic hypotension is the inability to reflexively compensate for the volume shift that occurs during a position change. This leads to symptoms such as dizziness, weakness, blurred vision, and syncope.

SECTION III: APPLYING YOUR KNOWLEDGE

Activity E   CASE STUDY

1. There are several factors that could be causing Josie's elevated blood pressure. She could be distressed because children this age are usually fearful of having their vital signs taken. If she has been taking her albuterol regularly this could also cause an increase in her heart rate. Also, both the presence of a fever and her inability to breath easily could be causing her a lot of anxiety which could lead to a higher heart rate.
2. With children who are Josie's age it is important to make them as comfortable with the process of taking vital signs as possible. Often, it does not work to

simply explain what you are doing. It does help to allow the child to play with the equipment before using them. You can also have their caregivers talk to them and comfort them.

SECTION IV: PRACTICING FOR NCLEX

Activity F MULTIPLE CHOICE

1. **Answer: a**
   RATIONALE: Inspiration is an active process. Muscles contract which result in increased intrathoracic volume as the lungs expand. Tidal volume, normally 500 mL/minute, is the amount of air moving in and out of the lungs with each breath. Internal respiration refers to the use of oxygen, the production of carbon dioxide, and the exchange of these gases between the cells and the blood.

2. **Answer: d**
   RATIONALE: Stridor is a harsh inspiratory sound that may be compared to crowing. It can indicate an upper airway obstruction. A high-pitched musical sound describes wheezing. Dyspnea is a term used to describe expirations that require excessive effort. Crackles are discontinuous popping sounds.

3. **Answer: a**
   RATIONALE: Diastolic blood pressure occurs when ventricular relaxation happens, blood pressure is due to elastic recoil of the vessels. Systolic blood pressure is measured during ventricular contraction. Systolic blood pressure is highest when the ventricles of the heart eject blood into the aorta and pulmonary arteries. Blood pressure in general is measured by taking the flow of blood produced by contractions of the heart and multiplying it by the resistance to blood flow through the vessels $(P = F \times R)$.

4. **Answer: b**
   RATIONALE: Glass mercury thermometers are no longer used due to the dangers of exposure to mercury.

5. **Answer: c**
   RATIONALE: Rate or frequency refers to the number of pulsations per minute. Rhythm refers to the regularity with which pulsation occurs. Quality refers to the strength of the palpated pulsation.

6. **Answer: a**
   RATIONALE: The sympathetic nervous system activation occurs in response to various stimuli, including pain, anxiety, exercise, fever, and changes in intravascular volume. Stimulation of the parasympathetic nervous system results in a decrease in the pulse rate.

7. **Answer: b**
   RATIONALE: A bounding pulse is stronger than normal and difficult to obliterate. A full or strong pulse is considered normal quality and can be palpated easily. Weak pulses are obliterated easily by the examiner's fingers and may be described as thready.

8. **Answer: a**
   RATIONALE: Evaporation causes heat loss as water is transformed to gas. An example of this is diaphoresis, or sweating.

9. **Answer: d**
   RATIONALE: In order to get an accurate reading, the patient should be in a warm, quiet environment. All the other answers, as well as exercise, would cause a false blood pressure reading.

10. **Answers: a, b, c, and d**
    RATIONALE: Oral temperature assessment is not safe for infants. Rectal temperatures are contraindicated in patients with cancer who are neutropenic.

CHAPTER 18

SECTION II: ASSESSING YOUR UNDERSTANDING

Activity A FILL IN THE BLANKS

1. Septicemia
2. Exotoxins
3. Environment
4. Influenza
5. Hand
6. Bactericidal
7. Tuberculosis
8. Sharps
9. Surgical
10. Toddler

Activity B MATCHING

1. 1 – E,   2 – B,   3 – D,   4 – A,   5 – C

Activity C ORDERING

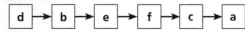

Activity D SHORT ANSWER

1. *Candida albicans* are part of the normal flora of the human skin and mucous membrane. When the normal mixture of flora is disrupted (i.e., during antibiotic use, high glucose levels in diabetics) certain microorganisms take advantage of the change in flora and grow out of control.

2. a. Infection prevention that includes the use of bundles to provide diligent care for vascular and urinary catheters and ventilators. b. Swift and precise diagnosis and treatment of the infectious organism. c. Accurate use of antimicrobials. d. Meticulous adherence to evidence-based transmission prevention strategies.

3. Puncture proof plastic containers, also known as "sharps" containers, should be easily accessible to immediately dispose of any needles or blades. Needles should never be recapped. Do not attempt to shove a needle or sharp into a full container; sharps containers should be emptied when they are 2/3 full.

4. Medical asepsis refers to measures taken to control and reduce the number of pathogens present. It is

also known as "clean" technique. Measures used to prevent the spread of organisms from place to place include hand hygiene, gloving, gowning, and disinfecting to help contain microbial growth. Surgical asepsis refers to "sterile" technique. To be sterile, an object must be free of all microorganisms. Sterile technique is used to prevent the introduction or spread of pathogens from the environment into the patient. Sterile technique is employed when a body cavity is entered with an object that may damage the mucous membranes, when surgical procedures are performed, and when the patient's immune system is already significantly compromised.

5. Inconsistency or lack of awareness regarding use of hand hygiene during clean activities such as taking vital signs or shaking hands with a patient. Misperception that gloves substitute for hand hygiene. Busy schedules leads to time saving measures. Irritation from alcohol-based sanitizers.

6. Wear clean gloves when touching blood, body fluids, secretions and excretions, mucous membranes, and nonintact skin. Perform handwashing immediately after removing gloves, when entering or leaving a patient room, and any time there is direct contact with blood, body fluids, secretions and excretions, or contaminated items. Wear a mask, eye protection, and face shield during procedures and patient care activities that are likely to generate splashes or sprays of blood, body fluids, secretions, and excretions. Wear a cover gown during procedures and patient care activities that are likely to generate splashes or sprays of blood, body fluids, secretions or excretions, or cause soiling of clothing. Remove soiled protective items promptly when the potential for contact with reservoirs of pathogens is no longer present.

SECTION III: APPLYING YOUR KNOWLEDGE

Activity E CASE STUDY

1. The most appropriate action is to reassign Vanessa to care for another patient. Certain infectious diseases can be detrimental to a fetus.

2. Both contact and respiratory precautions might be appropriate. Contact precautions are absolutely necessary. This means that anyone entering the room should wear a protective gown and gloves. Respiratory precautions may be necessary if the patient has a cough or signs of a upper respiratory infection, since a rash is often a symptom of an illness that is transmitted by respiratory means.

3. You must maintain ordered precautions even when performing a procedure. If the patient is in contact precautions, you should don your protective gown and gloves when entering the room. Sterile gloves can be placed over the protective clean gloves. You may find it easiest to set up a sterile field outside of the room and then wheel the tray into the room.

SECTION IV: PRACTICING FOR NCLEX

Activity F MULTIPLE CHOICE

1. **Answer: b**
RATIONALE: Pathogenicity is an organism's ability to cause infections.

2. **Answer: a**
RATIONALE: Contact may be either direct or indirect.

3. **Answer: a**
RATIONALE: Urinary catheters account for the highest percentage (26%) of hospital-associated infections.

4. **Answer: d**
RATIONALE: Hand hygiene is the most important way to prevent transmission of infection.

5. Answer: c
RATIONALE: A new gown should be used each time you enter the room.

6. **Answer: c**
RATIONALE: Active tuberculosis always requires a negative flow room.

7. **Answer: a**
RATIONALE: Hepatitis B is most virulent and most contagious of blood borne diseases. Without knowing Anita's vaccination status or the patient's history, this would concern you the most.

8. **Answer: a**
RATIONALE: Infection with rubella during the first trimester is of great concern as it frequently leads to congenital rubella syndrome. The later in the pregnancy that a woman develops rubella, a reaction is less likely and typically less severe.

9. **Answers: b, c**
RATIONALE: Artificial nails are never appropriate. Chewing of nails is not prohibited, but if the skin surrounding the nail is not intact, gloves should be worn.

10. **Answers: a, b, d**
RATIONALE: Tuberculosis would be a significant respiratory exposure, but it is not transmitted by blood.

11. **Answers: a, b, c**
RATIONALE: A respirator is typically reserved for patients with tuberculosis. A face shield is more appropriate for protection from influenza.

CHAPTER 19

SECTION II: ASSESSING YOUR UNDERSTANDING

Activity A FILL IN THE BLANKS

1. Generic
2. Trade (could also be Brand)
3. Prescription
4. Pharmacokinetics
5. Excretion

6. Therapeutic
7. Anaphylactic
8. Incompatibility
9. Teratogenic
10. Intradermal
11. Subcutaneous
12. Intramuscular
13. Controlled
14. Pharmacodynamics

Activity B MATCHING

1. 1 – B,   2 – C,   3 – D,   4 – A
2. 1 – C,   2 – A,   3 – B,   4 – E,   5 – D

Activity C CROSSWORD

Across
2. Metabolism
4. Distribution
6. Chemical

Down
1. Absorption
3. Transdermal
5. Botanical

Activity D SHORT ANSWER

1. The dangers of nonprescription medications lie in their misuse. Taken not as directed, they can produce dangerous side effects. Also, people may self-medicate with nonprescription medications and delay seeking professional help for a major problem. A third danger is in the risk for serious drug interaction if more than one nonprescription medication is taken at the same time.
2. It is important to ask about a person's utilization of herbal medications because many of these can have toxic effects. They can also cause drug interactions with other herbal medications as well as prescription and nonprescription, over the counter, medications.
3. Patients have the right to have medications appropriately and safely administrated to them. They trust that the person caring for them will adequately assess them for the appropriateness of a medication and whether they are the right person, the drug is the right drug, the dose is the right dose, it is given to them at the right time, and that the administration is documented appropriately.
4. Medication reconciliation is when medications that a person is taking is verified and documented. This occurs when a person is handed off between healthcare providers or agencies. Medication reconciliation is important because having an accurate and up-to-date list of what a person is taking prevents medication errors such as missed doses or the prescribing of contraindicated medications.
5. It is important to always assess a patient prior to giving a medication because the medication may not be appropriate for the patient at the time and can cause an adverse reaction. An example of this is

if a person's blood pressure is 99/65, giving their antihypertensive could cause a dangerous drop in their blood pressure.

SECTION III: APPLYING YOUR KNOWLEDGE

Activity E CASE STUDY

1. Before I give Tara her medications I will perform a thorough assessment. She has orders for insulin, lisinopril, and atorvastatin. My assessment of Tara would include a blood glucose check to assess whether or not she needs insulin and how much insulin to give her if she does need it. I would also check her blood pressure to make sure that she needs her lisinopril. Because I will be giving two oral medications, I will further assess whether she can swallow and if she has any motility issues, such as vomiting, that need to be addressed prior to administration.
2. Medication education for Tara should focus on insulin because it is a new medication for her and it is complex. As her nurse, I would provide information that is as clear and straight forward as possible. I would want to include the name of the medication, the reason she is taking it, how and when to take it, how long she should take the medication for, any foods or other medications that could interfere with the medication, and the usual adverse effects of the medication. Tara will also need to know how to check her blood sugar prior to taking her insulin and what the blood glucose values mean. She will further need to know how to safely handle and dispose of the needles used for administration. Also, I would encourage Tara to keep a log of what her blood glucose values are and how much insulin she is giving herself so that her primary care provider can alter the type of insulin she is getting as well as the doses if needed.

SECTION IV: PRACTICING FOR NCLEX

Activity F MULTIPLE CHOICE

1. **Answer: b**
   RATIONALE: The components of an order include the patient's name, the mediation's name, the amount and frequency of the dose, and the route of administration.
2. **Answer: d**
   RATIONALE: The National Formulary describes medication products according to their source, physical and chemical properties, tests for purity and identity, method of storage, category, and normal dosages.
3. **Answer: a**
   RATIONALE: Inotropes strengthen cardiac contraction, antiarrhythmics regulate heart rhythm, anticoagulants decrease clot formation, and diuretics increase urine production and elimination.

4. **Answer: b**
   RATIONALE: A PRN order is one that is given to a patient on an as needed basis.
5. **Answer: d**
   RATIONALE: Prescribing and dispensing medications are not legal practices for registered nurses, with the exception of nurses in advance practice roles.
6. **Answer: a**
   RATIONALE: Severe allergic reactions to medications include wheezing, dyspnea, angioedema of the tongue and oropharynx, hypotension, and tachycardia. These reactions occur immediately after the medication is administered.
7. **Answer: d**
   RATIONALE: The formula to calculate the correct medication amount is (Dose on hand/Quantity on hand = Dose desired/X). If you use this for this scenario you would have 30 g/45 mL = 20 g/X, where X = 30 mL.
8. **Answer: a**
   RATIONALE: Buccal medication is not chewed, swallowed, or placed under the tongue. Sublingual medications are placed under the tongue. Medications that are given through a nasogastric tube are oral. A medication that is designed to produce systemic effects and is absorbed through the skin is called transdermal.
9. **Answer: a**
   RATIONALE: Ophthalmic medications are administered in the eyes, parenteral medications are given by injection or infusion.
10. **Answer: a**
    RATIONALE: A synergistic reaction is one in which one drug increases the effect of another drug. Tylenol PM and oxycodone have a synergistic relationship. Doxycycline and calcium carbonate have an antagonistic relationship.
11. **Answers: a, b, d, e**
    RATIONALE: Patients have the right to expect safe and appropriate drug administration. Nurses must observe each of the above rights to ensure that the nurse accomplishes this.

CHAPTER 20

SECTION II: ASSESSING YOUR UNDERSTANDING

Activity A FILL IN THE BLANKS

1. Colloids
2. Peripheral
3. Decreases
4. Central
5. 15
6. 72
7. Air
8. Hour

9. Aseptic
10. Central

Activity B MATCHING

2. 1 – B,   2 – D,   3 – A,   4 – C

Activity C SHORT ANSWER

1. Isotonic solutions have the same osmotic pressure as that which is found in the cell. Isotonic fluids are used to provide intervascular volume, such as in cases of hypotension. Hypotonic fluids have osmotic pressure that is lower than that found in the cell. Hypotonic fluids are used when cellular dehydration is present because they will allow fluid to shift into the cell.
2. The five steps of the CCB are: a. hand hygiene, b. maximum barrier precautions during insertion, c. chlorhexidine skin antisepsis, d. optimal catheter site selection with subclavian vein preferred, and e. daily assessment of catheter necessity. Following these steps has dramatically reduced the incidence of catheter-associated blood stream infections (CABSI).
3. When intravenous solutions inadvertently leak into the subcutaneous tissues it is referred to as infiltration. If the fluid is a vesicant, it is referred to as extravasation.
4. The veins of an infant are small and difficult to cannulate. Umbilical veins may be used for neonates up to 2 weeks old (though usually only in the first few days of life). For infants younger than 9 months, scalp veins in the temporal region are often used. IV therapy delivered into a scalp vein can prove very upsetting for parents, so provide teaching, support, and comfort. Never ask parents to restrain a baby. Secure the IV site well so that the parents can hold and comfort the infant without fear of dislodging the IV.
5. Group A has anti-B antibodies; group B has anti-A antibodies; group AB has no A or B antibodies; and group O has anti-A and anti-B antibodies in the serum.
6. Fever can occur as a result of a hypersensitivity reaction to cell components or additives to the blood product. Allergic reactions, with symptoms such as flushing, urticaria (hives), wheezing, and a rash with itching can occur in response to the donor's plasma proteins. In each of these cases, the transfusion should be stopped and both the blood bank and a licensed provider notified. The most serious reaction is an acute hemolytic reaction in response to transfusion with an incompatible blood type. Hemolysis or destruction of RBCs occurs when the antibodies in the recipient's blood quickly react to the donor's blood cells. Symptoms, which are immediate, include facial flushing, fever, chills, headache, low back pain, tachycardia, dyspnea, hypotension, and blood in the urine. Prompt intervention is essential to prevent death.

SECTION III: APPLYING YOUR KNOWLEDGE

Activity D CASE STUDY

1. The patient receiving home IV or nutritional support is monitored by both a home care nurse and the physician. Be present to start the initial nutritional support at home, set up all equipment, and make sure that all supplies, including glucose monitoring equipment, are present.
2. PICC lines are used for patients who require intermediate- to long-term venous access. Because PICC lines can be left in place for several months, they are very useful for home, as well as acute, care. PICC lines have a small diameter, which makes them ideal for use in the very young and the elderly. The catheter flexibility does not restrict arm movement. These lines have been shown to be associated with fewer severe complications, such as pneumothorax, air embolism, and sepsis, than other central lines.
3. CABSI are the most common complication of home infusion therapy. Fever, malaise, and changes in blood pressure are indications of a CABSI. An elevated WBC is a laboratory sign of infection, though this is non-specific. A positive blood culture confirms infection. Phlebitis may be associated with a CABSI and would manifest as a reddened streak up the vein or a firm, cordlike vessel.
4. 33 drops/minute.

SECTION IV: PRACTICING FOR NCLEX

Activity E MULTIPLE CHOICE

1. **Answer: b**
   RATIONALE: Isotonic fluids are used to increase blood pressure secondary to hypovolemia.
2. **Answer: d**
   RATIONALE: This patient is both anemic and thrombocytopenic. Both red blood cells and platelets could be administered in this case.
3. **Answer: a**
   RATIONALE: Typical lumen size in an adult is between 18 and 22 gauge. The catheter should be the shortest possible length. Usually 1 to 1 ¼ inches is sufficient for IV therapy.
4. **Answer: c**
   RATIONALE: PICC lines are appropriate for long-term therapy and can easily be used in the home environment. A peripheral IV is rarely used for home therapy, especially when the patient will need infusions for more than 1 day. The tunneled catheter and implanted ports require an operation to place; this is too invasive for this patient.
5. **Answer: a**
   RATIONALE: This patient needs frequent IV access. A central port is easily accessed for chemotherapy

sessions, then the access is discontinued even though the port remains in place subcutaneously. A central port also allows for the infusion of chemotherapy into a central vessel; this is important because chemotherapy is caustic and severely damages peripheral vessels.

6. **Answer: a**
   RATIONALE: Under current regulations an IV dressing change is not a task that can be delegated.
7. **Answer: d**
   RATIONALE: Phlebitis occurs when the vessel is irritated from a caustic solution. Rotating the site helps to prevent this complication.
8. **Answer: c**
   RATIONALE: This is a sign of infiltration. Infiltration with PRBCs will give the appearance of a bruise.
9. **Answer: c**
   RATIONALE: Patients with type B blood have anti-A antibodies. This means they would attack any type A blood they receive, prompting a transfusion reaction.
10. **Answer: b**
11. **Answer: d**
12. **Answers: a, c, d**
    RATIONALE: Lowering the patient's extremity would increase the flow of the IV fluid.
13. **Answers: b, c, d**
    RATIONALE: The joints should be avoided because toddlers are often quite active and as a result may dislodge the IV.

CHAPTER 21

SECTION II: ASSESSING YOUR UNDERSTANDING

Activity A FILL IN THE BLANKS

1. Postoperative
2. Laparoscope
3. Antiembolic
4. Ileus
5. Pain
6. Stress
7. Preoperative
8. Autologous
9. Intestinal
10. Checklist
11. Circulating
12. Time-out
13. Moderate
14. Peristalsis
15. Eight
16. Asepsis
17. 200

Activity B MATCHING

1. 1 – C,   2 – E,   3 – B,   4 – D,   5 – A

Activity C SHORT ANSWER

1. Deep breathing exercises are the current standard of treatment for non-intubated postsurgical patients. An incentive spirometer is a tool used to promote deep breathing and is often used hourly in the post-operative period.

2. The stress of surgical procedures often leads to glucose instability in all patients, but particularly in patients with diabetes mellitus. As a result, patients often experience extremely high blood glucose levels. These elevated glucose levels encourage growth of opportunistic bacteria and set the patient up for surgical site or systemic infection. Tight control of glucose levels in the postoperative period is the current standard of practice for surgical patients.

3. Malignant hyperthermia is a hypermetabolic disorder of skeletal muscle that can be induced by some anesthetic agents, including certain inhalants and muscle relaxants. Malignant hyperthermia is manifested by masseter muscle rigidity and ventricular dysrhythmias. Tachypnea, cyanosis, skin mottling, and unstable blood pressure are signs of ventricular dysrhythmia. Fever is a late sign of malignant hyperthermia, and the body temperature may rise quickly if the condition goes untreated (possibly 1°C every 5 minutes if untreated).

4. Some religious beliefs prohibit the use of blood transfusions (Jehovah's Witness) or medications/organs derived from animal parts (pig, cow). Many religions consider the elective abortion of a fetus to be a sin. Families may wish to have members of the religious community perform procedures (circumcision). Families of infants or small children may request baptism or a spiritual ceremony prior to a planned surgical intervention.

5. Informed consent is required for all non-emergent surgical procedures. The surgeon is required to sit with the patient or the family and provide a description of the proposed surgery, the possible risks and benefits of the procedure, the reason the surgery is indicated, the probability of success, the consequences of nonsurgical treatment or no treatment, and any other information that will help the patient reach an informed decision. The surgeon, the patient, and a witness must sign and date the consent form. The bedside nurse often acts as the witness to consent. Do not administer any medications that might alter judgment or perception before the patient signs the consent form because many drugs commonly administered as preoperative medications, such as narcotics or barbiturates, can alter cognitive abilities and invalidate informed consent.

SECTION III: APPLYING YOUR KNOWLEDGE

Activity D CASE STUDY

1. School-aged children enjoy helping with tasks. Juan could assist you with marking the surgical site,

attaching his name band or applying electrodes for cardiac monitoring. Juan should also be present for explanation of the procedure and have the opportunity to ask questions.

2. The surgeon is required to sit with the legal guardian and provide a description of the proposed surgery, the possible risks and benefits of the procedure, the reason the surgery is indicated, the probability of success, the consequences of nonsurgical treatment or no treatment, and any other information that will help the patient reach an informed decision.

3. Apply the patient's name band. Surgical site and type of surgery. Location of valuables. Allergies. Appropriate dress of the patient. Surgical consent obtained. NPO status. Appropriate records and paperwork. Laboratory and diagnostic study results entered on the chart. Blood availability. Preoperative medication administration. The status of any additional physician's orders. At this time, IV access and, if necessary, an arterial line may be established.

4. Anxiety r/t planned operative procedure AEB patient fidgeting, increased HR.

SECTION IV: PRACTICING FOR NCLEX

Activity E MULTIPLE CHOICE

1. **Answer: c**
   RATIONALE: This request is beyond your scope of practice as a nurse. There are many ethical considerations in this case, including the fact that Avery is considered a minor and that her request will likely place her life in danger. An ethics team may help the patient and family arrive at a plan of care that upholds Avery's religious beliefs except in an extreme life-threatening emergency.

2. **Answer: a**
   RATIONALE: Patients should void a minimum of 8 hours after an operative procedure. Bed rest can make urination difficult because the patient is not positioned in a manner that promotes voiding. Trying to reposition the patient while maintaining bed rest is the best option here.

3. **Answer: b**
   RATIONALE: Delirium refers to acute confusion that is reversible. It is common in the acute postoperative period.

4. **Answer: d**
   RATIONALE: Toddlers are prone to separation anxiety. Allowing the child to be with the parents will lower anxiety levels for all members of the family. This will subsequently ease the care for the bedside nurse.

5. **Answer: d**
   RATIONALE: A type IV reaction is characterized by local inflammation, pruritus and erythema.

6. **Answer b**
   RATIONALE: Although choice A is technically correct, B is the better choice. Even in an emergency,

the patient or family should have the opportunity to ask questions IF it will not delay the procedure.

7. **Answer: a**
RATIONALE: Two hours is a standard NPO time for clear liquids, though the nurse should always check with their institutions policy.

8. **Answer: b**
RATIONALE: Rectal anxiolytics are commonly administered to toddlers prior to painful procedures such as blood draws and IV placement to help ease their transition. A toddler should spend as much time as they can with their caregiver to ease anxiety; the caregiver may meet you in the recovery room and may come back with them to the operating room. The patient may be allowed to bring a security item into surgery, but all of their stuffed animals are excessive.

9. **Answer: c**
RATIONALE: The procedural pause (time-out) must be done prior to any procedure to ensure patient safety and verify the patient identity, staff roles, and procedure being performed.

10. **Answers: a, c, d**
RATIONALE: The job of the circulating nurse is to manage the patient. This requires the nurse to be present in the operating room during the procedure.

11. **Answers: a, b, c, d**
RATIONALE: All of these substances may contain latex. Latex is found in the elastic of underwear.

12. **Answers: b, c, d**
RATIONALE: Morphine may be administered following painful procedures after less invasive nonpharmacologic techniques have failed.

CHAPTER 22

SECTION II: ASSESSING YOUR UNDERSTANDING

Activity A FILL IN THE BLANKS

1. Second
2. Ergonomics
3. Sentinel
4. Disaster
5. Avoidance
6. Toddlers
7. Asbestos
8. Bath
9. Lift
10. Restraint

Activity B MATCHING

1. 1 – B,   2 – C,   3 – E,   4 – A,   5 – D

Activity C SEQUENCING

1. c → a → d → b

Activity D SHORT ANSWER

1. Accidents are particularly of concern in this age group because curiosity is present but toddlers and preschoolers lack mature judgment and do not perceive danger. Safety measures should be in place so that toddlers can explore with minimal risk of injury. Water heaters should be set to 120 degrees or less. Nonskid mats should be present in bathtubs. Guardrails need to be placed at the top of steps, and windows should open from the top. Toys must be sturdy, free of sharp or rough edges and without small, removable, or breakable parts that the child could swallow or have lodge in his or her respiratory tract or that could damage an eye.

2. Older adults have a diminished sense of balance which could lead to falls into hot objects. Decreased sensitivity to touch and slowed reflexes results in delayed reaction to the touch of hot objects.

3. A bed or wheelchair with unlocked wheels. Oxygen at each bedside presents a potential fire hazard. Procedure errors such as not checking name bands or monitoring IV infusion rates or sites can cause direct patient harm. Contaminated needles, violent patients, and heavy lifting all pose risks to hospital personnel.

4. Neuropsychological testing can be used to determine the type and source of a cognitive abnormality. Blood pressure assessment, electrocardiogram (ECG) testing, and pulmonary function tests can be used to detect cardiopulmonary capacity and abnormalities. Specific blood tests can identify the presence of certain conditions, such as a complete blood count (CBC) and renal and hepatic function tests to detect an infection, kidney and liver disease, or the ability to eliminate toxins from the body. Laboratory tests can also measure the amount of alcohol, drugs or lead in a person's blood.

5. Ensure that the room is uncluttered and free of obstacles between the bed and the bathroom. Use of a night light and bedside rails is standard protocol. Instruct each patient and his significant others about activity limitations and assist with ambulation as needed. A nurse call light should be within reach. Patients should wear nonskid socks. Proper patient identification with two unique identifiers should be used for medication administration and laboratory sample collection. Use ergonomic positioning and a lift device or lift team when transferring patients.

SECTION III: APPLYING YOUR KNOWLEDGE

Activity E CASE STUDY

1. Luisa is 80 years old, which puts her at risk for age-related safety concerns: poor eyesight and hearing can diminish balance, reflexes slow and sensitivity to temperature decreases placing older adults at increased risk for exposure or injury. Medications

for Parkinson's disease in particular place Luisa at risk for falls due to orthostatic hypotension.

2. Two-year-old children lack experience and mature judgment. They are also high in energy and quite curious. This puts toddlers at particular risk for unintentional injury. Stairs need guard rails, cupboards need locks. Water heaters should be set to less than 120 degrees. Outlets must be covered and bathtubs should have nonstick surfaces. By the age of six, Sean has probably learned what is safe and unsafe around the house. Gun safety is a big concern at this age because children may believe they are toys.

3. Well lit and unobstructed hallways are key to preventing falls. Toys should always be cleaned and out of the walkways. Hand rails may be needed on stairs or uneven surfaces. Loose carpets should be removed. Nonskid surfaces in the bathtub used by both Luisa and Genevieve are helpful. Any cupboard that contains chemicals or dangerous materials should be locked. Fire and carbon monoxide detectors should be installed.

4. Ensure a well lit and unobstructed walkway. Assess for confusion; patients who are ill and in a new environment can have new onset of delirium. Delirium can cause patients to crawl over bed rails or fight against procedures. Ensure that Luisa has a call button within arm's reach. Minimize the use of tubing and catheters as these can present a fall risk.

SECTION IV: PRACTICING FOR NCLEX

Activity F MULTIPLE CHOICE

1. **Answer: a**
   RATIONALE: Windows pose a serious risk to toddlers. Screens can easily give way to the weight of a toddler. This is an unsafe behavior. Toddlers thrive in exploration. The parent must be fastidious in monitoring and helping the toddler accomplish tasks. The buddy system is a great safety tool for school age children.

2. **Answer: c**
   RATIONALE: All of these toys present a choking hazard except for the rocking horse. Rocking horses are a great toy for development of leg muscles.

3. **Answer: c**
   RATIONALE: Adolescence is a time of rapid physical growth and more sleep is required. Many adolescents try to balance after school curricular activities with jobs and school, resulting in sleep deprivation. This, in turn, poses a safety risk as adolescents have increased freedoms, such as driving.

4. **Answer: a**
   RATIONALE: Contributing factors include speeding, lack of defensive driving techniques, failure of bicycle riders and skateboarders to use helmets, fatigue, and the use of alcohol and other substances that cause impairment while driving.

5. **Answer: d**
   RATIONALE: Bruising in different stages of healing on non-bony prominences is highly suspicious for abuse. Small round burns are commonly cigarette burns, plus Anita has a broken arm. Most states require nurses to report suspected abuse for follow-up investigation.

6. **Answer: c**
   RATIONALE: Restraints can be placed emergently without the order of a licensed provider. However, a face-to-face assessment of the patient must be made within one hour of restraint placement.

7. **Answer: a**
   RATIONALE: Unintentional injuries are the fifth leading cause of deaths behind heart disease, cancer, stroke, and chronic obstructive lung disease.

8. **Answers: a, b**
   RATIONALE: Infants should remain in the infant seat up to the maximum weight limit or until their length exceeds the length of the seat. Children between 20 and 40 lbs should remain in a forward facing car seat.

9. **Answers: c, d**
   RATIONALE: The use of 4-point restraints and isolation would likely increase her agitation. These would be appropriate if her behavior was violent or if her behavior posed an immediate threat to herself or others, such as trying to climb out of the bed.

CHAPTER 23

SECTION II: ASSESSING YOUR UNDERSTANDING

Activity A FILL IN THE BLANKS

1. Self-care
2. Hygiene
3. Plaque
4. Xerostomia
5. Halitosis
6. Pediculosis
7. Alopecia
8. Dysphagia
9. Micturition
10. Commode
11. Urinal
12. Pannus
13. Capitis
14. Tartar

Activity B MATCHING

1. 1 – D,   2 – A,   3 – B,   4 – C
2. 1 – E,   2 – B,   3 – A,   4 – C,   5 – D

Activity C ORDERING

1. d → b → c → a → e

Activity D SHORT ANSWER

1. Characteristics of routine self-care in regards to hygiene include the ability to bathe, dress, feed,

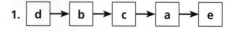

and toilet oneself. Bathing removes excess oil, perspiration, and bacteria from the skin. Grooming includes feet, nail, hair, oral, eye, ear, and nose care. All of these characteristics are important for maintaining a healthy person.

2. A person's ability to feed himself or herself is one of the most important self-care skills in terms of independence. Once a person looses this ability, they lose this sense of independence. This extends to being able to choose what they want to eat and when.

3. Because of poor circulation, the older adult is more at risk for foot problems. Decreased circulation can lead to skin breakdown and infection. The older adult may not be mobile enough to inspect their feet regularly.

4. It is important to use the physical exam to further assess what the patient has told you during your patient interview. Looking for lack of self-care, it is important to focus on an inability to manage self-care, such as poor grooming, body odor, skin lesions, and poor nutrition. Also important, is to assess for a person's ability to process sensory input, for any evidence of disabilities, for manual dexterity needed to complete certain self-care tasks, and for the use of sensory or mechanical aids.

5. Health promotion surrounding self-care can include education regarding the link between good hygiene and optimal health. This can be directly differently to different age groups. For example, in preschools a nurse can talk to a class about the importance of washing your hands after going to the bathroom.

SECTION III: APPLYING YOUR KNOWLEDGE

Activity E CASE STUDY

1. One possible nursing diagnosis for Al is Hygiene Self-care Deficit. Related factors could include muscle weakness, fatigue, physical limitations due to his recent procedure, and possibly some depression if this is a new state.

2. I would first assist the patient to remove their upper and lower dentures, handling both with a gauze pad to keep from dropping them. I would next wash the dentures with soap and warm water, using a soft bristled brush. To prevent them from getting broken or lost, I would place them in a container labeled with the patient's name.

SECTION IV: PRACTICING FOR NCLEX

Activity F MULTIPLE CHOICE

1. **Answer: d**
   RATIONALE: Self-care refers to a person's ability to perform primary care functions in bathing, feed-

ing, toileting, and dressing without the help of others.

2. **Answer: b**
   RATIONALE: Proper neuromuscular functioning is imperative for motor functioning. It controls both gross and fine motor movements as well as controls normal alignment and a person's awareness of the body's spatial position.

3. **Answer: a**
   RATIONALE: The most therapeutic response to Walt would be one that acknowledges his feelings and allows for him to talk about what he is experiencing.

4. **Answer: b**
   RATIONALE: In order to assess this patient's normal pattern of self-care while on her medications, it is important to assess what her expectations are? Once these expectations are established, the nurse can work with the patient to achieve them.

5. **Answer: c**
   RATIONALE: An internal resource is one that comes from within the patient. An external resource is one her environment and community offer her.

6. **Answer: b**
   RATIONALE: This patient is still able to bathe herself but has difficulty standing for long periods of time. In order to foster her independence and provide her with a safe bathing environment, a sit-down shower with shower chair would be most appropriate.

7. **Answer: a**
   RATIONALE: A sitz bath washes the pelvic area with warm water and can help to decrease inflammation after childbirth.

8. **Answer: b**
   RATIONALE: This describes of a corn. A callus is a flattened thickening of epidermis which is often found on the bottom or side of the food, over a bony prominence. A plantar wart is a round or irregular area that is flattened by pressure and is surrounded by cornified epithelium. A bunion is an inflammation and thickening of bursa the great toe joint which causes an enlargement of the joint and a displacement of the toe.

9. **Answer: b**
   RATIONALE: People who are at the greatest risk for foot problems are those with poor circulation and those with diabetes. Older age can also put you at risk but an active older adult is less at risk. A paraplegic could also be at risk for skin issues in general if they are not active.

10. **Answer: c**
    RATIONALE: If she is tired, it is best to cover the area that is soiled, in order to make her feel more comfortable, and wait until she has rested until changing her linens.

11. **Answer: a**
    RATIONALE: It is important to first close the patient's door or close the curtains to allow for privacy.

12. **Answer: b**
    RATIONALE: A back massage can be delegated to a medical assistant. Assessments and wound care must be done by the RN.
13. **Answers: a, b**
    RATIONALE: A person with poor circulation should never use sharp instruments to cut nails as they can cause damage to the foot itself. Further, they should always wear shoes to protect their feet. Soaking the feet causes them to dry out and can cause cracking.

CHAPTER 24

SECTION II: ASSESSING YOUR UNDERSTANDING

Activity A FILL IN THE BLANKS

1. Epiphysis
2. Relax
3. Legs
4. Aerobic
5. Phosphorus
6. Periosteum
7. Osteoarthritis
8. Contracture
9. Atrophy
10. Flexion

Activity B MATCHING

1. 1 – F,   2 – B,   3 – A,   4 – E,   5 – C,   6 – D
2. 1 – B,   2 – C,   3 – E,   4 – A,   5 – D

Activity C SEQUENCING

1.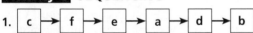

Activity D SHORT ANSWER

1. Balance is maintained by the vestibular apparatus in the inner ear consisting of the cochlear duct, the three semicircular canals, and two large chambers known as the utricle and the saccule. When the head moves, these hair cells are bent, pulled, or compressed, transmitting signals to the sensory nerves over the appropriate nerve tracts to the area that controls equilibrium and balance.
2. Remove any unnecessary equipment (i.e., IV poles or lines, tubing, monitoring equipment). Secure necessary equipment such as ventilators. Obtain assistance from other staff or a mechanical lift device. Adjust bed to appropriate height for staff (if patient is immobile) or patient (if patient will ambulate). Count "one, two, three" to coordinate movements. Provide non-skid slippers if patient is ambulatory.
3. A normal gait is composed of a stance phase and a swing phase. The stance phase is composed of heel strike, mid-stance and push-off. The nurse assesses where the heel strikes on the ground and how the foot rolls through to push-off. The stance phase is comprised of acceleration, swing through, and deceleration. The nurse watches for continuity and direction of the movements during this phase.
4. Muscle atrophy occurs during periods of prolonged immobility. An example of this is seen by comparing two extremities after a cast is removed. Atrophy leads to decreased activity tolerance. Unfortunately, atrophy can permanently alter the function of a particular muscle, even after immobility is reversed. Contractures occur when range of motion is not performed. Contractures limit movement and can disfigure a patient. If the patient is kept in a supine position, the workload of the heart is increased. Orthostatic hypotension can occur during position changes because of blood pooling secondary to gravity. Deep vein thrombosis is a risk of venous stasis. Decreased lung volume and metabolic rate, anorexia, osteoporosis, pressure ulcers, and urinary tract infections are also risks of prolonged immobility.
5. Some patients who are immobile do not want to bother others for a bedpan. Others have difficulty relaxing the perineal muscles in order to properly void. Chronic delay can lead to overstretching the detrusor muscle in the bladder wall, permanent changes in bladder tone, and causing small tears in the mucosa to which bacteria aggregate. The flushing action of urine through the urethra helps to prevent urinary tract infections. If this flushing is impaired, opportunistic bacteria will invade. Patients who do not fully void often require a catheter to empty their bladder increasing the risk of pathogen invasion.

SECTION III: APPLYING YOUR KNOWLEDGE

Activity E CASE STUDY

1. When trauma occurs, the loss of mobility is sudden. It is not expected or desired. Some patients find it difficult to cope with such loss. Depression, anxiety, and frustration are common among persons with altered mobility. However, it is important not to assume that Peter's feelings today are permanent or related to his injury. The nurse should engage in a discussion with Peter regarding his lack of desire to participate in PT today.
2. Anorexia is common in hospitalized patients. Patients who are supine find it difficult to eat in that position. Most patients do not prefer the taste of hospital food. Decreased metabolic need also leads to decrease demand. Osteoporosis is also a risk factor of prolonged immobility. Osteoblastic activity requires stress and strain on the bone. When this does not occur, there is an imbalance in osteoblastic and osteoclastic activities, and osteoclasts break down bone faster than osteoblasts restore it.

3. Impaired mobility r/t therapeutic amputation AEB patients continued need for physical therapy, stated decreased desire to mobilize. The risk for impaired coping r/t psychological impact of limb amputation.

4. Peter may require passive ROM on his affected leg. However, active ROM should be encouraged, particularly in the upper extremities. A trapeze bar above the bed can assist a patient with upper extremity ROM and isometric exercise and be a useful transfer tool. Isometric strengthening exercises should be done in both legs to help Peter prepare for ambulation. Use of ambulation aids, such as crutches or a prosthesis, should be encouraged because ambulation alone can improve physical and mental health.

SECTION IV: PRACTICING FOR NCLEX

Activity F MULTIPLE CHOICE

1. **Answer: c**
   RATIONALE: Isometric exercise isolates a specific muscle or muscle group and exercises it by holding the muscle steady and maintaining tension.

2. **Answer: a**
   RATIONALE: Exercise generally leads to an increased appetite.

3. **Answer: d**
   RATIONALE: The toddler years are a time of rapid longitudinal growth and rapid skill acquisition and refinement. Any regression in skill acquisition is indicative of a larger problem and must be evaluated.

4. **Answer: a**
   RATIONALE: Osteoporosis is not a normal part of aging, though it is more common in older adults, particularly women.

5. **Answer: b**
   RATIONALE: Elevation of the stump can result in contractures. Frequent position changes and protecting skin under bony prominences are preferred strategies to promote skin integrity.

6. **Answer: a**
   RATIONALE: Susan is exhibiting signs of a deep vein thrombosis (DVT). She also has several risk factors for developing a DVT (hormone use, smoking). Any patient with a DVT requires prompt treatment to prevent a pulmonary embolism (PE).

7. **Answer: d**
   RATIONALE: Eloise is engaging in weight-bearing activity. This is protective against osteoporosis. Smoking, Caucasian race, and post-menopausal age are all risk factors for osteoporosis.

8. **Answers: a, b, c**
   RATIONALE: Each of these activities will reduce the risk of falling and encourage the patient to increase his mobility.

9. **Answers: b, c, d**
   RATIONALE: Breath holding is a sign of muscle strain and an inefficient use of body mechanics.

10. **Answers: a, b, c**
    RATIONALE: The cerebral cortex initiates voluntary motor activity. The pyramidal tract (the direct corticospinal pathway) initiates transmission of impulses to the spinal cord for voluntary movements. The cerebellum has a special role in controlling movement: it controls muscles used to maintain steady posture and coordinated, detailed movements. The hypothalamus is primarily responsible for regulating temperature, controlling hunger, and thirst and regulating circadian rhythms.

11. **Answers: b, c**
    RATIONALE: The under-axilla lift technique should never be used because it exerts pressure on the brachial plexus that can affect the nerve function to the neck, shoulder, arm, and hands and can subluxate the shoulder. Safe transfers typically involve the use of extra trained personnel or use of assistive devices.

12. **Answers: a, b, c**
    RATIONALE: Gait disturbances, history of falls, certain medications, and weakness are highly predictive of a fall. Well-tacked carpeting can help prevent a fall in a home, while hardwood floors or loose rugs present a fall risk.

CHAPTER 25

SECTION II: ASSESSING YOUR UNDERSTANDING

Activity A FILL IN THE BLANKS

1. Bronchioles
2. Alveoli
3. Ventilation
4. Bronchospasm
5. Hemoptysis
6. Hypoxemia
7. Hypercapnia
8. Hypoventilation
9. Tracheostomy
10. Atelectasis
11. Eupnea

Activity B MATCHING

1. 1 – D, 2 – F, 3 – A, 4 – D, 5 – B, 6 – E

Activity C CROSSWORD

Across
1. Dyspnea
4. Diffusion

Down
2. Pneumonia
3. Cyanosis
5. Fremitus

Activity D ORDERING

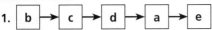

1. b → c → d → a → e

Activity E SHORT ANSWER

1. Oxygen is transported in one of two forms. Small amounts are dissolved in the plasma and transported away from the lungs. Most oxygen is transported by attaching to hemoglobin molecules on red blood cells.

2. The upper respiratory tract protects the rest of the system in a couple of different ways. First, it warms and humidifies the air entering into the respiratory system, which maintains the fluid character of the mucus in the lower respiratory tract. Second, it acts as a filter, trapping foreign particles within the nares and preventing them from entering the rest of the airway. The epiglottis also acts as a trapdoor to protect large particles from entering into the lower airway.

3. Adolescence is a time when people start smoking. Because of a sense of invulnerability that is inherent to this age group, they don't believe that the smoking they do now can have long term consequences such as lung cancer or heart disease. Once they start, it is very easy to become addicted.

4. An upright posture allows for greater lung expansion. Conversely, if someone is hunched over, the lungs can't expand to their greatest potential. When lying down, organs press into the diaphragm which then has to work harder to expand the lungs.

5. Many chronic respiratory illnesses, such as chronic obstructive pulmonary disease, may have a slow progression that allows for the person to adapt to the changes. A patient might state that their breathing is fine but have oxygen requirements above what a person with no respiratory problems might have.

6. Incentive spirometry is a device that both encourages the patient to breathe deeply and gives them objective information about how they are doing. All patients should be breathing deeply often but many are hindered by lying in bed, a respiratory illness, or by pain. By giving them an incentive spirometer, they are able to complete the task of breathing deeply at least 8 to 10 times per hour.

SECTION III: APPLYING YOUR KNOWLEDGE

Activity F CASE STUDY

1. One goal that is appropriate for this patient is that she will effectively cope with changes in self-concept. Possible outcome criteria included that within a week of having the tracheostomy surgery she will identify support people to provide emotional strength. Another possible outcome criterion is that before she is discharged she will demonstrate oxygen-conserving measures such as sitting while dressing and planning rest periods.

2. Because this is a new tracheostomy, I will be sure to change the dressing frequently so as to keep it clean and help prevent infection. I will also assess for blood loss and notify the surgeon if it is excessive. I am worried also about keeping this patient well hydrated so that they can mobilize and clear their secretions.

SECTION IV: PRACTICING FOR NCLEX

Activity G MULTIPLE CHOICE

1. **Answer: a**
   RATIONALE: Acute bronchitis is caused by inflammation. Inflammatory mediators such as histamine may directly stimulate nerve endings made hypersensitive by the disease process. This process causes a sensation of pain as air travels over those nerve endings. Patients with pneumonia often experience pain with deep breathing because each breath increases pressure on pain receptors that are already compressed and irritated by swollen, inflamed lung tissue. Coronary artery disease should be ruled out in anyone complaining of chest pain but Martins sensation of burning in his airway with each breath is more suspicious for a respiratory issue. Emphysema is a more chronic illness, which causes a slow progression of increasing shortness of breath. Martin is definitely at risk for this but is would not explain his worsening shortness of breath over the last 2 days.

2. **Answer: d**
   RATIONALE: The pharynx, mouth, and nose are major organs of the upper respiratory tract. The trachea, bronchi, and lungs are major organs of the lower respiratory tract.

3. **Answer: b**
   RATIONALE: One pack year is equal to smoking one pack of cigarettes for a day for 1 year. Based on Erin's information, Erin's has a 7.5 pack-year smoking history.

4. **Answer: a**
   RATIONALE: Cyanosis around the lips indicates serious hypoxemia. Cyanosis is caused by a desaturation of oxygen on the hemoglobin in the blood. Hypercapnia is caused by an abnormally high carbon dioxide in the blood. Hypoxemia is caused by low oxygen levels in the blood.

5. **Answer: b**
   RATIONALE: The lungs move only passively. They stretch and recoil in response to neuromuscular activity.

6. **Answer: d**
   RATIONALE: Peripheral and central chemoreceptors in the aortic arch and carotid arteries and the medulla are sensitive to circulating blood levels of carbon dioxide and hydrogen ions. Increased

carbon dioxide levels lead to more rapid and shallow breathing and decreased carbon dioxide levels lead to slower and deeper respirations.

7. **Answer: c**
   RATIONALE: Burt has all the risk factors of sleep apnea, which is multiple periods of apnea during sleep. These periods of apnea cause the person to move into a lighter sleep more often than someone without this disease, thus causing the daytime sleepiness.

8. **Answer: d**
   RATIONALE: Pulmonary function testing is used to measure lung size and airway patency. Chest x-rays are used to detect pathologic lung changes. Bronchoscopy allows the visualization of the airways directly. Skin tests are used to detect allergies. A PPD is used to test for tuberculosis exposures.

9. **Answers: a, b, c, d, e, f**
   RATIONALE: All of the characteristics are part of a normal breathing pattern.

CHAPTER 26

SECTION II: ASSESSING YOUR UNDERSTANDING

Activity A FILL IN THE BLANKS

1. Five
2. Automaticity
3. Output
4. Stroke volume (SV)
5. Perfusion
6. 3
7. 50
8. Hypertension
9. 20
10. Pulmonary embolism, stroke
11. 5
12. 30
13. Sodium
14. Blood pressure

Activity B MATCHING

1. 1 – F, 2 – B, 3 – A, 4 – E, 5 – C, 6 – D
2. 1 – A, 2 – D, 3 – B, 4 – E, 5 – C

Activity C SHORT ANSWER

1. The coronary arteries are located throughout the muscular layers of the heart itself. Their function is to provide the heart with oxygenated blood. These arteries fill when the heart is relaxed (during diastole).

2. Blood passively flows into the right atrium from the systemic circulation (superior and inferior vena cava) or the left atrium from the pulmonary circulation (pulmonary veins) during diastole. As the atria fill, the increased pressure causes them to contract and blood flows into the ventricles through the AV valves. The rising pressure in the ventricles causes contraction, and blood is pushed into the pulmo-

nary circulation (from the right side of the heart) or to the systemic circulation via the aorta (from the left side of the heart).

3. Women tend to develop heart disease later in life, typically post-menopause. Women are three times more likely to develop diabetes following a myocardial infarction (MI). Women are also 50% more likely to die as a result of an MI. This is likely because women often present with atypical symptoms such as nausea or back pain.

4. Type A personalities tend to be competitive and have higher stress levels. Type D, or distressed personalities, tend to have negative attitudes and be less involved in the surrounding community and with persons around them.

5. Early signs of decreased blood flow to the brain are a new onset of anxiety or restlessness. If obstruction of blood flow continues, symptoms will progress to confusion, listlessness, slurred speech, and fatigue. A blockage of blood flow to specific areas of the brain will cause more unilateral and specific symptoms such as one-sided weakness and disturbances in speech, vision, and mobility. These occur with transient ischemic attacks (TIA) or stroke.

6. Encourage patients to change position or ambulate frequently. Flexing of leg muscles can also promote venous return. Compression stockings will help promote venous return and can be used for patients who are on their feet most of the day (i.e., nurses, waitresses) or in specific high-risk situations (air travel). These stockings should always be used in bedridden patients unless a contraindication is present. Avoid clothing that constricts blood return to the heart, such as socks with tight elastic around the top. Avoid crossing legs which creates pressure points against veins. Also avoid sitting too far back in a chair because this can also put pressure behind the knees and impede blood flow.

SECTION III: APPLYING YOUR KNOWLEDGE

Activity D CASE STUDY

1. Food choices: Edgar admits that he often eats convenience foods. These foods are typically calorie dense and high in sodium and saturated fats, all of which can contribute to heart disease. Physical activity: Edgar discussed muscle building activities but has not discussed any cardiovascular activity. Weight: Edgar is obese (defined as BMI >30). Obesity is a risk factor for cardiovascular problems such as type 2 diabetes, hypertension, and elevated cholesterol and triglyceride levels. Obesity also puts increased strain on the heart muscle itself to adequately perfuse extra tissue. Edgar's age and ethnic background are examples of non-modifiable risk factors.

2. A complete blood count (CBC) would provide information about his blood's oxygen carrying capacity and clotting ability. A B-type natriuretic peptide

(BNP) is a specific marker for heart failure and would be drawn if this diagnosis was suspected. Blood urea nitrogen (BUN) and creatinine are checked to assess kidney function since kidneys are at increased risk for damage in patients with cardiovascular disease. A lipid panel provides information about risk factors for cardiovascular disease.

3. A baseline 12-lead EKG would be appropriate for Edgar. This test would provide clues about any previous damage that may have occurred without specific cardiac symptoms. It would also provide information about heart conduction and may detect any abnormal rhythms that are present.

4. (Answers will vary). Risk for activity intolerance r/t obesity and sedentary lifestyle.

5. Document the duration, activity during onset, and vital signs during the episode of pain. Report this information to the physician. Prompt transfer to a hospital is often indicated. Once in a hospital, a 12-lead EKG should be obtained, nitroglycerin administered and oxygen started. The patient should remain on bedrest.

SECTION IV: PRACTICING FOR NCLEX

Activity E MULTIPLE CHOICE

1. **Answer: a**
   RATIONALE: Pulse oximetry is often used as a measure of tissue perfusion. An oxygen saturation of >94% is typically indicative of good tissue perfusion.

2. **Answer: b**
   RATIONALE: Coronary arteries fill during diastole. A HR of 246 bpm is known as SVT, which does not allow adequate time for diastole and thus impedes filling of the coronary arteries.

3. **Answer: d**
   RATIONALE: A minimum systolic BP for Tyler's age is 70 + (2 × age) or 80 mm Hg. The ideal systolic BP is around 100. Thus, this BP is low for Tyler's age, probably due to dehydration.

4. **Answer: a**
   RATIONALE: Smoking cessation decreases the risk for cardiovascular disease by 50%. By 3 to 4 years after smoking cessation, the risk is the same as a nonsmoker.

5. **Answer: c**
   RATIONALE: Native American heritage is an example of a non-modifiable risk factor for heart disease.

6. **Answer: b**
   RATIONALE: Alcohol use has not been linked to increased risk of DVT formation.

7. **Answer: a**
   RATIONALE: The BNP is the only test specific to heart failure. Troponin and CK-MB are used to assess for ischemia and MI. A CBC is often used as an assessment of a patient's cardiovascular well-being but does not provide specific information about heart failure.

8. **Answers: a, b, c**
   RATIONALE: The incidence of risk factors of high blood pressure increases in low-income families due to diets that are focused on fried or salty foods and more individuals live a sedentary lifestyle.

9. **Answers: a, b, c**
   RATIONALE: According to the studies (see chapter), there is evidence that women develop hypertension and cardiovascular disease later in life than men; a link between the onset of menopause and cardiovascular events and heart failure has been established, and the risk for developing diabetes following a heart attack is three times higher in women than men.

10. **Answers: a, b, d**
    RATIONALE: Statins are used to lower LDL levels.

CHAPTER 27

SECTION II: ASSESSING YOUR UNDERSTANDING

Activity A FILL IN THE BLANKS

1. Intracellular
2. Interstitial
3. Osmolarity
4. Electrolytes
5. Diffusion
6. Acid
7. Hypertonic
8. Baroreceptors

Activity B MATCHING

1. 1 – C,   2 – A,   3 – B,   4 – D
2. 1 – A,   2 – D,   3 – C,   4 – B

Activity C ORDERING

1.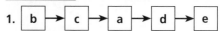

Activity D SHORT ANSWER

1. Older adults are at increased risk for electrolyte imbalances. This is especially true during and after bowel preparation for procedures such as a colonoscopy or barium enema. Fluid replacement may be needed to prevent vascular volume deficit and significantly less hypokalemia.

2. Water and electrolytes can be lost from the body in four ways. They can be lost from the kidneys as urine, from the skin as perspiration, from the gastrointestinal tract in stool or vomit, and from the lungs as insensible water loss.

3. It is important to ask patients about any recent illnesses which caused vomiting or diarrhea and to perform a good symptoms analysis of these if they occurred. It is also important to ask about chronic illnesses such as renal disease and cardiac disease, which could cause imbalances. Because medications can also cause imbalances it is important assess what the patient is taking.

4. It would be important, as a nurse, to monitor a patient's intake and output if either are found to be less than normal or there are known abnormal losses. It is also important to monitor a patient's intake and output if they are on IV therapy, if they have an illness which is known to cause imbalance, or if they are physiologically not stable.

5. Changes in the skin that indicate a fluid deficit include parched mucous membranes, a flushed appearance, dry skin, or tenting (an assessment of turgor). Skin changes that can signify a fluid volume excess include pitting edema or ascites.

SECTION III: APPLYING YOUR KNOWLEDGE

Activity E CASE STUDY

1. Because of John's congestive heart failure, his heart is not able to pump effectively. This causes a decrease in blood perfusion and a decrease in the amount of fluid that is pumped through the kidneys. Because of this, aldosterone and antidiuretic hormone secretion is stimulated which causes a resulting excess of extracellular volume and water. This extra fluid collects in the lungs, causing an increase in shortness of breath, and in there rest of the body, where it causes pitting or dependent edema.

2. One nursing intervention for John could be teaching him about restricting his oral fluid intake. This may be hard because John may feel thirsty if the fluid in his body has shifted from the intravascular space to interstitial spaces, but it is important that John doesn't exacerbate the problem by drinking more fluids. I could work with John to help him keep track of his daily fluid intake and help him to save his fluid intake for when he knows he likes to drink the most (i.e. at meal time). Ice chips may help with feelings of thirst without giving John too much extra fluids. Teaching the patient to avoid salty or very sweet fluids can also minimize his thirst.

SECTION IV: PRACTICING FOR NCLEX

Activity F MULTIPLE CHOICE

1. **Answer: a**
   RATIONALE: Buffers are substances that help to prevent large changes in pH by absorbing or releasing H + ions. Successful buffering causes extra H + ions from the weak acids of the buffer pairs to be released into the blood. The function of lungs being responsible for controlling the amount of carbon dioxide in the blood describes respiratory compensation. The function of kidneys influencing the maintenance of the normal acid-base balance describes renal compensation.

2. **Answer: b**
   RATIONALE: In addition to increased plasma levels of antidiuretic hormones, plasma levels of albu-

min decrease, so that the distribution of extracellular fluid changes, vascular volume decreases, and interstitial volume increases. Complications often lead to ascites. Complications from cardiac failure can be described as the secretion of aldosterone and antidiuretic hormone is stimulated due to a lowered blood pressure, which results in extracellular fluid volume and water excess. Hyperkalemia and hypocalcemia are common and metabolic acidosis occurs with renal failure. Complications associated to respiratory failure include a disruption of acid–base balance occurs and a disruption in this organ's ability to excrete carbon dioxide causes the pH of the person's blood to fall.

3. **Answer: a**
   RATIONALE: Chloride, along with sodium and bicarbonate, are the primary ECF electrolytes.

4. **Answer: c**
   RATIONALE: Chloride is a common anion, which is a negatively charged ion. Magnesium, potassium, and calcium are cations; positively charged ions.

5. **Answer: d**
   RATIONALE: When excess fluid cannot be eliminated, hydrostatic pressure forces some of it into the interstitial space.

6. **Answer: a**
   RATIONALE: In fact, the kidneys regulate magnesium levels by reabsorbing the ion when serum levels are low and excreting it when serum levels are high.

7. **Answer: b**
   RATIONALE: Normal serum sodium levels range from 135 to 145 mEq/L. Water usually follows sodium so if sodium is low, it means that there is too much water. Sodium along with chloride and a proportionate volume of water are regulated by the renin–angiotensin–aldosterone system and natriuretic peptides.

8. **Answer: d**
   RATIONALE: Normal serum potassium ranges from 3.5 to 5.0 mEq/L.

9. **Answer: a**
   RATIONALE: Approximately 99% of the body's calcium is found within the bones and teeth. The remainder is in the serum.

10. **Answers: a, d, e, f**
   RATIONALE: Calcium is important in wound healing, synaptic transmission in nervous tissue, membrane excitability and is essential for blood clotting.

CHAPTER 28

SECTION II: ASSESSING YOUR UNDERSTANDING

Activity A FILL IN THE BLANKS

1. Essential
2. Water
3. B

4. C
5. Processed
6. Iodine
7. High
8. Basal
9. Triples
10. 30
11. K
12. Prealbumin

Activity B **MATCHING**

1. 1 – C,   2 – A,   3 – E,   4 – D,   5 – B

Activity C **SHORT ANSWER**

1. Fat-soluble vitamins are absorbed with fat into the circulation. Since fat-soluble vitamins are stored in the liver and adipose tissue, consumption of too much can cause toxicity. Examples of fat-soluble vitamins are vitamins A, D, E, and K. Water-soluble vitamins are not stored anywhere in the body and therefore must be consumed on a daily basis. Examples include B-complex and vitamin C.
2. Infants, adolescents, and menstruating women are at highest risk for iron-deficiency anemia. Circulating hemoglobin is reduced and the body cannot meet the oxygen demands of the organs and tissues. Thus, symptoms of iron-deficiency anemia are excessive fatigue, lethargy, and poor resistance to infection.
3. Enjoy your food, but eat less quantity. Avoid over-sized portions of any food. Make fruits and vegetables half your plate portions. Switch to fat-free or low-fat (1%) milk. Make at least half your grains whole grains. Compare sodium in foods and choose foods with lower numbers. Drink water instead of sugary drinks.
4. Refined grains have undergone a process that removes the germ and bran from the product. This process also removes dietary fiber, iron, and many B vitamins. If a product is listed as "enriched," then selected B vitamins and iron have been added to replace those lost during milling.
5. Women require an increase in protein, calcium, folic acid, and iron during pregnancy. Caloric need also increases, but not by much. The adage "eating for two" does not apply; a pregnant woman who starts at an ideal body weight only requires about 200 extra calories per day to sustain healthy weight gain during pregnancy.
6. Rooms where eating will take place should be clean, well ventilated, and free of strong odors. The atmosphere should be relaxing. Oral care before eating promotes comfort and taste. Timing administration of medications to control nausea and pain will help patients achieve optimal relief at mealtimes. Food should be served in an attractive, appetizing manner and at the right temperature. Family members can bring favorite foods from home, as long as such food is permitted in the patient's diet. It is preferable

for patients to be out of bed and sitting in chairs for meals. This position facilitates chewing and swallowing and prevents reflux of stomach contents.

SECTION III: APPLYING YOUR KNOWLEDGE

Activity D CASE STUDY

1. Caloric need typically decreases as older adults become increasingly sedentary. However, the need for vitamins and most minerals remains high. Depending on where an older adult lives, they may have access to fresh fruits and vegetables or they may have difficulty obtaining groceries. Fixed incomes also contribute to the ability to purchase foods. Digestion is affected by a change in the contents of bile and pancreatic secretions, decreased peristalsis, and decreased blood flow to the GI tract. Impaired dentition can make chewing difficult. Poor dentition may make chewing difficult.
2. Women tend to need increased amount of calcium as they age to prevent osteopenia and osteoporosis. Women over age 50 typically need about 1,200 mg of calcium per day to prevent bone loss. Women also tend to need less iron when they are postmenopausal.
3. IBW for a woman who is 5'0" is about 100 lbs and about five additional pounds for every inch above 5'0". Using this formula, Ava's IBW is 110 lbs.
4. Ava is underweight and at increased risk for infections and osteoporosis. Skin, nail, and hair integrity are risk of being affected. Impaired skin integrity affects the body's first line defense against infection. Impaired mucous membranes increase the risk of poor dentition. If Ava is rapidly losing weight, she should be checked for a hypermetabolic state such as malignancy or hyperthyroidism.

SECTION IV: PRACTICING FOR NCLEX

Activity E MULTIPLE CHOICE

1. Answer: b
RATIONALE: Fiber promotes peristalsis to maintain normal bowel elimination.
2. Answer: a
RATIONALE: Normal blood glucose is 80 to 110 mg/dL.
3. Answer: d
RATIONALE: Severe vitamin D deficiency manifests as rickets, osteomalacia, poor dentition, and tetany.
4. Answer: b
RATIONALE: Vitamin B_{12} deficiency is most commonly found in vegetarians, particularly in strict vegans. Individuals who have such rigid dietary restrictions must take care to supplement this vitamin.
5. Answer: c
RATIONALE: Concurrent administration of vitamin C and iron helps with iron absorption. Orange

juice is a common and inexpensive dietary source of vitamin C.

6. **Answer: d**
   RATIONALE: Exercise increases metabolic demands beyond the basal metabolic rate.

7. **Answer: c**
   RATIONALE: Extra calcium, iron, and folic acid are often obtained via prenatal vitamins. Pregnant woman only need about 200 extra calories per day to sustain a pregnancy.

8. **Answer: c**
   RATIONALE: A body mass index (BMI) between 25 and 29.9 is considered overweight.

9. **Answer: b**
   RATIONALE: Spinach is high in vitamin K.

10. **Answer: c**
    RATIONALE: Water should comprise the majority of fluid intake. The remainder should come from food sources such as fruit or 100% fruit juices.

11. **Answers: a, b, d**
    RATIONALE: Pale mucous membranes might be a sign of anemia.

12. **Answers: b, c, d**
    RATIONALE: The level of HDL cholesterol, or "good" cholesterol, in the blood is lowered by trans fats.

13. **Answers: b, c, d**
    RATIONALE: Cutting carbohydrates is not necessary for long-term weight loss.

CHAPTER 29

SECTION II: ASSESSING YOUR UNDERSTANDING

Activity A FILL IN THE BLANKS

1. Incision
2. Macerated
3. Dermatitis
4. Abrasion
5. Friction
6. Granulation
7. Hematoma
8. Dehiscence
9. Fistula

Activity B MATCHING

1. 1 – A,   2 – A,   3 – B,   4 – C
2. 1 – D,   2 – F,   3 – A,   4 – E,   5 – B,   6 – C

Activity C ORDERING

1. d → c → a → b

Activity D SHORT ANSWER

1. Newborn skin is thinner and more sensitive than that of older infants. Active sebaceous glands may cause milia, small cysts that appear around the chin and nose. Lanugo, fine hair, may cover the newborn's skin.

2. Good nutrition is important for healthy skin by providing it with the nutrients it needs. Adequate protein and calorie intake prevents hair from becoming dull and dry as well as preventing hair loss. Many vitamins prevent abnormal skin changes and adequate intake of iron, copper, and zinc is important to prevent abnormal pigmentation and changes in nails and hair.

3. Shear force occurs when tissue layers move on each other, causing blood vessels to stretch as they pass through the subcutaneous tissue. This stretching of the blood vessels leads to torn vessels which, in turn, increases the risk for ulcer formation.

4. Wound healing may be decreased in obese patients because adipose tissue is relatively avascular. This means that it provides a weak defense against microbial invasion and impairs delivery of nutrients to a wound.

5. Health promotion should focus on maintaining intact skin, which is the body's first line of defense. Maintaining adequate hydration of the skin as well as maintaining adequate nutrition should be a part of this. Also, teaching about adequate circulation is imperative and can be maintained by exercise and frequent turning of patients who are immobile.

SECTION III: APPLYING YOUR KNOWLEDGE

Activity E CASE STUDY

1. Nursing management of pruritus aims at relieving the situations that cause it, decreasing the associated discomfort, and preventing additional trauma to the skin. This can be done by applying lotions regularly, limiting bathing which promotes skin drying, and by using a gentle soap which is rinsed off entirely. It would also be important to advise Soriah to keep her nails cut short and to not scratch the irritated area. Cool baths or compresses may help as well so this can be offered to her.

2. Because Soriah's abscess is deep and has moderate drainage, I might should a product such as alginate to place in the wound. This type of dressing would also help to prevent the wound from closing prematurely. I would then cover it with a protective pad and secure the dressing with a nonallergenic paper, silk, or nonwoven fabric tape so as not to irritate her skin further.

SECTION IV: PRACTICING FOR NCLEX

Activity F MULTIPLE CHOICE

1. **Answers: a, d**
   RATIONALE: The major cell of the dermis produces collagen and elastin and is the thickest skin layer. The dermis underlies the epidermis, which is the skin's outermost layer. The major cell of the epidermis produces keratin, while the basal cells of the epidermis produce melanin.

2. Answer: b
RATIONALE: Hair, the sebaceous gland and eccrine sweat glands are skin appendages that are formed with the enfolding of the epidermis into the dermis. The dermis is composed of connective tissue.

3. Answer: a
RATIONALE: Second-degree burns are moderate to deep partial-thickness burns that may be pink, red, pale ivory, or light yellow-brown. They are usually moist with blisters. First-degree burns are superficial and may be pinkish or red with no blistering. Third-degree burns are full-thickness burns and may vary from brown or black to cherry red or pearly white; bullae may be present; can appear dry and leathery.

4. Answer: c
RATIONALE: In partial-thickness wounds, in the third phase, the proliferative phase, epidermal cells reproduce and migrate across the surface of the wound in a process called epithelialization. The onset of vasoconstriction, platelet aggregation, and clot formation are part of the first phase of wound healing; hemostasis. The second phase, the inflammatory phase is marked by vasodilation and phagocytosis as the body works to clean the wound. Maturation is the final stage of full-thickness wound healing in which the number of fibroblasts decreases, collagen synthesis stabilized and collagen fibril become increasingly organized.

5. Answer: c
RATIONALE: Healing by secondary intention occurs in wounds with edges that do not readily approximate. The wound gradually fills with granulation tissue and, eventually, epithelial cells migrate across the granulation base. Wounds with minimal tissue loss, such as wounds with clean surgical incisions or shallow sutured wounds. The edges of the wound are approximated and the risk of infection is lower when a wound heals in this manner. Maturation is the final stage of full-thickness wound healing. Tertiary intention occurs when a delay happens between injury and wound closure. The delay may occur when a deep wound is not sutured immediately or left open until no sign of infection.

6. Answer: d
RATIONALE: Evisceration is the protrusion of viscera through an abdominal wound opening. Evisceration can follow dehiscence if the opening extends deeply enough to allow the abdominal fascia to separate and internal organs to protrude.

7. Answer: b
RATIONALE: Keratin is the primary material in the shed layer of cells. Melanin is what protects against the sun's ultraviolet rays.

8. Answer: a
RATIONALE: Local capillary pressure must be higher than external pressure for adequate skin perfusion.

9. Answers: a, b, c, e, f
RATIONALE: Sensory perception, nutrition, ability, and friction are all part of the criteria used in the Braden Scale. Age is not a graded criterion in predicting the risk for pressure ulcers.

10. Answer: c
RATIONALE: This describes serosanguineous wound drainage. Drainage that is pale yellow, watery, and like the fluid from a blister is called serous. Drainage that is bloody is called sanguineous and drainage that contains white cells and microorganisms is called purulent.

CHAPTER 30

SECTION II: ASSESSING YOUR UNDERSTANDING

Activity A FILL IN THE BLANKS

1. Skin
2. Warmth
3. Adolescence
4. Virus
5. Hyperglycemia
6. Latent
7. Bacteria, parasites
8. Four
9. Antibiotic
10. Allergic
11. Six
12. Opportunistic

Activity B MATCHING

1. 1 – C,   2 – A,   3 – B,   4 – D
2. 1 – E,   2 – B,   3 – A,   4 – C,   5 – D

Activity C SEQUENCING

1.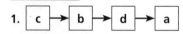

Activity D SHORT ANSWER

1. Active immunity is developed in response to antigen exposure. An example is immunity to a particular influenza virus strain after weeks of illness or after vaccination. Passive immunity bypasses the host's immune system by giving antibodies directly to the host. Infants acquire passive immunity from their mothers across the placenta and intravenous immunoglobulin (IVIG) can be given to protect an individual following exposure to a particular infection.

2. The skin becomes thinner, drier, and loses elasticity. This decreases its barrier function as the primary prevention against infection. White blood cell (WBC) counts do not always rise in response to infection and phagocytosis is stunted. Thus, patients do not mount a fever to infection and the body is unable to properly fight the invasion. Infections can quickly become widespread with little warning.

3. The incubation period spans the time of entry to the appearance of symptoms; thus this period is symptom free. During this time, the organism invades the body and multiplies. Incubation can last from hours to years depending on the offending pathogen. The prodromal phase is when vague symptoms manifest themselves, such as fever, pharyngitis or body aches. The prodromal phase is actually quite predictable for many illnesses and helps the nurse identify the offending organism.

4. Recent exposure to illness. Normal sleep and exercise patterns and any variance. Vaccination history and recent travel outside of the area. A list of medications the patient is currently taking. Recreational drugs, cigarette or alcohol use, all of which can depress the immune system or expose the individual to specific pathogens. Any chronic health conditions that increase patient's susceptibility to infection. Ability to function and perform activities of daily living (ADL).

5. Skin and environmental contaminants can easily grow in culture medium. This can lead to a false positive culture result and unnecessary treatment with antibiotics.

6. Warm broth and rest may ease feelings of malaise. A tepid sponge bath or cool cloth to the forehead may ease fever. Warm blankets can ease shaking chills.

SECTION III: APPLYING YOUR KNOWLEDGE

Activity E CASE STUDY

1. The risk for infection r/t impairment of skin integrity.

2. A WBC count of >12,000 or <4,000 with immature granulocytes (bands) >10%. ESR > 15 mm/hr. Lactate > 2.6 mmol/L. Temperature > 38.2 °C or < 36 °C, HR > 90 bpm, RR > 20. Alex's age may cause his WBC count to drop rather than increase. He may also develop a mild fever or have a drop in temperature rather than a high fever, even with a serious systemic infection.

3. Don sterile gloves. DO NOT clean the site prior to collection of the culture as you would remove the offending organism. Using a sterile cotton swab, collect an area of pus with the tip. Be careful not to touch the surrounding skin as to avoid collecting normal skin flora. Place the cotton swab in the culture medium.

4. Keep the incision and skin surrounding clean and dry. Apply dressings or medications as ordered. Maintain a therapeutic environment, minimizing noise and interruption. Remove invasive devices such as IVs and other catheters as soon as it is safe to do so. Ensure the patient receives adequate nutrition and advocate for enteral nutrition as the patient displays signs of readiness. Encourage ambulation when appropriate; if not appropriate, encourage the patient to sit up, take deep breaths and actively or passively move all extremities.

SECTION IV: PRACTICING FOR NCLEX

Activity F MULTIPLE CHOICE

1. **Answer: d**
   RATIONALE: Children can frequently have fevers over 40 °C. Young children are more prone to febrile seizures than adults. However, the overall percentage of children who have a febrile seizure is still relatively low. Young children frequently mount a high fever to an invading organism. A fever of 39.5 °C is not typical of a post-operative temperature elevation.

2. **Answer: a**
   RATIONALE: Mr. Porter is exhibiting signs of an infection: tachycardia, tachypnea, and diaphoresis, which likely indicates fever. Pneumonia is most common 2 to 5 days post-op. Mr. Porter is particularly at risk because, following a hip replacement, he is unable to ambulate. This can lead to pooling of respiratory secretions, which attracts microorganisms.

3. **Answer: a**
   RATIONALE: Ambulation helps to prevent the stasis of secretions. Invasive devices, breaks in skin integrity, and inadequate nutrition are all risk factors for infection.

4. **Answer: d**
   RATIONALE: Colonization occurs when microorganisms are introduced into a body surface and grow and multiply but do not invade or cause illness. In a vulnerable host, colonization can lead to infection.

5. **Answer: b**
   RATIONALE: The definition of a high-grade fever is anything above 38.2 °C and below 40.5 °C.

6. **Answer: a**
   RATIONALE: Nursing diagnoses should not convey judgment. Avoid using loaded words such as "promiscuous". There is no evidence of a knowledge deficit.

7. **Answer: a**
   RATIONALE: Peak levels are drawn shortly after the drug is administered. 3 PM is the best choice because it closely follows the time of infusion which is when the drug concentration would be highest.

8. **Answers: a, c, d**
   RATIONALE: It is not necessary for Pam to shower with harsh soaps. This may actually lead to drying of the skin and decreased skin integrity which is the first barrier to infection.

9. **Answers: a, b, c**
   RATIONALE: The thymus is critical in the development of T-lymphocytes. The tonsils and spleen are critical storage areas for lymphocytes, particularly in children and young adults.

10. **Answers: c, d**
    RATIONALE: A temperature greater than 38 °C and a WBC count greater than 12,000 or less than 4,000 are signs of septicemia. Other signs include a HR greater than 90 bpm and a RR greater than

20 bpm, chills, confusion, lethargy, mottling and decreased urine output.

CHAPTER 31

SECTION II: ASSESSING YOUR UNDERSTANDING

Activity A FILL IN THE BLANKS

1. Detrusor
2. Micturition
3. Diuresis
4. Hydronephrosis
5. Cystitis
6. Polyuria
7. Stress
8. Enuresis
9. Cystocele

Activity B MATCHING

1. 1 – B,   2 – D,   3 – A,   4 – C

Activity C ORDERING

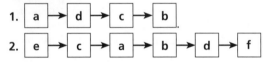

Activity D SHORT ANSWER

1. Loss of body fluid affects urination by causing the kidneys to increase reabsorption of water from the glomerular filtrate in order to maintain proper osmolarity of extracellular fluid. This increase in reabsorption causes urine output to be decreased.
2. A nurse can facilitate normal pattern identification by asking specific questions regarding a person's urination such as when they last voided, how many times per day do they usually void, what amount do they usually void, and whether they wake up during the night to void. The nurse can also facilitate the gathering of information by ensuring privacy and by being sensitive to the patient's feelings of embarrassment. It is also important to use words that the patient can understand such as "peeing" instead of "urination" which everyone might not know the meaning of.
3. In order to identify areas of risk for someone with urinary issues, it is important to ask about any previous renal or urinary tract problems and, if positive, how was it treated. It is also important to ask about any recent changes in a person's daily routine and the person's physical ability to reach the bathroom in time.
4. Urine output that is greater than fluid intake may indicate diuresis whereas urine output which is less than fluid intake could indicate a decrease in kidney perfusion, loss of body fluids from other sources, or a physiologic conservation of body fluids. If intake and output are not assessed for, it is harder to detect such issues and to further evaluate what might be happening.

5. The risks associated with catheterization are a risk for infection and a risk for trauma. In order to prevent infections from catheterization it is important use sterile technique during catheter insertion and to remove the catheter as soon as it is not indicated. Using securement devices can help reduce trauma.

SECTION III: APPLYING YOUR KNOWLEDGE

Activity E CASE STUDY

1. Nursing assessment of Tony's suprapubic catheter includes frequent observations of his urine noting color, clarity, and quantity. It also includes assessing his fluid intake, temperature, and level of comfort and the condition of the abdominal insertion site.
2. Home considerations for Tony include teaching him how to properly care for his device. It is also important that Tony knows how to recognize signs of infection and what to do if he notices them.

SECTION IV: PRACTICING FOR NCLEX

Activity F MULTIPLE CHOICE

1. **Answer: a**
   RATIONALE: By the age of 5, children should be continent both during the day and the night. Although most children in North America achieve daytime continence by 3 years of age, some can take a bit longer. Most children will achieve daytime urinary control by 3 to 4 years of age. The first voiding may be slightly pink-tinges. This is caused by uric acid crystals being excreted. School-age children should achieve urinary elimination habits that are similar to adults. This frequency and color are very normal.
2. **Answer: a**
   RATIONALE: Urine output of less than 30 mL per hour may indicate inadequate blood flow to the kidneys. In adults, the average amount of urine per void is approximately 200 to 400 mL. Adults generally have a urine output of 1500 mL per day, while children, depending on age, have a urine output between 500 and 1500 mL per day. Urine output can vary greatly, depending on intake and fluid losses.
3. **Answer: d**
   RATIONALE: Urine may appear cloudy, dark reddish-brown, or streaked with blood when a woman is menstruating.
4. **Answer: a**
   RATIONALE: A 24-hour urine specimen is required for accurate measurement of the kidney's excretion of substances that the kidney does not excrete at the same rate throughout the day. A clean-catch or midstream-voided specimen is used when a specimen relatively free from microorganisms is required. Random urine specimen collection is used when sterile urine is not required.

5. Answer: c
RATIONALE: Functional Incontinence is the inability of a normally continent person to reach the bathroom in time to avoid the unintentional loss of urine. Stress Incontinence is a state where the patient loses small amounts of urine with increased pressure on the abdomen. Urge Urinary Incontinence is when a patient experiences an involuntary loss of urine, when a specific bladder volume is reached. Total Urinary Incontinence is when a patient experiences continuous, unpredictable loss of urine.

6. Answer: a
RATIONALE: Untreated diabetes insipidus can cause an increase in the formation and excretion of urine without a concurrent increase in fluid intake. Renal disease often leads to oliguria and even anuria, a decrease in urine outputs. Urinary tract infections causes and increase in frequency but not necessarily an increase in the amount of urine that is produced. Renal calculi can cause hematuria.

7. Answers: a, b, c
RATIONALE: Older men experience urinary hesitancy and delayed urinary stream related to prostati hypertrophy. Older adults may attempt to manage incontinence by restricting fluid intake, using absorbent pads in clothing, and changing clothing. Kidney function decreases with age due to cardiovascular changes. Urinary incontinence is not usually a health problem in the early to middle adult years. Women have a higher risk of developing urinary incontinence due to lower estrogen levels and weakened perineal muscles.

8. Answers: c, d, e, f
RATIONALE: Alcohol and caffeine-containing foods irritate the bladder and contain a diuretic that can increase urine output when they are ingested in large amounts. If large quantities of salty foods, such as potato chips or pretzels are ingested without increasing water intake, urine outpot will decrease and the urine will be more concentrated.

9. Answer: d
RATIONALE: While the specimen can be collected at any time during the day, the first urine voided in the morning is preferred. The first urine is usually more concentrated because the patient does not usually consume fluid during the night and the effects of diet and activity are minimized.

CHAPTER 32

SECTION II: ASSESSING YOUR UNDERSTANDING

Activity A FILL IN THE BLANKS

1. Jejunum
2. Peristalsis
3. Parasympathetic
4. 75; 2,000
5. Incontinence
6. 72
7. Umbilicus
8. Duodenocolonic
9. Warm
10. Right
11. Enzymatic juices

Activity B MATCHING

1. 1 – C,   2 – A,   3 – E,   4 – D,   5 – B
2. 1 – C,   2 – E,   3 – B,   4 – B,   5 – D

Activity C SEQUENCING

1.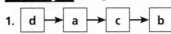

Activity D SHORT ANSWER

1. *Clostridium difficile* is the most common cause of hospital-acquired diarrhea in the United States. Normal gastrointestinal flora prevents the growth of the bacteria *C. difficile* in the intestines. However, when gastrointestinal flora are disturbed, typically by antibiotics, *C. difficile* spores replicate and release a toxin that causes profuse, foul-smelling diarrhea.

2. Paralytic ileus or an abdominal tumor can mechanically prevent stool and flatus from passing through the intestine and cause abdominal distention. Constipation can also mechanically block the evacuation of flatus. A decrease in activity, such as bed rest after surgery, can cause peristalsis to slow.

3. The history and other parts of the physical exam will dictate with what force the nurse presses on the abdomen. Palpation may also temporarily stimulate bowel tones and thus skew auscultation.

4. The FOBT looks for unseen (occult) blood in the stool. Blood in the stool can be a sign of upper or lower GI tract bleeding. If blood is occult, it is typically an ominous sign indicative of bleeding from an ulcer or a tumor. Bleeding from hemorrhoids or contamination from menstrual bleeding is typically visible, not occult. To perform this test, place a small smear of stool on the card, then apply the appropriate developer. A color change to blue indicates a "positive" test or the presence of blood. The American Cancer Society recommends annual FOBT screening for colorectal cancer in all persons age 50 and older.

5. Encourage five to six servings of high-fiber foods and 1.5 to 2 L of fluid intake daily. Daily exercises such as walking promote peristalsis. Isometric abdominal and pelvic floor exercises help to strengthen the Valsalva maneuver. Encourage the patient to make time for defecation at regular intervals (whatever is regular for the patient).

6. Low suction is 20 to 40 mm Hg. High suction is 80 to 120 mm Hg. If a nasogastric tube has a vent, continuous suction may be used. The vent prevents the stomach from being "caught" in the suction of the tube. This vent should be frequently irrigated with air to ensure patency. Intermittent suction is required when a nasogastric tube does not have a vent.

SECTION III: APPLYING YOUR KNOWLEDGE

Activity E CASE STUDY

1. The risk for impaired skin integrity r/t colonic diversion to the abdomen; the risk for infection r/t presence of invasive tubing.
2. Ensure accurate placement of the nasogastric tube. Extract a small amount of fluid from the tube using a syringe and test the pH. If it is placed properly, the pH should be <5. Note that some medications may alter the pH of the stomach. Instillation of air and auscultation of the air bubble can be used as a secondary process to assure confirmation.
3. The perfusion of the intestine should be assessed immediately post-op and frequently during the first days of hospitalization. The stoma should appear pink and moist, though exudates may be present post-op. A bluish discoloration indicates decreased perfusion. Skin integrity should also be assessed immediately post-op and on a regular basis throughout the hospitalization. A wound care nurse can assist in maintaining skin integrity by developing a method for stool and intestinal content collection. Stoma patency is also assessed; observation of regular discharge of gastric contents is often sufficient to ensure patency.

SECTION IV: PRACTICING FOR NCLEX

Activity F MULTIPLE CHOICE

1. **Answer: a**
   RATIONALE: Some vitamins and iron are absorbed in the ileum, along with a small amount of fluid. However, most of the fluid is absorbed in the large intestine. Electrolytes are predominantly absorbed in the duodenum, jejunum, and large intestine.
2. **Answer: c**
   RATIONALE: Contraction of the external sphincter is a voluntary reflex in response to the defecation reflex.
3. **Answer: d**
   RATIONALE: Antibiotics, such as Bactrim DS, iron, and immobility can cause constipation.
4. **Answer: b**
   RATIONALE: According to the Rome III criteria, symptoms must be present for 12 nonconsecutive weeks in the last 12 months for 25% of bowel movements.
5. **Answer: a**
   RATIONALE: A bluish or dark stoma indicates impaired circulation to the stoma. This requires intervention to improve circulation to avoid permanent damage to the stoma.
6. **Answer: d**
   RATIONALE: This patient is not currently experiencing diarrhea. He does not describe his stools as watery or loose. Rather, this patient's problem is with control of the bowel.

7. **Answer: a**
   RATIONALE: Children should not, but may, return to a school or daycare setting during the infectious phase of their illness. Hand washing is key to preventing the spread of infection.
8. **Answers: a, b**
   RATIONALE: Family members should never be substituted for a medical interpreter. Use of an interpreter who is of the same age and gender may be helpful in this situation. The presence of blood in the stool is always of concern and must be addressed that day.
9. **Answers: a, b, c**
   RATIONALE: It is unlikely that a patient who needs a bowel training program will regain their previous level of bowel independence. However, this does not mean that a patient cannot create a new, independent norm for themselves.
10. **Answers: a, b, c**
    RATIONALE: The risks for colorectal cancer increase after the age of 50, have a positive family history of colorectal cancer, and also has Crohn's disease. An important nursing responsibility is to teach patients about annual screening begin at 50, encourage endoscopic exam every 5 years, or colonoscopy every 10 years for normal-risk individuals.
12. **Answers: b, c, d**
    RATIONALE: Nonpharmacologic methods, including fiber supplementation, are often sufficient to promote healthy defecation pattern.

CHAPTER 33

SECTION II: ASSESSING YOUR UNDERSTANDING

Activity A FILL IN THE BLANKS

1. Rest
2. Polysomnography
3. Sleepiness
4. Circadian
5. Nocturia
6. Hypnotics
7. Narcolepsy
8. Parasomnias
11. Fatigue
12. Latency

Activity B MATCHING

1. 1 – B,   2 – A,   3 – E,   4 – C,   5 – D
2. 1 – C,   2 – A,   3 – D,   4 – B,   5 – E

Activity C SEQUENCING

1. b → a → e → c → d

Activity D SHORT ANSWER

1. Cultural considerations having to do with sleep include differences in beliefs and behavior. In some

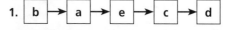

cultures naps are acceptable, whereas in other cultures the use of caffeine is more widely accepted in the middle of the day. Sleep hygiene varies from one cultural to another as well as beliefs surrounding "co-sleeping" within families.

2. A change in someone's sleep–wake schedule causes disruption in his or her internal circadian clock and sleep–wake cycle. Often times, people are not able to sleep at times that are misaligned with their body's circadian rhythm that causes a sleep deficit. This deficit, over a long period of time, causes an increase in health risk for effected individuals and leads to increased sleepiness, compromises clinical judgment, and decreases decision-making ability.

3. Sleep disordered breathing (SDB) is considered a major public health and safety issue because it results in chronic sleep disturbances. Chronic sleep disturbances lead to excessive daytime sleepiness and an increased risk for motor vehicle accidents. SDB is also hard to diagnose. Patients may complain of difficulty concentrating or poor memory and may not realize that these are symptoms of restless sleep.

4. Sleep hygiene consists of the common practices that effect sleep. This includes exercise, the use of stimulants, and having a routine at bedtime. Exercise can either positively affect sleep, by getting an adequate amount each day, or can negatively affect sleep, by performing strenuous exercise close to bedtime. The use of stimulants, especially closer to bedtime, would be considered poor sleep hygiene because it can increase sleep latency. Having a relaxing bedtime routine that prepares your mind for sleep would be considered good sleep hygiene.

5. Hypnotics are useful for treating insomnia in the short term. They can help someone sleep but they do not induce normal sleep, can impair waking function, and have side effects. Certain people should not take hypnotics because they can further depress someone's respiratory drive and may take longer to metabolize in some patients.

SECTION III: APPLYING YOUR KNOWLEDGE

Activity E CASE STUDY

1. Using the BEARS approach, I would assess the full extent of Virginia's insomnia and by including the spouse in the assessment I may be able to gather additional information about the issue. I would further want to identify Virginia's normal sleep–wake cycle to identify adequacy of her sleep. Once the problem is identified and fully illustrated, I would perform a physical assessment looking for signs of sleep deprivation such as the presence of dark circles under her eyes.

2. Interventions to promote sleep for Virginia would be based on redflags that were identified during her assessment. She might state, for example, that she can't fall asleep if she can hear any of her children making noise. Interventions would include environmental modifications and recommendations to improve sleep hygiene if appropriate. I would provide education on the importance of intimacy and security and how to manage sleep needs. This may be difficult with a 6 month old but we could work together to come up with a sleep ritual and her husband may be able to help with putting the children to bed, if he doesn't already, so Virginia can do her own routine that might include a relaxation exercise.

3. Use of a consistent routine, although harder to accomplish in the setting of a hospital, is important to maintain. I could implement a plan to help her go to bed and get up at the same time each day. I can help her fall asleep by teaching her relaxation exercises and stress management techniques. If medications are warranted, I could provide those to her once ordered and educate her on the side effects. I would also want to work with her to come up with a plan for getting enough sleep when she goes home.

SECTION IV: PRACTICING FOR NCLEX

Activity F MULTIPLE CHOICE

1. **Answer: c**
   RATIONALE: Susanna appears to be suffering from early-awakening insomnia. Because it has been longer than 1 month it is considered a chronic insomnia. Danielle appears to be suffering from insufficient sleep syndrome. She does not have an adequate amount of time for sleep each night, as seen with insomnia, but it is a self-imposed restriction of sleep. Mike is not getting enough sleep because he has some form of SDB. Although he might think he is allowing enough time for sleep, his quality of sleep is disrupted by these periods of apnea. John appears to be suffering from narcolepsy. Along with the two episodes of cataplexy, he is excessively sleepy throughout the day and falls asleep at inappropriate times.

2. **Answer: a**
   RATIONALE: Drinking a caffeinated beverage is not as energizing as a short 15-30 minute nap, stretching exercises, or taking a short walk.

3. **Answer: d**
   RATIONALE: Brain activity decreases from wakefulness. During SWS, muscles are relaxed, but muscle tone is maintained during NREM. Sympathetic nerve activity decreases from wakefulness and body temperature is regulated at a lower level from wakefulness.

4. **Answer: a**
   RATIONALE: By middle age, the frequency of nocturnal awakenings increases, and satisfaction with sleep quality decreases. Situational variables such as job-related stress, pregnancy, parenting, family caregiving responsibilities, and illness may explain these changes in sleep patterns.

5. Answer: b

RATIONALE: This outcome criterion addresses the goal by stating physical, objective, signs that the person is better rested. It also mentions a timeframe, which makes it measurable and easier to evaluate.

6. Answers: a, b, c

RATIONALE: Blood pressure and pulse rate show wide variations and may fluctuate rapidly, a person is unable to move during this stage, and theta waves often have a sawtooth or notched appearance. Muscles are relaxed but muscle tone is maintained and sleepwalking and bed-wetting are most likely to occur during NREM.

7. Answers: a, b, c, d, e

RATIONALE: All of these factors affect sleep and rest. Relationships can include parents frequent awakening while caring for infants contribute to chronic sleep loss and disturbances in a primary relationship may cause sleep loss. Food affects people differently, some people will awaken from hunger while others cannot fall asleep if they've just eaten. Vigilance is the perceived need to create a protective role, such as the parent that creates an arousal threshold so they can the small child wandering down the hall in the middle of the night. Shift work affects sleep as frequent changes in the sleep-wake schedule contributes to the mis-alignment of the internal circadian clock.

8. Answers: a, b, c, d

RATIONALE: Avoiding strenuous activities and caffeine for several hours before bedtime can help an individual who is having difficulty falling asleep. This patient could also benefit from removing any distractions in his bedroom, by improving his sense of security by decreasing any feelings of social isolation, and by creating a routine around bedtime. Teaching Torrance that shorter unbroken sleep periods are not normal not only provides him with false information but may also cause him to feel abnormal.

CHAPTER 34

SECTION II: ASSESSING YOUR UNDERSTANDING

Activity A FILL IN THE BLANKS

1. Sympathetic
2. Endogenous
3. Heighten
4. School
5. Somatic
6. Suffering
7. Children
8. Assessment
9. Multimodal
10. Patient

Activity B MATCHING

1. 1 – E,   2 – C,   3 – A,   4 – D,   5 – B
2. 1 – C,   2 – A,   3 – D,   4 – B

Activity C SEQUENCING

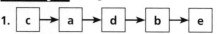

1. c → a → d → b → e

Activity D SHORT ANSWER

1. Pain in older adults can be disabling, leading to decreased mobility and resulting social isolation. Untreated pain increases the risk of depression and cognitive dysfunction, perhaps as a result of social isolation and decreased physical function. Untreated pain also increases the difficulty of self-care in the older adult population, since older adults are more likely to become disabled from chronic pain when compared to their younger counterparts.

2. Vital sign changes include increase in heart rate, respiratory rate, and blood pressure.

3. Tolerance is an adaptive function of the body. When the body is exposed to a substance over and over again, such as an opioid, the body will begin to need more to have the same effect. Addiction is a neurologic disease that is characterized by compulsive use, impaired control, and cravings despite physical harm.

4. Symptoms of physical withdrawal include diaphoresis, anxiety, tachycardia, or nausea. Patients can avoid these unpleasant symptoms by tapering their medications slowly over the course of days to weeks.

5. Heat, particularly moist penetrating heat, can relieve stiffness. Massage is effective for muscular pain. Strengthening and stretching will help to stabilize surrounding muscles. TENS and biofeedback are particularly useful to help patient's avoid narcotic use.

SECTION III: APPLYING YOUR KNOWLEDGE

Activity E CASE STUDY

1. The Wong-Baker FACES scale is often appropriate for children under the age of 8 years. You could also approach Sahib's family and ask for their input into his behavior.

2. Sahib is likely in severe pain. An IV opioid agonist or an epidural (if already placed) with opioid would be appropriate options.

3. Addiction is a complex cognitive process that involves cravings and use of a substance despite adverse consequences. Children can often develop physical tolerance to opioids. However, children this young are not cognitively developed enough to experience addiction.

4. Respiratory depression is the most serious side effect of opioid use, particularly in an opioid-naïve patient. Constipation is the most common side effect. All patients who are on opioid therapy should also have a bowel program laid out for them. Other side effects are dose related and include sedation, nausea, vomiting, pruritus, delirium.

SECTION IV: PRACTICING FOR NCLEX

Activity F MULTIPLE CHOICE

1. **Answer: c**
   RATIONALE: Herpes zoster is a common cause of hyperalgia.
2. **Answer: d**
   RATIONALE: Opioids are not contraindicated in older adults but are rarely used in chronic pain prior to nonpharmacologic measures.
3. **Answer: a**
   RATIONALE: Caucasian individuals most commonly rely on western medicine to treat chronic pain.
4. **Answer: a**
   RATIONALE: Depression and anxiety often lead to increase in pain sensation.
5. **Answer: d**
   RATIONALE: Kidney function would be temporarily suppressed by acute pain.
6. **Answer: a**
   RATIONALE: Pain should be addressed during your first encounter with the patient. However, you will probably want to start a professional conversation prior to addressing pain. Vital signs are often collected in the beginning of the patient visit. This would be the most appropriate time to address pain.
7. **Answer: b**
   RATIONALE: Gabapentin is used to treat nerve pain.
8. **Answer: b**
   RATIONALE: Tolerance is characterized by the need for increased dose of narcotic over time.
9. **Answer: c**
   RATIONALE: Respiratory depression is always a major concern in an opioid-naïve patient.
10. **Answers: a, c**
    RATIONALE: Rest, ice, and elevation are most appropriate immediately following injury. Heat can be applied for pain after swelling diminishes, usually after a few days. Range of motion should be started several weeks after injury when the patient is pain-free.
11. **Answers: a, b**
    RATIONALE: Assessment of pain a minimum of once per shift is a Joint Commission standard of care. More frequent assessment is required if pain is not controlled.
12. **Answers: b, c**
    RATIONALE: Artificial nails are never appropriate. Chewing of nails is not prohibited, but if the skin surrounding the nail is not intact, gloves should be worn.
13. **Answers: b, c, d**
    RATIONALE: Although peripheral nerves may be less sensitive to painful stimuli, older adults very much experience pain. However, this pain is often underreported.

CHAPTER 35

SECTION II: ASSESSING YOUR UNDERSTANDING

Activity A FILL IN THE BLANKS

1. Reticular
2. Receptors
3. Visceral
4. Special
5. Somatic
6. Sensoristasis
7. Overload
8. Hallucinations
9. Kinesthetic
10. After burn
11. Deprivation

Activity B MATCHING

1. 1 – C, 2 – B, 3 – E, 4 – A, 5 – D

Activity C SEQUENCING

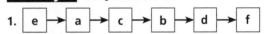

1. e → a → c → b → d → f

Activity D SHORT ANSWER

1. Adaptation occurs when sensory receptors adapt to repeated stimulation by responding less and less. Lead time and after burn are the ways in which a person processes new stimuli so that he or she can respond appropriately.
2. Internal factors, information, and the environment can all lead to sensory overload and a decrease in the amount of information that is actually relayed. If a patient is overwhelmed by a diagnosis or procedure in general or is impaired by a medication they are taking, they are less likely to comprehend what you are trying to teach. Likewise, if you give too much information at one time, people tend not to absorb a lot of it. By taking into account the environment that information is given in, the nurse is able to allow for adjustment in a new environment and may be able to decrease extraneous environment stimuli which can detract from someone's learning.
3. When someone is depressed they develop a sense of helplessness and a loss of self-esteem. This leads to a withdrawal from social interaction and sensory input from the world around them.
4. Subjective data provides important information about a person's sensory perception. Subjective data can identify someone's normal level of functioning. By asking someone how he or she spends a typical day, for instance, you can gain insight into the level of stimulation the person usually experiences. It can also be used to identify any risks and/or dysfunctions.
5. Patient teaching topics to address sensory perception should include ways to prevent sensory loss and to maintain general health. Health promotion

could include topics such as getting a regular eye examination and the importance of close control of chronic illnesses such as diabetes and hypertension. Another topic could be using protective eye and ear wear in appropriate situations to prevent vision and hearing loss.

Activity E CROSSWORD

Down
1. Adaptation
2. Kinesthetic
5. Overstimulation

Across
3. Delusions
4. Anxiety
6. Disturbed

SECTION III: APPLYING YOUR KNOWLEDGE

Activity F CASE STUDY

1. I know that she has total lack of sensory input in her lower extremities. I also know that she normally functions at a high level when in her own environment as she is able to complete much of her activities of daily living independently. I also know that because she lives in a skilled nursing facility she has access to assistance if she needs it and is probably provided transportation.

2. The biggest risk identified in this scenario so far is her inability to relax in this new environment with increased auditory stimuli. I would want to know how she has dealt with change in the past to find out if her anxiety has escalated in the hospital setting or if it passes with interventions and time. I would also want to know if she is taking any medications, either for her anxiety or otherwise, that would affect her sensory perception.

3. This patient is indicating that the increased noise and the lack of privacy are affecting her negatively. Because of this, as her nurse, I would want to work on stimulation reduction. I would focus on reducing the amount of information I give her at one time; I would work on changing the environment so there is less noise, and work on reducing internal factors causing her anxiety. If the sensory overload were causing her to neglect her activities of daily living than I would assist her in accomplishing those as well.

SECTION IV: PRACTICING FOR NCLEX

Activity G MULTIPLE CHOICE

1. **Answer: c**
   RATIONALE: A newborn's sensory perception is rudimentary. They see only gross patterns of light and dark or bright colors.

2. **Answer: d**
   RATIONALE: Laney is experiencing altered sensory reception because her progressive blindness is limiting her visual cues. Tracy, Marcus, and Lydia are experiencing a sensory deprivation because they are immersed in deprived environments.

3. **Answers: a, b, c, d**
   RATIONALE: Touch, pressure, vibration, and positioning are all somatic senses. Auditory acuity is associated with normal hearing. Odors are associated with normal smell.

4. **Answers: c, d, e**
   RATIONALE: Visual acuity at or near 20/20, full field of vision, and tricolor vision (red, blue, green) are all associated with normal vision. Extraocular movement refers to the movement of parts of eye and are assessed in a vision examination.

5. **Answers: a, b, c, d, e**
   RATIONALE: All of these sensory aids can help promote optimal function of the impaired sense and other available senses.

CHAPTER 36

SECTION II: ASSESSING YOUR UNDERSTANDING

Activity A FILL IN THE BLANKS

1. Cognition
2. Neurotransmission
3. Memories
4. Phonation
5. Articulation
6. Perceiving
7. Thinking
8. Delirium
9. Aphasia
10. Thought
11. Pasticity

Activity B MATCHING

1. 1 – A, 2 – C, 3 – B, 4 – E, 5 – D

Activity C SEQUENCING

1.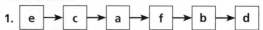

Activity D SHORT ANSWER

1. The hippocampi assist in retaining new knowledge and help determine which memories become long term.

2. Blood flow affects cognitive function because it supplies every cell in the body with oxygen. Lack of oxygen to the brain causes cellular damage and/or death and a change in cognition.

3. Sundown syndrome is an increase in confusion and agitation at the end of the day, specifically in the first hour of darkness. Sundowning occurs in people with significant cognitive impairment and often happens after a change in routine.

4. People with mild to moderate cognitive impairment are often embarrassed by their deficits. Often, they find ways to compensate so their impairment is not as noticeable.

5. A review of someone's medications should always be included in an assessment of a patient with a cognitive impairment as certain medications can cause altered thought processes. A medication review should include all medications, including those that you can buy over-the-counter, and their doses.

SECTION III: APPLYING YOUR KNOWLEDGE

Activity E CASE STUDY

1. Nursing interventions with this patient can start with providing the patient with as much structure as possible while he is in the hospital. Environmental restrictions can also be placed so as to decrease overstimulation. Next, communication must be clear and open. The patient's fluid intake and nutritional intake can be monitored to assure that both are adequate to prevent further confusion from electrolyte imbalance. By encouraging mobilization, I can help prevent deconditioning and possible improvement or maintain oxygenation to the brain and cardiovascular function. Safety would be of the utmost importance for this patient. Although he is fairly healthy, his recent fall with the episodes of forgetfulness suggests he is at risk for further injury. I would lastly want to give reassurance to his son and offer him community resources for help should he or his father need it.

2. Standardized tests, such as those that are used to measure intelligence, are standardized to white, middle-class Americans and often do not relate to the experience of other ethnic and socioeconomic groups. Thus, they cannot be used to measure this patient's intelligence compared to someone whose first language is English.

SECTION IV: PRACTICING FOR NCLEX

Activity F MULTIPLE CHOICE

1. **Answer: a**
   RATIONALE: The cochlea is part of the inner ear. The reticular activating system is a diffuse cluster of neurons that extends from the brain stem and projects upward and throughout the spinal cord. Broca's area is the section of the brain associated with word formation and speech.

2. **Answer: d**
   RATIONALE: Delirium results from one or more organic factors; is often recognized and can lead to death if not diagnosed. The sundown syndrome is an increase in confusion and agitation that occurs at the end of the day. Aphasia is a partial or total loss of language abilities.

3. **Answer: d**
   RATIONALE: Somatic receptors for pain, touch, and pressure in the skin are part of exteroceptors. Exteroceptors respond to stimuli from the external environment.

4. **Answer: a**
   RATIONALE: People with dementia experience a gradual decline in all cognitive processes. It is not associated with disturbance in level of consciousness, but it does interfere with social or occupational functioning.

5. **Answer: c**
   RATIONALE: Communicating is a process that is integrated within normal cognitive patterns. It is not a characteristic of cognition.

6. **Answer: b**
   RATIONALE: Movement of water and electrolytes via active and passive movement maintains a balance of each and protects cells, including brain cells, against cellular damage.

7. **Answer: a**
   RATIONALE: The acceleration of Jane's decline in cognitive functioning is multifactorial. Being in an unfamiliar environment is affecting her cognitive process of orientation. Being close to a nurse's station, which is typically noisy, adds to the amount of stimuli Jane is receiving and can decrease her ability to find meaning in what she is sensing. Also, depression interferes with cognitive function and can contribute to altered thought processes. The fact that Jane's daughter visits her every day at the same time can actually provide an orienting cue which may help decrease Jane's confusion.

8. **Answer: b**
   RATIONALE: Susan is experiencing anomia or problems retrieving certain words. Compared to Dan, Susan's anomia is mild and she is able to describe what she means even if she can't come up with the exact word. This is characteristic of anomic aphasia. Garrett is experiencing global aphasia where he can neither understand nor communicate with the outside world. Jenny is experiencing receptive aphasia and shows little insight into what is going on.

9. **Answers: a, b, c, d**
   RATIONALE: Pets, music, recreation and reminiscence are forms of socialization therapies. The purpose of these therapies is to encourage patients to expand contact with others in social settings in an effort to increase cognitive and sensory stimuli.

10. **Answers: a, b, c**
    RATIONALE: The larynx, nasal cavity, and tongue are all involved in speech production. Semicircular canals Are part of the inner ear and the organ of Corti. In response to vibration, hair cells of the organ of Corti generate nerve impulses that the cochlear nerve, in company with the vestibular nerve, carries to the central auditory pathway.

CHAPTER 37

SECTION II: ASSESSING YOUR UNDERSTANDING

Activity A   FILL IN THE BLANKS

1. Self
2. Self-concept
3. Self-perception
4. Self-esteem
5. Identity
6. Role
7. Ambiguity
8. Self-efficacy
9. Conflict

Activity B   MATCHING

1.   1 – D,   2 – A,   3 – C,   4 – B
2.   1 – C,   2 – D,   3 – A,   4 – B

Activity C   SEQUENCING

1.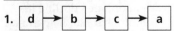

Activity D   SHORT ANSWER

1. Body image is how a person pictures and feels about their body. This can be both conscious and unconscious feelings about one's size, sex, sexuality, and the way someone looks in general. Everyone has a body image, whether it is a positive or a negative image. Body image is also driven by cultural and social contexts. It is important to consider all of this when creating a plan patient care because they might not have the same goals as you do based on their body image and their idealized body image.

2. Infants start to think of themselves as separate from others, a change from the newborns feeling of undifferentiated self. They start to recognize that their feelings are their own and self-concepts start to develop. Soon the infant begins to read the wants of others.

3. Often, people feel defined by what they do for work. When this period in your life is over, a huge shift occurs in role performance and self-esteem. A loss of self-esteem can occur for people who place great value on their working role.

4. Someone who is able to cope and weather stressors is more likely to have a healthy self-concept. Both internal and external resources enhance coping. On the other hand, poor coping and stress tolerance can lead to a damaged self-concept. This is especially true during times of illness.

5. It is important to consider the person's developmental stage, previous experience, intensity of a stressor or threat, and self-expectations when identifying their risk for self-concept dysfunction. A person's developmental stage can put them at greater risk depending on which stage they are in. For example, if the patient is a teen and their illness changes their body image, it is most likely going to have a bigger impact on their self-concept. Past experience can either assist with someone's coping or hinder it if, for instance, they have a history of unsuccessful coping mechanisms. Also, how intense a threat is and how that person believes themselves capable of dealing with that threat can either cause them to cope or cause a lack thereof.

SECTION III: APPLYING YOUR KNOWLEDGE

Activity E   CASE STUDY

1. Richard, because he is an adolescent, is going through many physical, emotional, and sexual changes. It would be normal for him to be attempting to assert himself as an adult, and as separate from his parents. His self-esteem is fragile and much of how he sees himself is dependent on how he is perceived by his peers. It is important to know Richard's developmental level in order to tailor your nursing interventions appropriately. A major illness can affect what developmental level a person is in and can cause someone to regress.

2. Richard is a teenager and considers him an adult at this point. It is important to be sensitive to these feelings and the discrepancy of him being on a pediatric floor. I would help him maintain his autonomy by offering him choices whenever possible. I would also provide feedback about his strengths and weaknesses to help him establish a realistic self-concept.

SECTION IV: PRACTICING FOR NCLEX

Activity F   MULTIPLE CHOICE

1. Answer: b
   RATIONALE: Jose is talking about self-evaluation, which is the conscious assessment of the self. Self-expectations are goals that someone sets. Self-knowledge is a basic understanding of oneself. Social self is how a person sees himself in relation to social situations.

2. Answer: a
   RATIONALE: Sex, height, weight, and appearance are all biological characteristics that affect self-concept.

3. Answer: c
   RATIONALE: A person with external locus of control perceives that outcomes happen because of luck, chance, or the influence of powerful others.

4. Answer: d
   RATIONALE: Situational transitions are associated with a change in relationships.

5. Answer: a
   RATIONALE: Role strain occurs when the person perceives himself or herself as inadequate or unsuited for a role and can occur when a person is forced to assume many roles. Role ambiguity occurs when a

person lacks knowledge of role expectations. This lack of knowledge causes anxiety and confusion. Role conflict is related to expectations concerning the role.

6. **Answer: b**

   RATIONALE: Objective data are what you can observe with your own eyes. Other objective data that may be collected include a missing body part, a concealment of a body part, or weeping.

7. **Answer: a**

   RATIONALE: A toddler needs an environment that allows them to practice newly developing skills, especially those related to movement. Providing this encourages the development of a positive body image and self-esteem. Assisting Austin's parents to accept their new role is most appropriate for the family of a newborn. Safety should be addressed with the parents of an infant. Preschoolers are more concerned with damage to their bodies so teaching them about good hygiene is important

8. **Answer: c**

   RATIONALE: Micah is using behavioral change to help his patient change her current behavior and to assist her with improving her self-concept problems.

9. **Answer: c**

   RATIONALE: Interrole conflict exists when a person is expected to fulfill two or more roles simultaneously.

10. **Answer: a**

    RATIONALE: An ascribed role is one in which the person has no choice such as to be born a male and therefore be someone's son. On the other hand, assumed roles are ones that are chosen. This includes the choice to be a nurse, a husband, or a mother.

11. **Answer: a**

    RATIONALE: According to Erikson, autonomy vs. shame should be the developmental level of a toddler.

CHAPTER 38

SECTION II: ASSESSING YOUR UNDERSTANDING

Activity A FILL IN THE BLANKS

1. Independence
2. Creativity
3. Doubled
4. Behavior
5. Sandwich
6. Emotional
7. Elderly
8. Family-centered
9. Caregiver
10. Multidisciplinary

Activity B MATCHING

1. 1 – D,   2 – A,   3 – E,   4 – B,   5 – C
2. 1 – D,   2 – C,   3 – A,   4 – E,   5 – B

Activity C SHORT ANSWER

1. Friends change as families move locations and individuals change careers or retire. Parents' food choices impact themselves and their child's nutritional status. Time spent on relaxation and exercise has direct benefit on physical health. A lack of affordable public services can leave children caring for aging parents and young children without adequate adult supervision.

2. Role strain occurs when an individual assumes a new role within a family. For example, a woman who was previously employed may have to leave her job to serve as the primary caregiver for an aging parent.

3. Persons caring for an individual with a chronic illness can experience anxiety, exhaustion, alterations in social contacts, and a new need to rely on others for help. The initial reaction is often denial but the family often adjusts to function as "normally" as possible.

4. Vague symptoms are often the only clues to child abuse. This is because the abused child may blame themselves and not discuss the abuse, or the abuser is skilled at hiding their abuse. Signs such as odd bruising patterns, a lack of visible attachment between parent/baby, or failure to thrive may be the only symptoms. Elderly who are financially or physically dependent on others are at increased risk for abuse. Elderly may be abused by their own children or by a third-party caregiver.

5. The nurse can clarify the conflict with the participants and help to identify contributing factors and correct misconceptions. The nurse can also provide objective feedback. Finally, the nurse can guide the family in decision making and support the decisions made by the family.

SECTION III: APPLYING YOUR KNOWLEDGE

Activity D CASE STUDY

1. Dysfunctional family process r/t job loss AEB Jim's admission that his job loss has affected his functioning; risk for dysfunctional family process r/t alcohol use.

2. Patient and family will achieve increased communication. Patient and family will explore means to address alcohol consumption.

3. Professional referrals and peer support groups are two ways by which nurses can support a family's decision to pursue change. In this case study, Jim and his family may benefit from both referrals. Marriage counseling is often an effective strategy to address interrelationship tension. A referral to a peer support group such as Alcoholics Anonymous may be appropriate if there is evidence that Jim will struggle to cut back on his alcohol use.

SECTION IV: PRACTICING FOR NCLEX

Activity E MULTIPLE CHOICE

1. **Answer: d**
   RATIONALE: Mrs. G. is is experiencing role strain because she is combining the roles of caregiver, wife, and employee. Role strain is a manifestation of family function when events and family developments force change roles.

2. **Answer: b**
   RATIONALE: Trust is the first of Erickson's stages of development which occurs during the first year of life.

3. **Answer: a**
   RATIONALE: Preschool age children rely on stability. When an inevitable family change occurs, such as the death of a loved one, children should be reassured that they are not to blame for this change. Children may benefit from play therapy to help them sort their feelings.

4. **Answer: b**
   RATIONALE: The role of the best friend typically develops during school age years. This is a time of industry, according to Erickson, and task-oriented behaviors are commonly enjoyed.

5. **Answer: b**
   RATIONALE: Children learn about life experience almost exclusively from their families of origin. Mrs. A's views on child rearing were directly affected by her learned experience from her mother.

6. **Answer: d**
   RATIONALE: Bruising and broken bones are normal injuries in active children. A child in the fifth percentile who maintains growth may just be small or may require supplementation.

7. **Answer: c**
   RATIONALE: An "enabler" is often a family member of a person who abuses substances. The enabler will take on the tasks that the substance abuser cannot in order to keep the family functioning at an altered level.

8. **Answers: a, b**
   RATIONALE: Judgment should not be conveyed in the nursing diagnosis, as is done by using the term "dead beat dad". Exhaustion is not an NANDA-I nursing diagnosis, nor is the diagnosis properly formatted.

9. **Answers: a, b, c**
   RATIONALE: Bruising on bony prominences such as elbows and knees is more often sign of an active and curious child than abuse.

10. **Answers: a, b, c**
    RATIONALE: Unemployment, substance abuse, and chronic illness are all risk factors for abuse. Other risk factors include inadequate housing, lack of education, and lack of resources.

CHAPTER 39

SECTION II: ASSESSING YOUR UNDERSTANDING

Activity A FILL IN THE BLANKS

1. Grief
2. Bereavement
3. Mourning
4. Anticipatory
5. Dysfunctional
6. Hospice
7. Death
8. Dying
9. Loss

Activity B MATCHING

1. 1 – D,   2 – C,   3 – A,   4 – B
2. 1 – A,   2 – C,   3 – B,   4 – D

Activity C ORDERING

1.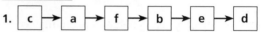

Activity D SHORT ANSWER

1. The two main categories of loss are material loss and psychological loss. Material loss is the loss of a tangible object such as a car when it is stolen or a family heirloom that is lost in a fire. Psychological loss is that of something that has no physical form but has some important symbolic meaning. An example of a psychological loss is when someone gets a divorce and they go through the experience of losing a relationship.

2. According to Parkes, there are four stages of grief; numbness, yearning, disorganization, and reorganization. Disorganization is characterized by severe depression, social withdrawal, and an overall lack of interest in people and activities.

3. Toddlers 18 to 24 months experience a keen sense of loss that manifests itself as separation anxiety. During this period, the toddler's developmental task is to gain a sense of autonomy. However, the inability to reconnect with a caregiver periodically can lead to fear of abandonment.

4. For the early school-aged child, death is perceived as unnatural, reversible, and avoidable. As the child grows older, they start to think of death more realistically, as irreversible, universal, inevitable, and natural. This is a dramatic step for the child.

5. It is important to reflect on one's own beliefs and traditions surrounding grief and loss so as to avoid imposing your personal beliefs and practice on your patients who might have other ways of coping. Having this self-reflection allows a caregiver to accept other cultural norms and thus facilitate this for patients.

SECTION III: APPLYING YOUR KNOWLEDGE

Activity E CASE STUDY

1. Hospice care is appropriate for this patient for many reasons. Not only can hospice help with pain management, but it further offers both the patient and the family support to help them cope with this difficult time. It affirms life and regards dying as a normal process, it integrates the psychological and spiritual aspects of patient care, and it supports the patient to live as actively as possible until death. Further, it uses a team approach to address the needs of the patient and enhances quality of life.

2. As the nurse, you need to be able to talk to patients and families about dying, pain, and other symptoms control techniques. You also need to be familiar with comfort care nursing interventions so as to properly implement them. A third skill is the ability to work within a multidisciplinary team to address the multitude of issues that arise in end of life care.

SECTION IV: PRACTICING FOR NCLEX

Activity F MULTIPLE CHOICE

1. **Answer: b**
   RATIONALE: The functions of grief include to make the outer reality of the loss into an internally accepted reality, to alter the emotional attachment to the lost person or object, and to make it possible for the bereaved person to become attached to other people or objects.

2. **Answer: b**
   RATIONALE: Lila is exhibiting a symptom of bereavement which includes emotional, physical, social, and cognitive responses.

3. **Answer: d**
   RATIONALE: The four stages of the grief cycle model are shock, protest, disorganization, and reorganization. Physical manifestations of protest include a feeling of pain in one's heart, sleep and appetite problems, weight loss, neglect of appearance, fatigue, lethargy, and poor hygiene.

4. **Answer: d**
   RATIONALE: According to Parke, progression through the four stages of grief normally takes 2 years or longer. The last stage, reorganization, usually begins 6 to 9 months after the loss and lasts the duration.

5. **Answer: a**
   RATIONALE: Adults tend to grieve more intensely and more continuously, but for a relatively shorter period of time than children. Having a good social network helps with this process, as well as having a stable lifestyle.

6. **Answer: b**
   RATIONALE: When assessing someone for their reaction, both physically and psychologically, to loss, it is important to get a sense for what part this person played in their life. If she was not close her to father, the impact might not be so great. On the other hand, if he was an important person in her life her response might be greater. Other things to initially ask about include whether the loss was expected and whether or not the person feels a sense of responsibility for the loss.

7. **Answer: c**
   RATIONALE: During this stage it is important to keep the person safe and to help them begin accept the reality of the loss. During the protest phase, nursing interventions should focus on encouraging the patient to express their emotions. During the disorganization phase, interventions started in the shock phase should be continued and the person may need assistance reorganizing their life. During the reorganization phase, assistance is needed to help the person create new patterns of behavior that are efficacious.

8. **Answer: b**
   RATIONALE: Her proposed stages of grief are denial, anger, bargaining, depression, and acceptance.

9. **Answer: a**
   RATIONALE: Higher-brain death results in a vegetative state with independent respirations. Irreversible cessation of heart–lung function describes death.

10. **Answer: e**
    RATIONALE: It is important to be very careful when labeling someone with dysfunctional grieving. Grief can manifest itself and many ways. If the manifestations of grief are not harmful, or potentially harmful, to either the patient or someone else and they are not lasting for more than 3 years, it is not necessarily dysfunctional.

11. **Answers: a, c, d, e**
    RATIONALE: Factors affecting grieving include meaning of loss, circumstances of loss, religious beliefs, personal resources and stressors, and sociocultural resources and stressors.

12. **Answers: a, c, e**
    RATIONALE: When preparing a child for death, it is important to know your own feelings and beliefs, be honest, begin at the child's level, include the child in family rituals related to death and mourning, encourage expression of feelings, provide security and stability, encourage remembrance of the deceased, recognize that children grieve differently than adults, expect the child to alternate between grieving and normal functioning, talk openly about death and the feelings it generates, and introduce death concepts into conversations naturally.

CHAPTER 40

SECTION II: ASSESSING YOUR UNDERSTANDING

Activity A FILL IN THE BLANKS

1. Homeostasis
2. Adaption
3. Stressors
4. Hippocampus
5. Immune
6. Neurogenesis
7. Activity or exercise
8. Physiologic
9. Lifestyle
10. Relaxation
11. Chronic

Activity B MATCHING

1. 1 – D,   2 – A,   3 – F,   4 – C,   5 – B,   6 – E

Activity C SHORT ANSWER

1. The hypothalamic–pituitary–adrenal (HPA) axis is the neuroendocrine regulator of stress. When the limbic system perceives stress, signals are sent to the hypothalamus. The hypothalamus secretes cortico-trophin-releasing hormone causing the anterior pituitary to secrete adrenocorticotropic hormone (ACTH). Corticosteroids are then released from the adrenal glands. It is these corticosteroids that increase glucose levels and regulate electrolytes.
2. Cortisol is the primary glucocorticoid released from the adrenal gland. Under acute stress, cortisol is protective of mood. Under chronic stress, cortisol can lead to anxiety and depression.
3. Epinephrine and norepinephrine cause excitatory actions during stress. These include pupil dilation, increased heart rate and force of contraction, bronchial dilation, and the conversion of glycogen to glucose. They also contribute to feelings of excitement and heightened awareness. Epinephrine and norepinephrine also have inhibitory effects during times of stress, such as decreased digestive function, insulin secretion, and the urge to urinate.
4. An increased resting heart rate, blood pressure, or respiratory rate. Auscultation of ectopic heart beats. A feeling of pounding in the chest. Air hunger, dizziness, or tingling in the extremities. Headaches or tightness in the shoulders, neck, or back. Loss of appetite, nausea, vomiting, or diarrhea secondary to increased peristalsis. Diaphoresis (sweating) or arrector pili (goose flesh).
5. The first step is identification of what one says when the situation occurs. This is termed identification of self-talk. It is the internal verbalizations that occur in response to excitement or disappointment. Everyone engages in self-talk. The second step is to analyze how rational or irrational those internal messages are. The third step is to replace the negative and/or irrational statements with supportive statements and find a way to integrate them into daily life.
6. Guided imagery or relaxation tapes can be used prior to a painful procedure. Rooms can be modified to reduce stress by dimming the lights or eliminating noxious smells and aggravating sounds.

SECTION III: APPLYING YOUR KNOWLEDGE

Activity D CASE STUDY

1. David may report any of the following: headache, back pain, change in appetite (increase or decrease), nausea, vomiting or diarrhea, chest pain, pressure or palpitations. Feelings of lightheadedness or dizziness. On exam, David may have an elevated heart rate, respiratory rate, or blood pressure and you may auscultate palpitations or "extra" beats. He may feel diaphoretic. You may note tense muscles in his shoulders or neck.
2. Fear r/t change in family dynamics AEB David stating that he feels he needs to be "perfect" in order to maintain his job; the risk for caregiver role strain r/t change in family dynamics.
3. One key health promotion activity is to work on perfection reduction. Work with David to help him set realistic work goals that will help him with job security. David may also benefit from a stress-reduction activity such as exercise or a relaxation activity like yoga or meditation. The nurse could engage David in a discussion about his interest in such activities and then facilitate initiation.

SECTION IV: PRACTICING FOR NCLEX

Activity E MULTIPLE CHOICE

1. **Answer: d**
   RATIONALE: Environmental stress is common when individuals move to a new location, even if that move is voluntary. It is associated with a lack of familiarity with the sights, smells, and sounds of the location. Relocation also requires alteration in daily routine which is in itself stressful.
2. **Answer: a**
   RATIONALE: Introjection is when an individual adapts a characteristic of someone else.
3. **Answer: b**
   RATIONALE: Aleah is exhibiting denial by refusing to accept something as is.
4. **Answer: c**
   RATIONALE: Music may be helpful for some, but is not essential for meditation.
5. **Answer: a**
   RATIONALE: This is an example of magical thinking. Magical thinking is a common reaction to stress in a school-aged child.

6. **Answer: a**
   RATIONALE: Collectivistic culture views the self as an interdependent part of others.
7. **Answer: d**
   RATIONALE: Alcohol abuse is a common altered coping pattern for individuals with poor coping skills. It is legal and easily accessible. Phrases such as "I just cannot cope" and "I need to numb the pain" are common among those who abuse alcohol.
8. **Answers: a, b**
   RATIONALE: Assertiveness, not aggressiveness, is a preferred health promotion strategy. CBT is a treatment, not health promotion.
9. **Answers: a, c**
   RATIONALE: There is no evidence that this family is ready to change their family process. There is also no evidence of anxiety.
10. **Answers: a, b, c**
    RATIONALE: Cesarean section is not a contraindication to holding an infant. Many women successfully bond with their infants following a cesarean.
11. **Answers: b, c, d**
    RATIONALE: Palpitations are a common manifestation of stress. They may be auscultated during exam or detected on an EKG. Tension headaches frequently come on in the evening and are always relieved. A headache that does not go away is an ominous sign. A blood pressure of 110/68 is normal for an adult man. Problems with distance vision are not associated with stress.

CHAPTER 41

SECTION II: ASSESSING YOUR UNDERSTANDING

Activity A FILL IN THE BLANKS

1. Sexuality
2. Prepuce
3. Menstruation
4. Transgendered
5. Menarche
6. Climacteric
7. Impotence
8. Vaginismus
9. Menopause

Activity B MATCHING

1. 1 – B, 2 – A, 3 – D, 4 – C
2. 1 – A, 2 – C, 3 – B

Activity C ORDERING

1.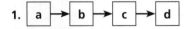

Activity D SHORT ANSWER

1. Breasts are considered sexual organs because they are directly influenced by reproductive organs and they are lactation organs.

2. Sexual expression differs from person to person. People may present themselves outwardly in terms of their sexuality. They may also choose to engage in coitus using different positions and with varying frequencies. Some people prefer more foreplay than others. Some people engage in masturbations while others may not. Still others may choose to abstain from sexual intercourse.
3. During fertilization, an organism's chromosomal formation is determined. A combination of chromosomes, one from the mother and one from the father, leads to the development of either female or male genitalia. A variation in this process can also lead to ambiguous genitalia which can cause problems in the parent–child relationship.
4. Everyone is biased by their own family's influences, religious beliefs, and personal experience when it comes to issues of sexuality. It is important to keep these in mind when working with patients who fall outside of these biases.
5. Someone who has a low self-concept may experience a decreased sexual drive or may attempt to compensate for this by overemphasizing involvement in sexual relations.

SECTION III: APPLYING YOUR KNOWLEDGE

Activity E CASE STUDY

1. Even though Sasha is young, it is important that issues of sexuality be addressed in an open manner. Statistically, Sasha is at great risk for contracting STDs and getting pregnant so she should be well informed about her decision to be sexually active and be empowered to protect herself. Sasha is going through a very turbulent time so it is also important to assess for how she is dealing with her changing body as well as hormonal changes.
2. Sasha is still young. Although it is possible that Sasha has chosen to become a sexually active being because she is secure in herself, it is also possible that she is compensating for a negative self-concept by overemphasizing involvement in sexual relations. It is important that a nurse be open and nonjudgmental but that they also are alert for dysfunctional and self-destructive behavior.

SECTION IV: PRACTICING FOR NCLEX

Activity F MULTIPLE CHOICE

1. **Answer: a**
   RATIONALE: Estrogen along progesterone inhibits milk production. Estrogen and progesterone are necessary for the stimulation of the target organs in preparing the body for possible pregnancy.
2. **Answer: d**
   RATIONALE: There are many causes why women have difficulty achieving orgasm. Lack of information, lack of adequate stimulation, or problems in an

intimate relationship may cause difficulty attaining orgasm.

3. Answer: a

RATIONALE: Cervical culture or urine analysis is used to diagnose *Chlamydia*. A pap smear is performed to detect cellular changes in cervix, cervical cancer. Blood work is used to detect various abnormalities. Wet preparation with KOH is used to detect *Candida, Gardenrella, and Trichomonaus.*

4. Answer: b

RATIONALE: During the plateau phase, the circumference of the penis thickens at the coronal ridge. The size of the testes also increase by 50% and a few drops of fluid appear at the urethral meatus.

5. Answer: c

RATIONALE: Many sexual response patterns have been documented in women. During the excitement phase, the clitoris becomes larger. Women do not experience a refractory period and are, therefore, able to experience multiple orgasms in a small period.

6. Answers: a, b, c, d

RATIONALE: The mons pubis, labia majora, clitoris, and skene's glands are external organs. The ovaries are internal organs.

CHAPTER 42

SECTION II: ASSESSING YOUR UNDERSTANDING

Activity A FILL IN THE BLANKS

1. Spirituality
2. Holistic
3. Faith
4. Families
5. Crisis
6. Ethics
7. Pluralism
8. Health
9. Distress
10. Build
11. Spirituality

Activity B MATCHING

1. 1 – A, D,   2 – A, C,   3 – A, B, E,   4 – A, C, E,
   5 – A, B, F,   6 – B, C, E

2. 1 – D,   2 – C,   3 – A,   4 – B

Activity C SHORT ANSWER

1. Religion is a formal doctrine of beliefs that are preached by a particular organization. Spirituality is a person's own ideas about the deeper meaning of life and provides meaning for life and life's journey. Religious affiliation may strengthen an individual's spirituality. Thus, the two may be interrelated, but the terms are not interchangeable.

2. A spiritual crisis occurs when an individual calls into question their spiritual belief system. This cri-

sis can trigger rejection of beliefs or anger toward a higher power. A spiritual crisis can also result in a renewed acceptance of beliefs and traditions that have fallen by the wayside. Separation from spiritual ties tends to occur because of geography. When an individual relocates temporarily during hospitalization or permanently by entering a retirement community, that person is forced to find a new source of religious practice. Some individuals choose to temporarily stop religious practice.

3. Stoll's (1979) *Guidelines for Spiritual Assessment* is a widely used tool to identify a patient's normal spiritual practice. Questions attempt to clarify the following: (1) concept of God or deity, (2) source of hope and strength, (3) religious practices and rituals, and (4) relationship between spiritual beliefs and state of health.

4. The patient expresses connectedness with someone/something other than self. The patient expresses meaning or purpose in life. The patient expresses connectedness with spiritual beliefs or spiritual leaders.

5. Toddlers thrive on ritual and routine. Nurses can offer toddlers' assistance in daily religious rituals such as mealtime or evening prayer. Nurses can also assist with celebration of important religious holy days by engaging the child in arts and crafts projects or singing simple songs.

Activity D CASE STUDY

1. Hospitalization itself can disrupt spiritual practice by interfering with the ability to attend worship services or engage with a person's spiritual community. Persons who are hospitalized or who receive a grim diagnosis are also at risk for developing a spiritual crisis.

2. Spiritual distress r/t diagnosis of significant medical condition AEB patient stating "no God would allow this to happen".

3. Listen to Paul and provide support by holding a hand or touching a shoulder while listening. Let Paul know that the hospital has spiritual support available but respect Paul's decision to decline this visit. If Paul does decide to resume religious practice, the nurse can help provide an environment to worship.

SECTION III: APPLYING YOUR KNOWLEDGE

Activity E MULTIPLE CHOICE

1. Answer: a

RATIONALE: A spiritual crisis can occur with an acute illness, sudden loss, or a new challenging diagnosis. These turning points often result in the questioning of one's beliefs.

2. Answer: c

RATIONALE: Separation from spiritual ties occurs when an individual changes location and does not have an access to spiritual services or feels uncomfortable joining a new group. This separation can be temporary or permanent.

3. **Answer: d**
   RATIONALE: These nurses working together to understand a wide variety of religious beliefs is a form of pluralism.

4. **Answer: a**
   RATIONALE: The most appropriate action is to work with Mr. V to maintain practice that is important to him. If Mr. V decided to suspend religious practice for medical reasons, it would be appropriate to support this decision.

5. **Answer: c**
   RATIONALE: Life support is appropriate as long as measures are not heroic.

6. **Answer: b**
   RATIONALE: Ritualistic care of the body following death is an important piece of the Muslim culture.

7. **Answer: b**
   RATIONALE: A patient's current religious practice is not necessarily indicative of lifelong practices. Talk with Mr. Z about his lifelong religious practice. As a result, you may uncover useful information that will help to guide the plan of care.

8. **Answers: a, b, c**
   RATIONALE: Stories and religious symbols are best introduced to children during the school-age years.

9. **Answers: a, b, d**
   RATIONALE: A spiritual and religious assessment attempts to identify and document any practices or beliefs that are important for the patient to maintain or that may alter medical or nursing treatment.

10. **Answers: a, b, c**
    RATIONALE: Biblical legends are more appropriate for school-age children.